TCRN
The Trauma Nurse Certification Review

Ann J. Brorsen
RN, MSN, PHN, CCRN, CEN

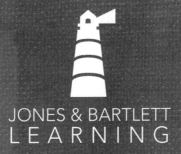

JONES & BARTLETT
LEARNING

World Headquarters
Jones & Bartlett Learning
5 Wall Street
Burlington, MA 01803
978-443-5000
info@jblearning.com
www.jblearning.com

Jones & Bartlett Learning books and products are available through most bookstores and online booksellers. To contact Jones & Bartlett Learning directly, call 800-832-0034, fax 978-443-8000, or visit our website, www.jblearning.com.

Substantial discounts on bulk quantities of Jones & Bartlett Learning publications are available to corporations, professional associations, and other qualified organizations. For details and specific discount information, contact the special sales department at Jones & Bartlett Learning via the above contact information or send an email to specialsales@jblearning.com.

11916-9

Production Credits

VP, Executive Publisher: David D. Cella
Acquisitions Editor: Teresa Reilly
Editorial Assistant: Anna-Maria Forger
Production Manager: Carolyn Rogers Pershouse
Senior Vendor Manager: Sara Kelly
Marketing Communications Manager: Katie Hennessy
Product Fulfillment Manager: Wendy Kilborn
Composition: S4Carlisle Publishing Services

Project Management: S4Carlisle Publishing Services
Cover Design: Michael O'Donnell
Rights & Media Specialist: Wes DeShano
Media Development Editor: Troy Liston
Cover Image (Title Page, Part Opener, Chapter Opener):
    © Happy person/Shutterstock
Printing and Binding: Edwards Brothers Malloy
Cover Printing: Edwards Brothers Malloy

Library of Congress Cataloging-in-Publication Data
Names: Brorsen, Ann J., author.
Title: TCRN certification review / Ann J. Brorsen.
Other titles: Trauma certified registered nurse certification review
Description: Burlington, Massachusetts : Jones & Bartlett Learning, [2019] |
    Includes bibliographical references and index.
Identifiers: LCCN 2017032883 | ISBN 9781284119152 (pbk. : alk. paper)
Subjects: | MESH: Wounds and Injuries--nursing | Emergency Nursing | Critical
    Care Nursing | Certification | Test Taking Skills | Examination Questions
Classification: LCC RC86.7 | NLM WY 18.2 | DDC 617.1/026--dc23 LC record available at https://lccn.loc.gov/2017032883

6048

Printed in the United States of America
21 20 19 18 17   10 9 8 7 6 5 4 3 2 1

Contents

About the Author

Ann J. Brorsen, RN, MSN, PHN, CCRN, CEN

Ann is a nationally known speaker and has presented certification review courses for adult and pediatric CCRN, CEN, PCCN, and trauma. She has helped thousands of nurses attain certification. Ann has authored multiple texts about advanced certification and physiology. She is a member of Sigma Theta Tau, the American Association of Critical-Care Nurses, the Society of Critical Care Medicine, and the Emergency Nurses Association. Ann also works as a consultant for educational program development and management training for healthcare facilities. She presents programs as diverse as advanced hemodynamics and trauma care to best practice models for hospital corporations. She continues clinical practice in the ICU, ED, and critical care transport. Ann is also currently the COO and Director of Clinical Applications for Pro Ed in Menifee, California.

Contributors

Melissa R. Christiansen, RN, MSN, NP-C, CCRN, CNRN

Melissa has over 25 years' experience as a critical care nurse in neurological, cardiac, and trauma ICUs. She is currently working as a family nurse practitioner in Southern California. Melissa has presented programs on neurologic and neuroscience topics, adult critical care, and emergency nursing certification reviews, as well as courses in post-anesthesia nursing. Melissa is a member of Sigma Theta Tau, the American Association of Critical-Care Nurses, the American Association of Neuroscience Nurses, and the American Academy of Nurse Practitioners.

Jacque E. Jackson, RN, PhD, APRN

Jacque has over 30 years of clinical nursing experience. In addition, he has been an educator, manager of cardiovascular and surgical ICUs, emergency departments, CNO, and a multi-hospital administrator. He has been a staunch advocate of certification for nurses and utilization of clinical ladders and best practice models for healthcare.

Keri R. Rogelet, RN, MSN, MBA/HCM, CCRN, RNC-NIC

Keri has presented national programs for adult health issues, the Neonatal CCRN, Pediatric CCRN, and Developmental Care. Keri is a regional NRP mentor/trainer for the American Academy of Pediatrics and a lead instructor for the S.T.A.B.L.E. program. Keri's professional associations include Sigma Theta Tau, the American Association of Critical-Care Nurses, and the Academy of Neonatal Nursing. Keri also works as a consultant for pediatric and neonatal product applications. Keri is currently attending Rush University College of Nursing's DNP Neonatal Clinical Nurse Specialist program. In addition to working full-time as the NICU Clinical Practice Coordinator in a Level II/III NICU, she is the CFO and Director of Clinical Development for Pro Ed in Menifee, California.

Reviewers

Brian N. Ingram, MD
Fairfax, Virginia

Randall C. Jackson, RN, MSN, CNS, CCRN
Pittsburgh, Pennsylvania

Acknowledgments

Mary Margaret Forsythe, RN, and Nancy O. Roberts, RN

Mary Margaret and Nancy were two instructors who were ultimate professionals and who believed in their students and the profession of nursing. These women were incredible individuals and will live in the hearts of hundreds of nurses. They passed before their time and are desperately missed.

Karen S. Ehrat, RN, PhD

Karen saw potential in a new grad and made education a joy and a privilege. Her untimely death stole a piece from every soul she touched.

The Editorial Staff at Jones & Bartlett Learning

The author would also like to express gratitude to the editorial staff at Jones & Bartlett Learning. Thank you for years of support and expertise in publishing to help nurses attain certification, improve patient care, and build individual and professional self-confidence.

The author is also grateful to all the nurses who provided suggestions for content of this book and to the contributors who worked unselfishly and through many a long night. Thank you to the reviewers who gave their time, effort, and suggestions to enhance the content of this manuscript.

A.J.B.

Preface

Congratulations! You have embarked on a journey to achieve certification as a trauma nurse. Research studies have shown that simply by studying for certification, nurses improve patient care. Achieving certification helps you grow professionally and personally by increasing self-confidence and knowledge, while refining your skills.

This textbook is an invaluable resource to help you successfully pass the TCRN certification exam. This text is actually two books in one. This written text contains over 900 questions with rationale which cover the topics from the new, 2017/2018 and beyond, TCRN Content Outline. The questions in this text are representative of the type of questions you will find on the actual examination.

The current trend for item writers is to present a question in such a way as to not state any identifiable characteristics, such as a name, age, or gender (if possible). Any name or patient condition presented here is for educational purposes only. Any resemblance to any person, living or dead, is purely coincidental.

All of us who contributed to the content of this book are dedicated to helping you successfully pass this exam and achieve recognition as a trauma care nurse. Please feel free to contact us if you have any questions or if you would like to schedule a TCRN review course for your facility or group.

Ann Brorsen
Contact: Pro Ed
Website: www.forproed.com
Email: info@forproed.com
Facebook: Pro Ed Healthcare Education

How to Use This Text to Pass the TCRN Certification Examination

If you have downloaded the TCRN Content Outline, you will notice it is divided into major sections. The book is formatted in much the same way, except the content in each section varies somewhat. In addition, the headings differ in places.

This author created a new section titled, "Special Populations I" to include Pediatric, Geriatric, and Bariatric content. Rather than adding Obstetrical to this mix, there is a section titled "Special Populations II," with Obstetric and Neonatal content to facilitate study.

Questions are written in the same style that appears on the exam. Not all questions involve complicated scenarios or explanations. There are very straightforward questions that involve recall, but also critical thinking. Rationales may also be simple or complex. A question may be written in different ways and appear in multiple sections. A variety of presentations allow the reader to stay engaged.

There is a computer code provided with the book. The code will allow access to the same questions as found in the written text. You can review the material on a variety of devices. In addition, you can mix and match questions to customize a practice exam. Keep reviewing the questions until you can confidently answer 80% correctly.

Remember, you can pass the TCRN exam. Take your time, be confident!

Test-Taking Strategies

When preparing for the TCRN exam, the first thing to do is be absolutely honest with yourself about how you study. If you have good study habits and plenty of time, you are very fortunate. If you are a procrastinator, studying a little bit at a time might help. Nurses have to juggle so many roles that take up their time: parent, child, employee, student, teacher, and so on. One of the biggest struggles is simply finding the time and a place to study. Discovering your learning style will help you find a better way to absorb information. Three types of learners are commonly identified: visual, auditory, and kinesthetic. There is no perfect strategy for learning because every person is unique. Not everyone has a single style of learning; you may use a mix of styles depending on your situation.

Visual learners learn better from reading and writing than from hearing and talking about information. Background noise, such as music or television, is distracting to these types of learners. Finding a quiet space is a problem for some people. You may have to stay awake after family members have gone to bed. Flashcards often work, and some people use colored markers to highlight important information.

Auditory learners learn information effectively by listening and talking. Playing music, listening to audiotapes, or being part of a study group often works.

Kinesthetic learners prefer to learn via a "hands-on" approach. Nurses often learn this way because we have to listen to lectures and then demonstrate skills. This approach focuses on the use of models, manikins, or patients and works well for many healthcare providers. Kinesthetic people are often "antsy" and cannot sit still for long periods of time, so lectures may be difficult for them without frequent breaks. If you are a kinesthetic learner, some of the things that might help while studying include taking frequent breaks, walking around, or riding a stationary cycle.

No matter what your personal learning style, your test-taking skills can be improved. How? Practice! That is why this book was written in a question-and-answer format. Keep practicing the questions until you can answer at least 80% correctly. Research has shown that two-thirds of study time should be spent taking sample tests and only one-third of study time should be spent reviewing content.

Studying, like regular exercise, is good for the brain. As nurses, we must always keep abreast of the professional literature and spend time studying to keep our knowledge and skills up-to-date. In addition, many states require continuing education to renew a professional license. Anything worthwhile takes time, effort, and sacrifice.

There is no way around studying for this certification. There are no shortcuts! If you have been out of school for a while, don't despair! It may be slow going at first, so take things a little at a time. Just like going to the gym, you should make a plan to study in one particular place and at the same time, if possible. This is your space and your time—claim it. Have all your books, tapes, and other study materials handy. If you need snack food, make sure it is not all sugar and include some salty food. Caffeine tends to make people jittery, but if you need it, it may be right for you.

The TCRN Content Outline is a blueprint of the exam's content. The major sections are broken down into subheadings and topics. If you study only a little at a time, you will be fine. One day you may feel like studying wound care; the next day you may want to focus on chest tubes. You may download the current content outline at www.bcencertifications.org/Get-Certified/TCRN/Study/TCRN-Content-Outline.aspx. The current content outline is not included in this book because the exam changes frequently; as such, you should have a copy of the current information.

If you study with a group, you can save a lot of time and effort by breaking up the topics for that study period and having each person present his or her topic(s) and provide handouts and practice questions for the rest of the group. When you can make up a test question about a subject, you really will be prepared. Study for short periods of time, say 30 to 45 minutes, and then take a break. Set small goals, and after you have accomplished each one, reward yourself!

EXAM CONTENT

The TCRN certification exam consists of 175 multiple-choice test questions. One hundred fifty are scored. Twenty-five questions do not count; they are there to be validated. Every question is tried first to see if it is written well and if a certain percentage of people answer it correctly. At this point in the process, those 25 questions can still be "tweaked" for use on future exams, depending on how the test-takers performed on these questions.

Your results are determined by how many answers you get correct and the version of the examination used. Some questions are a bit more difficult than others. If you do not know an answer, take your best guess, because you have at least a chance of guessing correctly. You get points only for questions answered correctly.

STUDY TIPS

A multiple-choice test question consists of three parts: an introductory statement, a stem (question), and options from which you must select the correct answer. The introductory statement provides information about a clinical issue, pathophysiology, or a nursing action or duty.

Stems are worded in different ways. Some stems are in the form of a question; others are in the form of an incomplete statement. Additionally, a stem usually requests one of two types of responses: a positive response or a negative response. The questions you will practice from in this book may have an occasional negative stem to facilitate learning. There are no longer any multiple-multiple-choice questions on the exam!

Key words are important words or phrases that help focus your attention on what the question is asking. Examples of key words include *always, most, first response, earliest, priority, first, on admission, common, best, least, not, immediately*, and *initial*.

You should always be looking for a therapeutic response, as the nurse is always therapeutic. In other words, your initial response as a nurse is always the therapeutic response—you must acknowledge and validate the patient's feelings. Communication skills learned in Nursing 101 are important components of successful test-taking strategies. More than one option may contain a therapeutic response. When in doubt, validate, validate, validate. Always validate feelings before you present information. A medical emergency would, of course, take precedence.

Who is actually the focus of the question? You need to be able to identify this person. Sometimes questions are asked about a friend, a relative, or a significant other instead of a patient. A lot of information in the question may be deliberately distracting. Also, you must, when applicable, validate that person's feelings first.

WHEN IN DOUBT

When answering questions on the examination, remember Maslow's hierarchy of needs and the ABCs (airway, breathing, circulation). When these goals are met, then safety is the priority. After safety, the psychological needs are a priority. Assessment always comes before diagnosis and treatment (intervention). Learning takes place only if the learner is motivated.

Eliminate incorrect options. This gives you a 50% chance of guessing the correct answer. Here are some hints:

- Select the most general, all-encompassing option.
- Eliminate similar options or those that contain words such as *always* or *never*.
- If two options say essentially the same thing, then neither is correct. If three of the four options sound similar, choose the one that sounds different.
- Look for the longest option. It is usually the correct answer.
- Watch for grammatical inconsistencies between the stem and options.

IT'S TIME TO TAKE YOUR TCRN CERTIFICATION EXAM!

Well, you are finally ready! The night before the exam, get a good night's sleep. Do not cram the night before, although that is easier said than done. Do something relaxing and enjoyable, like going to a movie or out to dinner. Try to avoid caffeine or any other stimulant. Please email or call when you pass the exam so you can be congratulated.

REFERENCES

Board of Certification for Emergency Nursing. Retrieved from www.bcencertifications.org

Kobel Lamonte, M. (2007). Test-taking strategies for CNOR certification. *Association of periOperative Registered Nurses Journal, 85*(2), 315–332.

Ludwig, C. (2004). Preparing for certification: Test-taking strategies. *Medical-Surgical Nursing, 13(2),* 127–128.

Special Considerations

- Biomechanics of Trauma
- Multiple Organ Dysfunction Syndrome (MODS)
- Shock
  - » Cardiogenic
  - » Distributive
  - » Hypovolemic
  - » Neurogenic
  - » Septic
- Systemic Inflammatory Response Syndrome (SIRS)

INTRODUCTION

Understanding how to interpret arterial blood gases (ABGs) is essential for the trauma nurse. On the TCRN examination, you will be asked to interpret ABGs. The first chart that follows is designed to assist you in determining the correct answer by reminding you of the normal values for ABG interpretation.

The second chart assists with critical thinking regardless of how a question might be presented. The chart contains common causes of respiratory and metabolic issues you will likely find on your TCRN exam.

Ordinarily, questions about ABG interpretation are presented one of two ways. First, you are asked to choose a set of numbers that match a given physiologic state, say respiratory acidosis. A second type of question may provide you with a set of numbers, then ask for the interpretation. A new type of question sometimes provides information that will lead you to identify the patient's problem, you are then asked to match a set of ABG results to that entity. This third type of question may be quite difficult to answer. The chart simplifies learning and saves time.

As an example, if your patient is in the compensatory stage of shock, the patient will exhibit respiratory alkalosis because of tachypnea and blowing off carbon dioxide. In late stages of shock, the patient will exhibit metabolic acidosis.

If a patient suffers from a flail chest, it is extraordinarily painful. The patient is unlikely to breathe normally, and will retain carbon dioxide.

Normal Values for ABGs

> pH (acidosis) 7.35 − 7.45 (alkalosis)
>
> CO_2 (alkalosis) 35 − 45 (acidosis)
>
> HCO_3 (acidosis) 23 − 27 (alkalosis)
>
> PO_2 80 − 100

If compensated, pH of 7.35 − 7.40 = acidosis

If compensated, pH of 7.40 − 7.45 = alkalosis

The third chart is a review of classifications of blood loss in hemorrhagic shock.

hypoventilation — hyperventilation

Respiratory Acidosis—Retention of Carbon Dioxide	Respiratory Alkalosis—Hyperventilation
Common Causes	**Common Causes**
Abdominal Distention	Anxiety/Fear/Pain
Aspiration	ARDS
Asthma	Asthma
Bronchiectasis	Atelectasis
Central Nervous System Disorders	Cerebrovascular Accident
Chest Trauma	CNS Disorders
Drug Overdose	Congestive Heart Failure
Emphysema	High Altitude
Flail Chest	Hypoxemia
Head Trauma	Infections/Sepsis/Fever
Mechanical Hypoventilation	Pneumonia
Neuromuscular Disorders	Pulmonary Embolism
Obesity	Salicylate Overdose
Oversedation/Anesthesia	Tumors
Pneumonia	
Pneumothorax	
Pulmonary Edema	
Restrictive Lung Disease	
Sleep Apnea	

Metabolic Acidosis—Gain of Metabolic Acids or Loss of Base	Metabolic Alkalosis—Gain of Base or Loss of Metabolic Acids
Common Causes	**Common Causes**
Administration of Exogenous Acids	Administration of Steroids and/or Diuretics
Anaerobic Metabolism (Lactic Acidosis)	Cushing Syndrome
Carbon Anhydrase deficiency	Excess Administration of Sodium Bicarbonate
Diabetic Ketoacidosis	Excess Ingestion of Antacids
Diarrhea	Increased Levels of Aldosterone
Drainage of Pancreatic Juices	Low Potassium and/or Chloride
Drug Overdose	Massive Blood Transfusions (Increased Citrate)
Ethylene Glycol	Nasogastric Suctioning/Lavage
Methanol	Vomiting
Overwhelming Sepsis	
Paraldehyde	
Renal Failure	
Rhabdomyolysis	
Salicylate Overdose	
Starvation	

Hemorrhagic Shock in Injured Patients				
	Class I	**Class II**	**Class III**	**Class IV**
Blood loss (ml)	Up to 750	750–1500	1500–2000	> 2000
Blood loss (%)	Up to 15%	15–30%	30–40%	> 40%
Pulse rate	< 100	> 100	> 120	> 140
Blood pressure	Normal	Normal	Decreased	Decreased
Pulse pressure	Normal or increased	Decreased	Decreased	Decreased
Respiratory rate	14–20	20–30	30–40	> 35
Urine output (ml/hour)	> 30	20–30	5–15	Negligible
Central nervous system	Slightly anxious	Mildly anxious	Anxious; confused	Confused; lethargic
Fluid replacement (3:1 rule)	Crystalloid	Crystalloid	Crystalloid and blood	Crystalloid and blood

American College of Surgeons, Committee on Trauma (2012). *Advanced trauma life support* (9th ed.). Chicago, IL: ENA.

SECTION 3: QUESTIONS

1. **Which of the following statements is true about vehicle versus pedestrian injuries?**
   A. Adults are likely to turn toward the vehicle just before impact
   B. The adult victim tends to be thrown away from the impact, striking the ground
   C. The adult victim tries to turn away from an impact
   D. The adult victim tends to be thrown onto the street immediately

2. **A sympathetic response to stimuli results in**
   A. Heightened awareness, increased blood pressure, bronchial dilation, and increased glucogenosis
   B. Dilated pupils, bronchial relaxation, increased gastric motility, normal urine output
   C. Vasodilatation, increased blood pressure, decreased gastric secretions, pupils at 3 mm
   D. Increased respiratory depth, increased heart rate, decreased gastric motility, sphincter dilation

3. **When evaluating a patient for possible hemorrhagic shock, the three primary areas to consider are**
   A. Isolated head injuries upper thigh, and abdomen
   B. Chest, upper thigh, and isolated head injuries
   C. Abdomen, pelvis, and chest
   D. Isolated head injuries, abdomen, and chest

4. **Your patient is a construction worker who was seen in the ED after falling into a trench. He sustained a left fractured tibia and fibula and a fractured left scapula. He required a splenectomy and was just admitted to your care. The nursing supervisor tried to get a bed in the ICU, but none was available. Your initial assessment results are as follows:**
   EKG: ST at 126 with isolated PVC
   BP: 84/50
   Skin pale, cool, clammy
   RR 26, breath sounds clear, slightly diminished RLL
   O_2: 2 L/min via NC
   Mentation: Responds to questions slowly, oriented to self and time CVP 4
   Which of the following conditions do you believe this patient is developing?
   A. Cardiogenic shock
   B. Hypovolemic shock
   C. Septic shock
   D. Left ventricular failure

5. **Which of the following would be considered a cause of distributive shock?**
   A. Neurogenic shock
   B. Cardiac tamponade
   C. Aortic stenosis
   D. Pregnancy

6. **The main components of the Trauma Triad of Death include**
   A. Hypotension, bradycardia, and progressive shock
   B. Coagulopathy, hypothermia, and metabolic acidosis
   C. Progressive, autoregulation, and hypoperfusion
   D. Anaphylaxis, resuscitation, and decompensated

7. By definition, systemic inflammatory response syndrome (SIRS) must be composed of two or more variables identified by the American College of Chest Physicians (ACCP) and the Society of Critical Care Medicine (SCCM). Which of the following variables was not identified in the definition of SIRS?
   A. Fever of more than 38°C (100.4°F) or less than 36°C (96.8°F)
   B. Respiratory rate of more than 20 breaths per minute or arterial carbon dioxide tension (PaCO$_2$) of less than 32 mmHg
   C. Abnormal white blood cell count (greater than12,000/µL or less than 4,000/µL or greater than 10% immature [band] forms)
   D. A heart rate of more than 80 beats per minute

8. When describing the amount of exterior deformation of a vehicle sustained in a collision, the commonly used term is
   A. Crush
   B. Intrusion
   C. Incursion
   D. Collision two

9. When considering the use of permissive hypotension during resuscitation, which statement below is a risk factor that must be considered prior to implementation of the therapy:
   A. The therapy increases the likelihood of hypothermia
   B. Permissive hypotension will exacerbate a head injury
   C. Risks associated with acidosis will increase
   D. Coagulopathies will likely increase

10. Administration of one unit of platelets elevates the platelet count approximately
    A. 1,000–40,000 u/dl
    B. 5,000–10,000 u/dl
    C. 3 g/dl
    D. 5%

11. When assessing your trauma patient for possible development of hemorrhagic shock, the areas that are prone to hemorrhage are
    A. Isolated head injuries, upper thigh, and abdomen
    B. Chest Zone II in the neck upper thigh, and isolated head injuries
    C. Abdomen, pelvis, and chest
    D. Isolated head injuries, abdomen, and chest

12. The ratio of heart rate in bpm to systolic blood pressure measured in mmHg is known as the
    A. Pulse pressure
    B. Systemic vascular resistance
    C. Shock index
    D. Impedance

13. There are multiple impacts that take place during a motor vehicle collision. When a victim sustains head, chest, and abdominal injuries, the injuries usually occur during the
    A. First impact
    B. Second impact sequence
    C. Third impact sequence
    D. Fourth impact sequence

14. In trauma patients, the INR may be useful in identifying trauma-induced coagulopathy early. The INR value that would indicate this condition is an
    A. INR of 3.5
    B. INR of 1.5
    C. INR of 2.7
    D. INR of 2.3

15. Administering uncrossed blood in an emergency has always been controversial. Recommendations now include Massive Transfusion Protocols that suggest the resuscitation rooms are stocked and reserved prior to patient arrival with
    A. O negative blood for males
    B. O positive blood for females
    C. O negative blood for females and children
    D. Only O positive blood

16. Which of the following arterial blood gases would likely be found in a patient with early hypovolemic shock:
    A. Respiratory alkalosis
    B. Respiratory acidosis
    C. Metabolic acidosis
    D. Metabolic alkalosis

17. While participating in a cardiac arrest on your unit, you note a colleague is performing chest compressions on an adult at a rate of approximately 90 per minute. According to the 2015 American Heart Association Guidelines for CPR and ECC Update, the correct rate for performing chest compressions is
    A. 80–90 per minute
    B. 80 per minute
    C. 100–120 per minute
    D. At least 100 per minute

18. Determine the pulse pressure for a patient who has a pulse of 78, a BP of 115/85, and a respiratory rate of 12.
    A. 42
    B. 37
    C. 30
    D. 103

19. What is the mean arterial pressure (MAP) for a patient with a blood pressure of 134/60 and a heart rate of 70?
    A. 64
    B. 52
    C. 85
    D. 47

20. An adult patient has fallen from the balcony of a sixth-floor apartment to the street below. Falls from this height usually result in a mortality rate of
    A. 100%
    B. 70%
    C. 50%
    D. 35%

21. Calculate the cardiac output for a patient with a heart rate of 76 and a stroke volume of 65 ml.
    A. 57%
    B. 4.94 L/min
    C. 1,285 ml/min
    D. 2.85 L

22. **Blood component replacement therapy for DIC may include all but which of the following?**
    A. FFP
    B. Cryoprecipitate
    C. Amicar
    D. Platelets

23. **How does low-molecular-weight heparin (LMWH) differ from unfractionated heparin?**
    A. It is more difficult to administer
    B. There are more side effects with LMWH
    C. LMWH is more stable
    D. Unfractionated heparin is easier to administer

24. **Hemoglobin is primarily phagocytized in the**
    A. Liver
    B. Gallbladder
    C. Spleen
    D. Pancreas

25. **Due to a data entry error an 18-year-old mother with A negative blood type received a transfusion of Rh-positive platelets following a placental abruption. As a trauma nurse, you know it would be appropriate to administer**
    A. Neostigmine
    B. FFP
    C. RhoGAM
    D. CuroSurf

26. **Your patient was practicing Parkour and attempting to jump across the roofs of buildings about 30 feet in the air, but then missed, and fell to the ground. Other than the head, what is the second deadliest part of the body this patient might land on when striking the street between the buildings?**
    A. The back
    B. The buttocks
    C. The calcanea
    D. The left side

27. **A function of a red blood cell is**
    A. Cell humoral mediation
    B. To function as a macrophage
    C. To initiate hemostasis
    D. Carbonic acid dissociation

28. **Use of the colloid Hetastarch may affect your patient in which of the following ways?**
    A. Hetastarch may elevate serum amylase levels
    B. Hetastarch may decrease serum potassium levels
    C. Hetastarch may increase capillary permeability
    D. Hetastarch may cause acute tubular necrosis

29. **Which of the following fluids can accelerate systemic inflammation in trauma patients by activating neutrophils?**
    A. Colloids
    B. Crystalloids
    C. Osmotic diuretics
    D. Hypertonic saline

30. **Which of the following IV fluids actually suppresses inflammation?**
    A. Hypertonic saline
    B. Normal saline
    C. Hetastarch
    D. D₅W

31. **Which of the following statements is true regarding the administration of colloids?**
    A. As hydrostatic pressure decreases, pores increase in size to let particles through
    B. You can give smaller amounts of fluid (about 250 ml) and achieve the same effect you would with 4 L of crystalloids
    C. Edema takes a much shorter time to resolve
    D. Colloids are neuroprotective

32. **Patients who are stung by bees numerous times are in danger of developing**
    A. Kidney failure
    B. Anemia
    C. Long QT interval
    D. Hydrocephalus

33. **Emergency medical services have radioed your ED and are in route with a victim of a police shooting. When the patient arrives, the patient is found to have been shot in the hip and mid abdomen. You ask what type of ammunition was used and the police officer states, "frangible." As a trauma nurse, you know this type of bullet**
    A. Is identical to a full metal jacket bullet
    B. A soft nose bullet
    C. A hollow point bullet
    D. Designed to break apart on impact

34. **Stroke volume is comprised of which of the following factors?**
    A. Viscosity, blood volume, and impedance
    B. Cardiac output, heart rate, and compliance
    C. Contractility, preload, and afterload
    D. Systemic impedance, heart rate, and compliance

35. **You are using the PQRST method of pain assessment for your patient complaining of chest pain. The "S" in this mnemonic stands for**
    A. Sensitivity
    B. Severity
    C. Standard
    D. Symptoms

36. **During inspiration your patient has a paradoxical rise in jugular venous pressure. This phenomenon is commonly associated with**
    A. Mitral stenosis
    B. Right heart failure
    C. An anterior wall MI
    D. Increased ventricular compliance

37. **Stimulation of the parasympathetic nerve fibers in the heart will result in**
    A. An increased heart rate
    B. An adrenergic response, causing a decreased blood flow to the extremities
    C. An increase in conduction and a major effect on the force of ventricular conduction
    D. The release of acetylcholine

38. **Dobutamine is used to improve cardiac output primarily by**
    A. Causing profound peripheral vasodilation
    B. Acting on alpha-adrenergic receptors in the heart
    C. Acting on beta-1 adrenergic receptors in the heart
    D. Acting on both alpha- and beta-adrenergic receptors in the cardiovascular tissue

39. **Alpha-adrenergic effects of norepinephrine include**
    A. Increased force of myocardial contraction
    B. Peripheral arteriolar vasoconstriction
    C. Increased AV conduction time
    D. Central venous vasodilation

40. **Which of the following blood types is the universal donor for packed red blood cells (PRBCs)?**
    A. Type AB negative
    B. Type A
    C. Type B
    D. Type O negative

41. **Which of the following would be an appropriate definition of anaphylactic shock?**
    A. Systemic vasodilation that causes low blood pressure, which is by definition 30% lower than the person's baseline or below standard values
    B. Anaphylaxis is the recurrence symptoms within 1–72 hours with no further exposure to the allergen
    C. Anaphylactic shock does not involve an allergic reaction but is due to direct mast cell degranulation.
    D. An overreaction and misdirection of immune responses

42. **In sepsis, endotoxins stimulate production of tumor necrosis factor (TNF). The TNF, in turn, stimulates**
    A. Neutrophil activation and platelet aggregation
    B. Parathyroid hormone production
    C. Increased CO_2 retention
    D. Increased CPP

43. **Which of the following statements about anaphylaxis is correct?**
    A. The condition of anaphylaxis requires the patient to be sensitized
    B. Anaphylaxis does not need IgE antibodies for a hypersensitivity reaction to occur
    C. There are five classifications of anaphylaxis, all are extreme emergencies
    D. An anaphylactoid response is identical to anaphylaxis

44. **It is critical to rapidly identify septic patients. They are defined as those with infection that has been confirmed or suspected by an experienced care provider, and the presence of two or more criteria for systemic inflammatory response syndrome. These criteria include a heart rate above 90 beats per minute, temperature below 36°C or above 38°C, either a respiratory rate above 20 breaths per minute or a CO_2 partial pressure less than 32 mmHg, and a WBC count either less than 4,000 cells/mm^3 or with greater than 10% immature (band) forms. To meet the criteria for septic shock, the patient would have a systolic blood pressure below 90 mmHg after a 20–30 ml/kg fluid bolus and a lactate level above**
    A. 4 mmol/L
    B. 20 L
    C. 35 mmHg
    D. 15 mm^3

45. **In trauma patients, the INR may be useful in identifying trauma-induced coagulopathy early. The INR value that would indicate this condition is an**
    A. INR of 3.5
    B. INR of 1.5
    C. INR of 2.7
    D. INR of 2.3

46. **The term *Massive Transfusion* generally means a patient who**
    A. Has received greater than 10 units of PRBCs within 24 hours of admission
    B. Has received at least five units of PRBs and five additional blood components
    C. Received three combinations of one unit PRBCs, three units of plasma, and three units of platelets
    D. Received at least five different blood components in the last four hours since admission

47. **Calculate the shock index (SI) for a patient with the following vital signs; HR: 120, RR: 22, BP 84/60.**
    A. 2
    B. 1.43
    C. 0.39
    D. 0.70

48. **Airbag injuries commonly associated with motor vehicle crashes are**
    A. LeFort I and II fractures
    B. Blowout orbital injuries
    C. Facial lacerations
    D. Tympanic membrane rupture and tinnitus

49. **Packed red blood cells will elevate hemoglobin levels by _____ and hematocrit levels by _____ per unit.**
    A. 3 grams per dl; 4%
    B. 5 grams per dl; 5%
    C. 2 grams per dl; 2%
    D. 1 gram per dl; 3%

50. **Your adult patient fell from a ladder and has sustained a closed femur fracture. Which of the following values closely represents the estimated blood loss for this patient?**
    A. 3,000 ml
    B. 500 ml
    C. 1,000 ml
    D. 2,000 ml

51. **When a patient receives banked blood, it is treated with citrate to prevent coagulation. Which of the following statements is true about the use of this preservative?**
    A. Citrate binds with calcium and makes it inactive
    B. The liver is unable to metabolize citrate
    C. The patient is likely to develop hypercalcemia
    D. Blood with citrate must always be warmed

52. **After a successful resuscitation, the patient has achieved ROSC but is comatose (lacking meaningful response to verbal commands). Which of the following TTM interventions is recommended for this patient?**
    A. Maintain a constant temperature between 32°C and 35°C (89.6°F and 95.2°F) for at least 24 hours
    B. Maintain oxygen saturation levels of at least 93%
    C. Waveform capnography reading of 10
    D. Transport to Cath lab immediately

53. **When performing CPR on an adult, it is optimal to target your compression depth from**
    A. 1.5 to 2.5 inches
    B. 2 to 2.4 inches
    C. 2.5 to 3 inches
    D. A minimum of 1.5 to 2 inches

54. **Your patient exhibits ST segment depression on his EKG along with moderate, substernal chest pain. These findings indicate a possible**
    A. Anteroseptal MI
    B. Myocardial ischemia
    C. Lateral wall MI
    D. Pericardial tamponade

55. **A low CVP reading may actually represent**
    A. Pulmonary hypertension
    B. Increased contractility
    C. Biventricular failure
    D. Cardiac tamponade

56. **You are caring for a patient who will be admitted for observation for a possible pulmonary contusion sustained from a bicycle accident. The patient refused to wait for a wheelchair. While ambulating, the patient suddenly complains of chest pain. You note that while describing the pain, the patient clenches his fist over the sternal area. This gesture is commonly associated with ischemic chest pain and is known as**
    A. Prinzmetal's sign
    B. Frazier's sign
    C. Homans' sign
    D. Levine's sign

57. **The fluid of choice for trauma resuscitation is**
    A. 5% albumin
    B. Lactated Ringer's
    C. 0.9% normal saline
    D. 0.45% normal saline

58. **Your patient was an unrestrained passenger in a lateral impact car crash. The patient was a "far side" impact victim. Which of the following statements is true regarding the injuries likely to be suffered by this patient?**
    A. This patient is unlikely to suffer an intrusion injury
    B. This patient is likely to suffer rotational and lateral injuries
    C. This patient is very likely to suffer shear injuries
    D. The severity of lateral injury will increase

59. **Which of the following fluids can accelerate systemic inflammation in trauma patients by activating neutrophils?**
    A. Colloids
    B. Crystalloids
    C. Osmotic diuretics
    D. Hypertonic saline

60. **An IV fluid not considered to be a colloid would be**
    A. 0.2% normal saline
    B. Mannitol
    C. Dextran
    D. Hetastarch

61. **Which IV fluid listed below is least likely to be used for resuscitation?**
    A. 5% albumin
    B. 25% albumin
    C. Dextrose 5% in water (D_5W)
    D. Lactated Ringer's

62. **A patient suffering from spinal shock would be expected to exhibit which of the following symptom:**
    A. Loss of autonomic function
    B. An increase in urine production
    C. Loss of reflexes above the site of injury
    D. Heightened proprioceptive sensation

63. **Which of the following statements is true regarding the use of damage-control resuscitation:**
    A. The amount of crystalloid use will be reduced
    B. Only packed red blood cells may be used
    C. Hemodilution is a likely result
    D. The risk of disease transmission is increased

64. **Usually, the earliest measureable sign of shock is considered to be**
    A. Deterioration of level of consciousness
    B. Tachycardia
    C. Restlessness
    D. Dysrhythmias

65. **The shock state best described as decreased cellular perfusion resulting from failure of a central pump is known as**
    A. Obstructive shock
    B. Hypovolemic shock
    C. Distributive shock
    D. Cardiogenic shock

66. **Which of the following substances will not initiate an anaphylactoid reaction?**
    A. Dextran
    B. Thiamine
    C. Opiates
    D. Milk

67. **On occasion, intraosseous placement is necessary. To ensure the needle is placed correctly**
    A. The needle needs to be held at 90° perpendicular to the injection site
    B. There must not be a return of marrow when aspirated
    C. Extravasation of fluid will occur when 40 ml of fluid is pushed
    D. The needle will stand up unassisted

68. **The universal donor for plasma is blood**
    A. Type B negative
    B. Type O positive
    C. Type AB negative
    D. Type O negative

69. **Fresh frozen plasma must be given within what period of time to be effective?**
    A. 2 hours
    B. 30 minutes
    C. 6 hours
    D. 3 hours

70. **Type II HIT patients are at great risk for developing**
    A. Generalized bleeding
    B. Pericarditis
    C. Thrombosis
    D. Limb amputation

71. **Which organ is responsible for the disposal of heme with RBC destruction?**
    A. Liver
    B. Gallbladder
    C. Spleen
    D. Pancreas

72. **A microbial phenomenon characterized by an inflammatory response to the microorganisms or the invasion of normally sterile tissue by those organisms is known as**
    A. Septicemia
    B. SIRS
    C. MODS
    D. Infection

73. **An elderly female is admitted to your unit with tachycardia (HR 132), RR 30, BP 90/65, T 96.4°F. Her white count is 17,600. The patient states she was treated for a "kidney infection" two weeks ago. She denies pain at this time. This patient probably is suffering from**
    A. MODS
    B. A kidney stone
    C. SIRS
    D. Appendicitis

74. **The systemic response to infection defined as the presence of SIRS in addition to a documented or presumed infection is known as**
    A. A SIRS sustained response
    B. Sepsis
    C. Bacteremia
    D. A mediated response

75. **The presence of bacteria within the bloodstream is known as**
    A. Bacteremia
    B. An inflammatory response
    C. Septic shock
    D. Septicemia

76. **A state of physiologic dysfunction in which two or more organ systems are not capable of maintaining homeostasis is known as**
    A. Cell-mediated sepsis
    B. Cellular ischemia
    C. End-organ hypoperfusion
    D. Multiple organ dysfunction syndrome

77. **A sepsis-induced state with hypotension, despite adequate fluid resuscitation, is called**
    A. Secondary sepsis-induced hypotension
    B. Severe sepsis
    C. Primary sepsis-induced hypotension
    D. Septic shock

78. **The pH of banked blood is**
    A. 6.5
    B. 7.3
    C. 6.8
    D. 7.1

79. **Classification of a moderate collision would include all but one of the characteristics listed below. As a trauma nurse, you know characteristics of a moderate collision would not include**
    A. A door might be jammed, but no entrapment exists
    B. An undrivable vehicle
    C. Door intrusion of less than four to six inches
    D. Minimal wheelbase reduction

80. **What is one cause of autonomic hyperreflexia?**
    A. Diarrhea
    B. Suctioning
    C. Constipation
    D. Warm breeze

81. **The presence of a systolic blood pressure of less than 90 mmHg or a reduction of more than 40 mmHg from baseline in the absence of other causes of hypotension is known as**
    A. Septic shock
    B. Secondary hypotension
    C. Sepsis-induced hypotension
    D. End-organ hypoperfusion

82. **An important nursing consideration when administering mannitol to your patient is**
    A. Higher doses are required for patients suffering from rhabdomyolysis
    B. Mannitol is not to be used in head-injured patients
    C. Mannitol must be administered using an inline 5 micron filter
    D. Mannitol causes ototoxicity if administered rapidly

83. **If your patient is hypokalemic, what changes would you expect to see on an EKG tracing?**
    A. Peaked T waves
    B. U waves
    C. Shortened QT intervals
    D. Absent P waves

84. **Lactate is a marker for cellular hypoxia. Certain conditions that cause inadequate oxygen delivery may elevate the lactate level. Which of the following conditions should not cause an elevation in lactate levels?**
    A. Septic shock
    B. Seizures
    C. Diabetes mellitus
    D. Hypothermia

85. **Epinephrine and norepinephrine may be used in the ED to treat hypotension. Which of the following actions of these vasopressors will increase blood glucose?**
    A. Lower peripheral insulin resistance
    B. Increase insulin secretion
    C. Decrease lipolysis
    D. Increase liver glycogenolysis

86. Your patient was stung by a bee and had an anaphylactic reaction. She has received epinephrine both via EpiPen and intravenously because she had severe airway obstruction due to swelling. Epinephrine is given for anaphylactic reactions because
    A. It prevents localized edema
    B. It promotes temporary changes in ST segments
    C. It prevents third space fluid loss
    D. It promotes bronchodilation and inhibits additional mediator release

87. Which of the following medications would you anticipate using to improve the pumping action of the heart when a patient is developing cardiogenic shock?
    A. Dobutamine
    B. Epinephrine
    C. Diltiazem
    D. Isoproterenol

88. Generalized myocardial depression usually occurs when
    A. The potassium level reaches 5.2
    B. The sodium level is 145
    C. The pH is less than 7.20
    D. The magnesium level is 4.0

89. Use of whole blood in damage-control resuscitation
    A. Is not likely to cause hypothermia
    B. Decreases the risk of disease transmission over packed cells
    C. Must be used within 24–48 hours to assure maximum effectiveness
    D. Has a universal donor

90. If a victim is ejected from a vehicle involved in a motor vehicle crash, the victim is _____ times more likely to be killed than if the victim was restrained in the vehicle at the time of the crash.
    A. 10
    B. 25
    C. 5
    D. 30

91. Which of the following statements is false about the concept of preload?
    A. Preload is increased by sympathetic stimulation
    B. Preload is a systolic phenomenon
    C. Hypervolemia increases preload
    D. Renal problems increase preload

92. Which of the following statements about motor vehicle crashes involving older adults is true:
    A. The MVCs are primarily related to speed and alcohol consumption
    B. Merging into traffic is smoother due to the experience of the driver
    C. Normal age-related physiological changes significantly contribute to MVCs
    D. There are less sternal fractures in older adults because of increased seatbelt use

SECTION 3: ANSWERS

1. **Correct answer: C**
   Adult victims of vehicle versus pedestrian collisions tend to turn away from the impact. They often are thrown onto the hood and windshield of the vehicle before sliding to the ground with potentially additional injuries. Impact is usually lateral and posterior. Children tend to turn toward the point of impact, suffering a combination of head, chest, and/or lower extremity injuries.

2. **Correct answer: A**
   A sympathetic response to stimuli results in heightened awareness, increased blood pressure, bronchial dilation, and increased glucogenosis. Other responses include dilated pupils for increased visual acuity, increased heart rate, increased myocardial contractility, increased blood pressure, increased respiratory rate, decreased gastric motility, decreased gastric secretion, decreased urine output, decreased insulin production, and decreased renal blood flow.

3. **Correct answer: C**
   When assessing a patient for the possibility of hemorrhagic shock, there are three primary areas to consider: the chest, abdomen, and pelvis. Isolated head injuries are unlikely to cause hemorrhagic shock.

4. **Correct answer: B**
   This patient appears to be decompensating and developing hypovolemic shock. He is in sinus tachycardia and his systolic blood pressure is only 84 and his CVP is 4, RR is 26, skin is cool and clammy, and his mentation is diminished.

5. **Correct answer: A**
   Neurogenic, septic, and anaphylactic are types of distributive shock. In distributive shock, there is a maldistribution that does not allow for normal flow to peripheral tissues, resulting in decreased cellular perfusion. Cardiac tamponade, pregnancy, and aortic stenosis are causes of obstructive shock.

6. **Correct answer: B**
   The main components of the Trauma Triad of Death include coagulopathy, hypothermia, and metabolic acidosis. When patients are hypothermic, thrombin production is impaired and platelet function is inhibited. A state of acidosis also impairs thrombin production. Due to hemodilution, the body's ability to produce clotting factors is diminished.

7. **Correct answer: D**
   A heart rate of more than 80 beats per minute was not identified as a variable for the definition of SIRS.

8. **Correct answer: A**
   When describing the amount of exterior deformation of a vehicle sustained in a collision, the commonly used term is *crush*. This term describes the description of dispersal of energy. The more crush, the greater the amount of energy that is absorbed by the vehicle and a lesser amount of energy transferred to occupants.

9. **Correct answer: B**
   Use of permissive hypotension will exacerbate a head injury by decreasing perfusion and thus oxygen and nutrient delivery. Also, permissive hypotension should never be used for elderly or pediatric patients. In actuality, permissive hypotension decreases the likelihood of hypothermia, reduces risks associated with hypothermia, and decreases coagulopathies.

10. **Correct answer: B**
    One unit of platelets elevates the platelet count approximately 5000–10,000 u/dl.

11. **Correct answer: C**
    When assessing a trauma patient for the possible development of hemorrhagic shock, areas to consider: the chest, abdomen, and pelvis. Zone II neck injuries and isolated head injuries are unlikely to lead to hemorrhagic shock.

12. **Correct answer: C**

The ratio of heart rate in bpm to systolic blood pressure measured in mmHg is known as the shock index (SI). Some clinicians use it to assess blood loss and degree of hypovolemic shock and the potential need for transfusions. The most commonly used scale is

Group I	= SI < 0.6	No Shock
Group II	= SI ≥ 0.6 to < 1	Mild Shock
Group III	= SI ≥ 1 to < 1.4	Moderate Shock
Group IV	= SI ≥ 1.4	Severe Shock

For example, a patient with a heart rate of 130 and a systolic blood pressure of 90, would have a shock index of 1.44, indicating severe shock. 130 ÷ 90 = 1.44.

13. **Correct answer: B**

There are multiple impacts that take place during a motor vehicle collision. When a victim sustains head, chest, and abdominal injuries, the injuries usually occur during the second impact. The victim continues in motion and will collide with the interior of the vehicle unless acted on by resistance such as an airbag or seatbelt.

Front seat occupants may sustain one of two types of injury patterns. If the victim sustains an "up and over" path, the head and chest strike the dashboard and windshield. The victim may also travel "down and under" the steering wheel or dashboard, suffering lower extremity or pelvic injuries. Many times, this type of injury occurs because the seatbelt is placed over the abdomen.

14. **Correct answer: B**

In trauma patients, the INR may be useful in identifying trauma-induced coagulopathy early. The INR value that would indicate this condition is an INR of 1.5.

15. **Correct answer: C**

Administering uncrossed blood in an emergency has always been controversial. Recommendations now include Massive Transfusion Protocols that suggest the resuscitation rooms are stocked and reserved prior to patient arrival with O negative blood for females and children, and O positive blood for male traumas. There is a larger donor pool for O positive and a much smaller pool for O negative donors.

16. **Correct answer: A**

Patients in the early stage of hypovolemic shock demonstrate respiratory alkalosis primarily due to tachypnea. CO_2 is blown off resulting in an alkalotic state.

17. **Correct answer: C**

While participating in a cardiac arrest on your unit, you note a colleague is performing chest compressions on an adult at a rate of approximately 90 per minute. The correct rate for performing chest compressions on an adult is 100–120 per minute, according to the 2015 American Heart Association guidelines for CPR and ECC. It is also good practice to allow the chest to fully recoil after each compression.

18. **Correct answer: C**

A pulse pressure is the difference between the systolic blood pressure and the diastolic blood pressure—in this case, 30. This measurement is significant because if the patient has a narrow pulse pressure, it would indicate systemic compensatory vasoconstriction due to a decrease in arterial pressure (the stroke volume falls and the systolic pressure decreases). Another way to look at this phenomenon is to think of the high systemic vascular resistance causing an increase in diastolic pressure.

19. **Correct answer: C**

The MAP is a mean pressure that takes into account that the diastolic phase of the cardiac cycle comprises two-thirds of the cycle. The calculation for the MAP is MAP = 2(DBP) + (SBP)/3; in this case, 85. If you took the average of the two pressures, it would not account for the importance of the diastolic phase. The heart rate is not entered into this calculation. Patients should maintain a MAP of at least 60 to ensure perfusion to the brain and kidneys.

When the heart rate is over 100, the diastolic phase may be less than one-half the cardiac cycle. Electronic machines are calibrated to take variables into consideration, and the digitally displayed MAP readings are highly accurate.

20. **Correct answer: C**
An adult patient has fallen from the balcony of a fourth floor apartment to the street below. Falls from this height usually result in a mortality rate of 50%. A fall is rated as severe if greater than three times the height of a victim. Children have a 50% mortality rate for falls from the sixth floor.

According to the CDC and 2011 Guidelines for Field Triage of Injured Patients, any victim meeting the following criteria needs to be transported immediately to a trauma center:

- falls
  - » adults: greater than 20 feet (one story = 10 feet)
  - » children: greater than 10 feet or two to three times the height of the child
- high-risk auto crash
  - » intrusion, including roof: greater than 12 inches occupant site; greater than 18 inches any site
  - » ejection (partial or complete) from automobile
  - » death in same passenger compartment
  - » vehicle telemetry data consistent with a high risk for injury
- automobile versus pedestrian/bicyclist thrown, run over, or with significant (greater than 20 mph) impact or
- motorcycle crash greater than 20 mph

21. **Correct answer: B**
Normal cardiac output should be 4 to 8 L/min. The formula for calculating this value is: CO = HR × SV. In this case, 76 (HR) × 65 (SV) = 4,940 ml/min. Converted to liters, this value would equal 4.94 L/min.

22. **Correct answer: C**
Blood component (factor) replacement therapy for DIC does not include aminocaproic acid (Amicar). Amicar is used to inhibit fibrinolysis, not replace clotting factors. It is used in the treatment of DIC, but it may change a simple bleeding issue into DIC. It must be used in combination with heparin. DIC is usually treated with FFP, cryoprecipitate, and platelets. Cryoprecipitate contains more than 5–10 times more fibrinogen than FFP. A good rule of thumb is to give 10 units of cryoprecipitate for every 3 units of FFP. If the patient is actively bleeding, platelets are commonly used.

23. **Correct answer: C**
Low-molecular-weight heparin is more stable than unfractionated heparin. LMWH (i.e., Lovenox) is so stable and predictable that PTTs are not required. It is also easy to administer at home.

24. **Correct answer: A**
Hemoglobin is phagocytized primarily in the liver. Hemoglobin is comprised of two parts. The first part is "heme" that causes the reddish color and contains iron and porphyrin. The second part is a protein called "globin." Hemoglobin combines with oxygen to form oxyhemoglobin. Hemoglobin also binds with CO_2 and carries it to alveoli to be expired. When the hemoglobin is phagocytized in the liver, it breaks down into the heme and globin.

25. **Correct answer: C**
Due to a data entry error an 18-year-old mother with A- blood type, received a transfusion of Rh-positive platelets following a placental abruption, and it would be appropriate to administer RhoGAM®. Assuming that the mother was not given RhoGAM® after her last pregnancy and the father of this fetus is Rh positive, then there is a 50% possibility that the fetus will be Rh positive and the mother may have developed IgG antibodies to this pregnancy. The risk of maternal memory B cells being triggered to produce antibodies to the Rho(D) antigen increase with the introduction of Rh positive blood. Antigen presenting cells like neutrophils, monocytes, macrophages, B cells and T_h cells take that antigen and

present it on the surface to T_h cells. These T_h cells present the antigen to primary B cells that create an IgG antibody to match the antigen and create memory cells or antibody factories that go dormant until exposed to that antigen again. With subsequent exposures, the anti-Rho(D) factories (plasma B cells) can go into production faster than before because the maternal immune system (memory cells) already recognizes the problem and has the blueprint for the solution (antibody). This would not be a problem, but the very thing we like about IgG (able to cross the placenta to provide immunity to the fetus) is the very thing that in this case will kill the fetus. As the antibodies for the Rho(D) antigen (found on all fetal RBCs) cause the fetal RBC to lyse, and the fetus becomes severely anemic. The massive destruction of RBC leads to hyperbilirubinemia as hemoglobin is released into vascular circulation with the potential of causing neurologic injury. As oxygen-carrying capacity decreases, hypoxemia increases hypoxia at the tissue level. All of these elements increase the risk for fetal death.

RhoGAM® is a Rh immune globulin. It is thought to attack the Rho(D) antigen on RBC in the maternal bloodstream. This would prevent activation of maternal immune response and resultant Rho(D) antigen antibody production. The method of action is either that the cells are destroyed before detection, hidden with globulin/antigen binding before detection, or the binding of the globulin to the antigen blocks T_h cells from binding and initiating the immune response cascade.

With each exposure to Rh positive blood, the immune response becomes faster with higher production of antibodies. This mother should be carefully monitored throughout this and any subsequent pregnancy for any possible change in fetal status indicating hemolytic anemia.

26. **Correct answer: B**
Your patient was practicing Parkour and attempting to jump across the roofs of buildings about 30 feet in the air, missed, then fell to the ground. Other than the head, the second deadliest part of the body to land on would be the buttocks. Energy would be transmitted to the pelvis, then the abdomen, followed by the thorax. There is the possibility of injury to so many vital structures. If the patient had landed on the back, some of the energy would dissipate and potentially reduce severity. If this patient had fallen feet first, energy would be absorbed by the lower extremities, limiting damage to vital structures. If this patient had landed on the side, there certainly could have been damage to the pelvis, and some vital structures, but the patient would have a better chance of survival.

27. **Correct answer: D**
A red blood cell has multiple functions, including carbonic acid dissociation to form bicarbonate ions. The RBC provides oxygen transport via hemoglobin and carbon dioxide transport via carboxyhemoglobin. The RBC buffers protons by binding with hemoglobin to form acid hemoglobin.

28. **Correct answer: A**
Hetastarch may elevate serum amylase levels, but the levels will return to normal within a week after administration. Hetastarch will not increase serum potassium levels or increase capillary permeability. Hetastarch must be used with caution in patients in anaphylactic or septic shock because capillary permeability is already increased. Dextran may cause acute tubular necrosis.

29. **Correct answer: B**
Crystalloids, particularly lactated Ringer's solution, can accelerate systemic inflammation in trauma patients by activating neutrophils. These neutrophils destroy surrounding tissue by way of oxidative burst, then release hydrogen peroxide into the tissue, leading to acute respiratory distress syndrome (ARDS) and multiple organ failure (MOF/MODS).

30. **Correct answer: A**
Hypertonic saline suppresses inflammation, helps correct electrolyte imbalances, and pulls water back to the intravascular space from the cells and interstitial spaces.

31. **Correct answer: C**
Colloids are used for volume expansion. Particles suspended in colloids don't break down into smaller pieces in water and most won't fit through most capillary pores, so therefore they stay in the vascular bed.

32. **Correct answer: A**

Patients who are stung by bees numerous times are in danger of developing kidney failure. Bee stings have proteins in the venom that act as enzymes. The enzymes lyse the cells, and the cellular debris accumulates very quickly and actually clogs the kidneys. The patient then dies from kidney failure. Any patient who has been stung multiple times needs to be monitored for at least two weeks after the incident.

33. **Correct answer: D**

A frangible bullet is designed to break apart on impact. The bullet shatters or disintegrates. The result is a projectile that can help eliminate over penetration because it does not expand or deform like a hollow point bullet.

34. **Correct answer: C**

Stroke volume is comprised of contractility, preload, and afterload. Viscosity, blood volume, and impedance represent the components of afterload. Myocardium is sensitive to changes, especially increased afterload. With only minute changes in afterload, the stroke volume can fall significantly.

35. **Correct Answer: B**

The PQRST pain assessment method is used to collect assessment data regarding chest pain in a logical manner that ensures complete assessment data is gathered.

- The P in the acronym stands for "provokes." Does any activity specifically provoke the pain?
- Q represents the "quality of the pain." Typical adjectives used include *sharp*, *stabbing*, *squeezing*, *pressure*, *tightness*, *dull*, *indigestion-like*, and *pulsating*.
- R is "radiation," meaning that pain starts at one location and ends at another location. For example, pain may radiate from the chest to the jaw, a specific arm, the back, and/or abdomen.
- S stands for "severity of the pain." Some patients may have altered pain sensation from other disease processes such as diabetes, neuropathies, and multiple scleroses and may not present with typical symptoms for a myocardial infarction.
- T stands for "time." The duration of the pain is important when considering antithrombolytics as treatment, because this is highly time sensitive and will impact success of the treatment.

36. **Correct answer: B**

During inspiration your patient has a paradoxical rise in jugular venous pressure. This phenomenon is commonly associated with right heart failure. Blood flow to the right ventricle is impaired because of a decrease in compliance or possibly fluid in the pericardial space. Blood backs up into the venous system, causing the increase in jugular venous pressure.

37. **Correct answer: D**

Stimulation of the parasympathetic nerve fibers in the heart will result in the release of acetylcholine. The acetylcholine binds to parasympathetic receptors. These receptors are classified into two types: muscarinic and nicotinic. Muscarinic parasympathetic receptors are located in the heart and smooth muscle. Nicotinic receptors are found at the neuromuscular junction, the central nervous system, and adrenal medulla.

38. **Correct answer: C**

Dobutamine is used to improve cardiac output by acting on beta-1 adrenergic receptors in the heart. It may cause minimal peripheral vasodilation but primarily acts to increase contractility, coronary blood flow, and heart rate to improve cardiac output. Dopamine acts on alpha-adrenergic receptors in the heart. Norepinephrine is a catecholamine that acts on both alpha- and beta-adrenergic receptors in the cardiovascular tissue.

39. **Correct answer: B**

Alpha-adrenergic effects of norepinephrine include peripheral arteriolar vasoconstriction. Increased force of myocardial contraction and increased AV conduction time are the effects of beta-adrenergic sympathetic stimulation.

40. Correct answer: D

The blood type that is the universal donor for packed red blood cells (PRBCs) is type O negative. Keep in mind that a patient with Rh negative blood and who may carry children in the future must receive Rh negative blood. A patient with Rh positive blood may receive both Rh negative and Rh positive blood.

41. Correct answer: A

Anaphylactic shock is one of three classifications of anaphylaxis. It is a systemic vasodilation that causes low blood pressure, which is by definition 30% lower than the person's baseline or below standard values.

Biphasic anaphylaxis is the recurrence of symptoms within 1–72 hours with no further exposure to the allergen. Pseudoanaphylaxis or anaphylactoid reactions are a type of anaphylaxis that does not involve an allergic reaction but is due to direct mast cell degranulation. *Nonimmune anaphylaxis* is the current term used by the World Allergy Organization.

42. Correct answer: A

In sepsis, endotoxins stimulate production of tumor necrosis factor (TNF). TNF, in turn, stimulates neutrophil activation and platelet aggregation. In addition, TNF stimulates increased capillary permeability and promotes the release of IL-1, IL-6, and IL-8.

43. Correct answer: A

The condition of anaphylaxis requires the patient to be sensitized by exposure to the antigen at least once and their reaction mediated through immunoglobulin E (IgE) antibodies. An anaphylactoid reaction doesn't need the presence of IgE-3. Examples of substances causing anaphylactic reactions include: antibiotics (penicillin, cephalosporins), foods (milk, egg whites, shellfish, nuts, chocolate, grains, beets), and foreign proteins (latex, venom, glue). Other potential causes of anaphylaxis may include anesthetics, egg-based vaccines, exercise, and cold.

44. Correct answer: A

Keep in mind that the half-life of lactate is around 20 minutes, even in septic patients. If the lactate is persistently elevated, it's not because the body can't get rid of it, but because the body continues to produce it.

It is critical to rapidly identify septic patients. They are defined as those with infection that has been confirmed or suspected by an experienced care provider, and the presence of two or more criteria for systemic inflammatory response syndrome. These criteria include a heart rate above 90 beats per minute, temperature below 36°C or above 38°C, either a respiratory rate above 20 breaths per minute or a CO_2 partial pressure less than 32 mmHg, and a WBC count either less than 4,000 cells/mm^3 or with greater than 10% immature (band) forms. To meet the criteria for septic shock, the patient would have a systolic blood pressure below 90 mmHg after a 20–30 ml/kg fluid bolus and a lactate level above 4 mmol/L.

45. Correct answer: B

In trauma patients, the INR may be useful in identifying trauma-induced coagulopathy early. The INR value that would indicate this condition is an INR of 1.5.

46. Correct answer: A

The term *Massive Transfusion* generally means a patient who has received greater than 10 units of PRBCs within 24 hours of admission. Having said that, several trauma surgeons have recently recommended changing the definition to include patients who have received 10 units of PRBCs within 6 hours.

47. Correct answer: B

The shock index (SI) for a patient with the following vital signs; HR: 120, RR: 22, BP 84/60 is 1.43. Heart rate of 120 divided by systolic BP of 84 = 1.43. This patient is in severe shock.

48. Correct answer: D

Tympanic membrane rupture and tinnitus are airbag injuries commonly associated with motor vehicle crashes. Keep in mind that patients with respiratory compromise, such as asthmatics, may develop issues secondary to the powder used in airbags. Patients may also sustain alkali injury in the eyes.

49. **Correct answer: D**
Use of packed red blood cells during resuscitation will raise hemoglobin levels by 1 gram per dl and hemoglobin by 3% per unit.

50. **Correct answer: C**
Your adult patient fell from a ladder and has sustained a closed femur fracture. A loss of 1,000 ml closely represents the estimated blood loss for this patient because this is an average for a patient with a closed femur fracture. The blood volume for an adult range between 4,700 and 5,500 ml.

51. **Correct answer: A**
When a patient receives banked blood, it is treated with citrate to prevent coagulation. The citrate binds with calcium, making it inactive, possibly worsening bleeding. The patient may become hypocalcemic, evidenced by dysrhythmias, tremors, and seizures. Usually about three grams of citrate is added per unit of blood. The liver can metabolize about 3 grams of citrate every 5 minutes. If the patient receives blood more often, they may suffer from citrate toxicity and hypocalcemia, so the patient must be carefully monitored. Calcium gluconate or calcium chloride may need to be administered.

52. **Correct answer: A**
Your patient suffered a cardiac arrest and has achieved ROSC but is comatose (lacking meaningful response to verbal commands). According to the 2015 American Heart Association guidelines for CPR and ECC, targeted temperature management (TTM) is to maintain a constant temperature between 32°C and 35°C (89.6°F and 95.2°F) for at least 24 hours.

53. **Correct answer: B**
Chest compressions tend to be too shallow or too deep. If too shallow, the compression may be ineffectual. If too deep, the compression may actually cause an injury. According to the 2015 American Heart Association guidelines for CPR and ECC, compression depth should be targeted at 2 to 2.4 inches.

54. **Correct answer: B**
ST segment depression usually indicates myocardial ischemia. This patient also exhibited substernal chest pain, another finding seen with ischemia.

55. **Correct answer: B**
A low CVP reading may represent increased contractility. The heart is able to eject its contents more easily, reducing the pressure in the right atrium.

56. **Correct answer: D**
You are caring for a patient who will be admitted for observation for a possible pulmonary contusion sustained from a bicycle accident. The patient refused to wait for a wheelchair. While ambulating, the patient suddenly complains of chest pain. You note that while describing the pain, the patient clenches his fist over the sternal area. This gesture is commonly associated with ischemic chest pain and is known as Levine's sign. It is thought that the clenched fist occurs because pain is referred primarily to the left forearm. Patients suffering from acute coronary syndrome, an MI, or angina pectoris often produce this gesture.

57. **Correct answer: B**
The fluid of choice for trauma resuscitation is Lactated Ringer's (LR). LR is an isotonic crystalloid solution, so the fluid is similar to extracellular fluid. The lactate in the LR is converted to bicarbonate in the liver and helps buffer acidosis.

58. **Correct answer: A**
Your patient was an unrestrained passenger in a lateral impact car crash. The patient was a "far side" impact victim. This patient is unlikely to suffer an intrusion injury. The energy may be partially absorbed by the car interior and the seatbelt. If the patient was the driver and suffered a "near side" crush from intrusion, possible injuries could include shearing injuries, fractured clavicle; lateral pelvic, head, and neck injuries; and abdominal injuries.

59. **Correct answer: B**
    Crystalloids, particularly Lactated Ringer's solution, can accelerate systemic inflammation in trauma patients by activating neutrophils. These neutrophils destroy surrounding tissue by way of oxidative burst, then release hydrogen peroxide into the tissue, leading to acute respiratory distress syndrome (ARDS) and multiple organ failure (MOF/MODS).

60. **Correct answer: A**
    An IV fluid not considered to be a colloid would be 0.2% normal saline. Colloids include human albumin (a natural protein that's separated from plasma) and hetastarch (HES), a synthetic starch derived from hydroxyethyl glucose. Additional colloids include mannitol (an alcohol sugar) and dextran (a polysaccharide).

61. **Correct answer: C**
    Dextrose 5% in water (D_5W) is not used for resuscitation because its glucose is metabolized and quickly becomes hypotonic. In fact, D_5W is a good source of free water.

62. **Correct answer: A**
    A patient suffering from spinal shock would be expected to exhibit a loss of autonomic function. Urine production would decrease, loss of reflexes would be noted below the site of injury, and there would be a decrease of proprioceptive and possibly cutaneous sensation.

63. **Correct answer: A**
    When utilizing damage-control resuscitation, the amount of crystalloid use will decrease. Damage-control resuscitation may utilize plasma, platelets, and packed red blood cells.

64. **Correct answer: B**
    Usually, the earliest measureable sign of shock is considered to be tachycardia. When the MAP decreases, it in turn stimulates the sympathetic nervous system via the baroreceptor reflex. To maintain the cardiac output, the heart rate is increased.

65. **Correct answer: D**
    The shock state best described as decreased cellular perfusion resulting from failure of a central pump is known as cardiogenic shock.

66. **Correct answer: D**
    Milk will not initiate an anaphylactoid response, but will cause an anaphylactic response. An anaphylactoid reaction can occur following a single, first-time exposure to certain agents in nonsensitized patients. Anaphylactoid substances cause a direct breakdown of the mast cell and basophil membranes. An anaphylactoid reaction doesn't need the presence of IgE antibodies for a hypersensitivity reaction to occur. Substances which may cause an anaphylactoid response include NSAIDS, aspirin, radiopaque contrast media, fluorescein opiates, thiamine, and dextran. Additional triggers include sulfites, perfumes, bleach, wine, and beer.

67. **Correct answer: D**
    On occasion, intraosseous placement is necessary. To ensure the needle is placed correctly, it should stand up on its own. A lack of bone marrow presence does not necessarily mean failed placement, but if no marrow is present, placement is confirmed. A small push (5–10 ml) should result in minimal resistance and no extravasation.

68. **Correct answer: C**
    The universal donor for fresh frozen plasma is blood type AB negative.

69. **Correct answer: C**
    Fresh frozen plasma must be used within six hours. FFP takes 20 minutes to thaw.

70. **Correct answer: B**
    Type II HIT patients are at great risk for developing pericarditis. Type II HIT is sometimes called "white clot syndrome." Thrombi are primarily venous in origin and can lead to DVT, pulmonary emboli, thrombotic stroke, limb ischemia, and myocardial infarction.

71. **Correct answer: A**

The liver is responsible for the disposal of heme from RBC destruction. Hemoglobin is comprised of two parts. The first part is "heme" that causes the reddish color and contains iron and porphyrin. The second part is a protein called "globin." Hemoglobin combines with oxygen to form oxyhemoglobin. Hemoglobin also binds with CO_2 and carries it to alveoli to be expired. When the hemoglobin is phagocytized in the liver, it breaks down into the heme and globin.

72. **Correct answer: D**

A microbial phenomenon characterized by an inflammatory response to the microorganisms or the invasion of normally sterile tissue by those organisms is known as infection.

73. **Correct answer: C**

SIRS is a systemic infection that can present in the elderly with hypothermia and even a WBC of 4,000 or 12,000. MODS is usually the result of a direct injury to an organ. A kidney stone or appendicitis should present with pain and tenderness.

74. **Correct answer: B**

The systemic response to infection defined as the presence of SIRS in addition to a documented or presumed infection is known as sepsis.

75. **Correct answer: A**

The presence of bacteria within the bloodstream is known as bacteremia. An individual with bacteremia does not necessarily develop sepsis or SIRS.

76. **Correct answer: D**

A state of physiologic dysfunction in which two or more organ systems are not capable of maintaining homeostasis is known as multiple organ dysfunction syndrome (MODS).

77. **Correct answer: D**

A sepsis-induced state with hypotension despite adequate fluid resuscitation is called septic shock.

78. **Correct answer: D**

The pH of banked blood is 7.1. The acidosis may contribute to the development of dysrhythmias.

79. **Correct answer: B**

As a trauma nurse, you know a moderate collision has a lower risk of severe injuries. Door intrusion is a maximum of 4–6 inches, there is little or no wheelbase reduction, and occupants are not trapped.

80. **Correct answer: C**

Autonomic hyperreflexia, also known as autonomic dysreflexia, is caused by numerous stimuli such as bowel or bladder dysfunction, cool breezes, a clogged urinary catheter, and constipation.

81. **Correct answer: C**

The presence of a systolic blood pressure of less than 90 mmHg or a reduction of more than 40 mmHg from baseline in the absence of other causes of hypotension is known as sepsis-induced hypotension.

82. **Correct answer: C**

An important nursing consideration when administering mannitol to your patient is mannitol must be administered using an inline 5 micron filter. Mannitol may crystalize at low temperatures. The filter is also required if using mannitol with greater than 15 g/100 ml (0.15%) solutions. Be cautious when giving mannitol to a patient in renal failure because the mannitol may cause hyperosmolarity.

83. **Correct answer: B**

A U wave is seen in patients who are hypokalemic. A peaked T wave, a shortened QT interval, and an absent P wave are seen with hyperkalemia.

84. **Correct answer: D**

Lactate is a marker for cellular hypoxia. Certain conditions that cause inadequate oxygen delivery may elevate the lactate level. Conditions that cause inadequate oxygen delivery may elevate the lactate level are septic shock, profound dehydration, diabetes mellitus, seizures, hyperthermia, trauma, and prolonged tourniquet application. A level above 4.0 mmol/L is associated with a 27% mortality rate, compared with a mortality rate of 7% for patients with a lactate level of 2.5–4.0 mmol/L and a death rate below 5% for those with a lactate level below 2.5 mmol/L.

85. Correct answer: D

Epinephrine and norepinephrine may be used in the ED to treat hypotension. The following actions of these two vasopressors will increase blood glucose by increasing liver glycogenolysis and stimulating glycogenesis. In addition, epinephrine and norepinephrine increase peripheral insulin resistance, increase lipolysis, and suppress insulin secretion.

86. Correct answer: D

Epinephrine is given for anaphylactic reactions because it promotes bronchodilation and inhibits additional mediator release. Epinephrine counteracts the bronchoconstrictive and vasodilator actions of histamine by stimulating alpha, beta-1, and beta-2 receptors. Epinephrine is also useful in treating hay fever and urticaria.

87. Correct answer: A

Dobutamine is an inotrope and will improve the pumping action of the heart. This alpha-, beta-1, and beta-2 agonist will increase contractility and cardiac output, with little or no concomitant increase in myocardial oxygen consumption. Dobutamine has a very mild vasodilatory effect, though high doses can cause ischemia.

88. Correct answer: C

Generalized myocardial depression usually occurs when the pH is less than 7.2. It is not recommended that the patient be treated with bicarbonate. Rather, fixing the underlying injury is more beneficial.

89. Correct answer: C

Whole blood must be used within 24–48 hours to assure maximum effectiveness. Whole blood does lack a universal donor, and increases the risk of disease transmission. Whole blood is not used in large quantities in DCR, so there is less likelihood of hypothermia and issues with coagulopathy.

90. Correct answer: B

If a victim is ejected from a vehicle involved in a motor vehicle crash, the victim is 25 times more likely to be killed than if they were restrained in the vehicle at the time of the crash. Other considerations with victims who are ejected are that the victim may suffer greater injury by striking the ground or other object after ejection. About half of ejected victims sustain spinal injuries. The distance between the vehicle and the patient may indicate how fast the vehicle was traveling and may be used to calculate how much energy was absorbed by the victim.

91. Correct answer: B

As a trauma nurse, you know preload is a diastolic phenomenon. It is modulated by a variation in intravascular volume. The inertia of flowing blood fills the heart chambers during diastole and, as a consequence, stretch the myocardial fibers, storing mechanical energy in them.

Frank-Starling Law

An increase in stretched fibers during diastole have more mechanical energy stored in them and, therefore, contract with a higher force during the following ejection phase. This can be caused by pharmacologic agents (inotropes). Positive inotropes increase the contractility during the entire electromechanical systole (pre-ejection period + ejection phase). Negative inotropes decrease the contractility of the entire electromechanical systole (pre-ejection period + ejection phase).

Preload

Increases Preload
- Decreased muscle stretch after heart surgery
- Heart failure
- Hypervolemia

- Renal problems
- Sympathetic stimulation
- Vasoconstriction

Decreases Preload
- Decreased fill time
- Diuresis/Dehydration
- Hemorrhage
- Hyperthermia and sepsis must also be considered
- Hypovolemia
- Surgery
- Vasodilation
- Vomiting/Diarrhea

Afterload

Afterload is the impedance, or resistance a ventricle must overcome to eject its contents.

Increases Afterload
- Aortic stenosis
- Effects of vasopressive agents
- Hypertension
- Hypervolemia
- Hypothermia
- Vasoconstriction

Decreases Afterload
- Effects of nitrates
- Hyperthermia
- Low BP
- Sepsis
- Vasodilatation

92. **Correct answer: C**

Normal age-related physiological changes significantly contribute to MVCs. Primarily, these changes include vision, perception, hearing, and flexibility.

Clinical Practice: Head and Neck

- Maxillofacial
- Neurologic Trauma
- Ocular

SECTION 4: QUESTIONS

1. **A patient requiring definitive airway management would have a GCS score of**
   A. 12
   B. 9
   C. 8
   D. 11

2. **The type of ICP monitoring device that is inserted below the skull and above the dura mater is a(n)**
   A. Subdural catheter
   B. Epidural catheter
   C. Subarachnoid bolt
   D. Intraventricular catheter

3. **If a patient is suffering from acute neurological deterioration, the patient will require**
   A. Long-term hyperventilation to achieve a $PaCO_2$ less than 32 mmHg
   B. The SBP to be maintained greater than 90 at all times
   C. A limited use of hyperventilation to prevent herniation
   D. The administration of low-flow oxygen

4. **What patient parameters does the Adult Glasgow Coma Scale measure?**
   A. Verbal response, orientation, and activity
   B. Eye opening, motor response, and verbal response
   C. Eye opening, orientation, and motor response
   D. Verbal response, orientation, and eye opening

5. **High doses of methylprednisolone sodium succinate (Solu-Medrol) for the treatment of spinal cord injuries**
   A. Is the first treatment used for reduction of swelling in cases of neurogenic shock
   B. Helps reduce ICP
   C. May lead to loss of sympathetic tone
   D. Is no longer recommended

6. **Normal intracranial pressure is in the range of**
   A. 0–5 mmHg
   B. 4–15 mmHg
   C. 16–20 mmHg
   D. 20–40 mmHg

7. **Which of the following mechanisms decreases intracranial pressure?**
   A. CO_2 retention
   B. PaO_2 less than 50 mmHg
   C. Increased cerebrospinal fluid absorption
   D. Increased metabolic activity

8. **What is autonomic hyperreflexia?**
   A. Malfunction of the autonomic nervous system seen with a head injury
   B. Malfunction of the autonomic nervous system seen with a spinal cord injury
   C. Malfunction of the autonomic nervous system seen with pituitary tumor removal
   D. Malfunction of the autonomic nervous system seen with epidural bleeds

9. **Your patient has a gunshot wound to his T11-12 spine. Upon assessment, you find motor paralysis on the same side as the gunshot wound but loss of pain and temperature sensation on the opposite side. This phenomenon is known as**
   A. Grey-Turner's syndrome
   B. Cushing's syndrome
   C. Syndrome X
   D. Brown-Sequard syndrome

10. **A young woman was injured in a motor vehicle accident, and she is now demonstrating decerebrate posturing. As a trauma nurse, you know decerebrate posturing displays as**
    A. One arm flexed, one flaccid, legs flaccid
    B. Both arms fully extended and internally rotated, legs flaccid
    C. Both arms fully extended and internally rotated, legs fully extended with toes pointed
    D. Flaccid arms and legs extended

11. **Your patient suddenly develops right pupil dilation. What significance does this change indicate?**
    A. A basilar skull fracture
    B. Uncal herniation
    C. Brainstem herniation
    D. Cerebrovascular accident

12. **Damage to which of the following cranial nerves will result in a loss of vision and disruptions in the visual fields?**
    A. Cranial nerve II (Optic)
    B. Cranial nerve IV (Trochlear)
    C. Cranial nerve III (Oculomotor)
    D. Cranial nerve VI (Abducens)

13. **What effect is seen with a normal response to the doll's eyes maneuver?**
    A. Disconjugate gaze with head turn
    B. Conjugate gaze in the opposite direction as the head is turned
    C. Conjugate gaze in the same direction as the head is turned
    D. Nystagmus with head turning

14. **Cerebrospinal fluid is formed in which of the following locations in the brain?**
    A. Lateral ventricles
    B. Choroid plexus
    C. Subarachnoid space
    D. Pia mater

15. **Your new patient has been diagnosed with meningitis and will be undergoing a lumbar puncture. As his trauma nurse, you know the cerebrospinal fluid (CSF) should be**
    A. Hazy with a glucose level of 85
    B. Clear with RBCs present
    C. Clear and colorless with less than 45 mg/dl of protein
    D. Clear and colorless with a white blood cell count greater than 150 cells/mm^3

16. **Which of the following medical diagnoses should not be considered as a cause of any patient's seizures?**
    A. Alcohol abuse and hypertension
    B. Psychological illness
    C. Panic attack and transient ischemic attack
    D. Cardiac arrhythmias and hypertension

17. Your assessment of a patient indicated an abnormal response when the patient was tested for pronator drift. This response indicates that the patient probably has
    A. A forearm fracture
    B. Myasthenia gravis
    C. Upper motor neuron disease
    D. A skull fracture

18. In a patient with a complete transection of the spinal cord at the C2-3 level, you would expect which of the following findings?
    A. Full sensation of the face, intermittent breathing, shoulder shrug
    B. Some sensation on the occiput, face, and ears, no diaphragm movement
    C. Complete loss of sensory and motor function below the level of the injury
    D. No movement of the diaphragm, shoulder shrug

19. What is the highest level of cervical spinal cord injury at which a patient can survive without ventilator assistance?
    A. C3-4
    B. C7-8
    C. C5-6
    D. C1-2

20. A motorcyclist skidded on the road, lost control of the motorcycle, then hit a curb. EMS reported that the patient lost consciousness for approximately three minutes and had been wearing a helmet at the time of the accident. The patient regained consciousness while being placed in the ambulance. At that time the patient was alert and oriented with a GCS of 15 and had no motor or sensory defects. About 20 minutes after arrival in the ED, the patient's GCS was only 10. The patient was confused, opened his eyes to painful stimuli, and demonstrated flexion withdrawal to pain. This patient is probably suffering from
    A. A brainstem herniation
    B. A basilar skull fracture
    C. A diffuse axonal injury
    D. An epidural hematoma

21. The first step in conducting a neurological assessment is to determine the patient's level of consciousness. A patient who is obtunded will demonstrate which of the following symptoms:
    A. Drowsiness, but awakened easily with sluggish mental, verbal, and motor responses
    B. Aroused only by vigorous, continuous external stimuli and verbal responses may be incomprehensible. Motor responses may be quite minimal
    C. No verbal response, minimal withdrawal to pain, no voluntary neural response with vigorous stimulation—awareness and arousal absent
    D. Drowsy, follows simple directions with minimal external stimuli, indifferent to surroundings

22. Trauma that affects the lower half of the face tends to occur more often between the
    A. C1 and C4 vertebrae
    B. C3 and C6 vertebrae
    C. C4 and C7 vertebrae
    D. T1 and T6 vertebrae

23. Your patient slipped down a flight of stairs, landing on the buttocks. The patient suffered a fractured coccyx and a severe shoulder sprain. As a trauma nurse, you know the patient is also likely to suffer from
    A. Central cord syndrome
    B. Brown-Sequard syndrome
    C. Cauda equina syndrome
    D. Posterior cord syndrome

24. **Which section of the spinal cord contains the ascending sensory neurons for light touch, proprioception, and vibration?**
    A. The lateral cord
    B. The posterior cord
    C. The anterior cord
    D. The central cord

25. **Your patient was involved in an altercation and was struck in the lower jaw with a golf club. After ruling out other injuries, it was determined the patient suffered from a mandibular fracture. The appropriate bandage used as a temporary treatment for this fracture would be**
    A. No bandage is necessary for this type of fracture
    B. A Barton bandage
    C. A Williams' bandage
    D. A Bainbridge bandage

26. **Where does the dermatome for the fifth thoracic spinal nerve cross the anterior portion of a patient's body?**
    A. At the level of the axilla
    B. At the level of the xiphoid process
    C. At the level of the clavicular line
    D. At the nipple line

27. **Today you are precepting a nursing student and demonstrating an assessment of pupillary function on your patient. Which of the following statements about pupillary function is true?**
    A. Parasympathetic pupil control initiates pupillary dilation
    B. Parasympathetic control of the pupil is via innervation of the ocular motor nerve (CN III)
    C. When sympathetic fibers are stimulated, the pupil constricts
    D. Pinpoint pupils are the result of stimulation of parasympathetic control

28. **Your patient was an unrestrained driver in a motor vehicle crash where he struck and fractured the windshield. He has a left frontal lobe injury. Which of the following symptoms would you expect in this patient?**
    A. Hearing and balance impairment
    B. Sensory and memory problems
    C. Personality changes, poor short-term memory
    D. Loss of motor function, hearing problems

29. **One way to check for low calcium levels is to tap over a branch of the facial nerve. If the patient is hypocalcemic, the upper lip on the same side (ipsilateral) will twitch. This response is known as**
    A. Trousseau's sign
    B. Chvostek's sign
    C. Grey-Turner's sign
    D. Homan's sign

30. **A positive Babinski or plantar reflex indicates**
    A. Malfunction of the hypothalamus
    B. Normal neurologic functioning
    C. Upper motor neuron lesion of the pyramidal tract
    D. Lower motor neuron lesion of the pyramidal tract

31. **What volume of cerebrospinal fluid is produced each day in the average adult?**
    A. 1000–1200 ml
    B. 600–700 ml
    C. 400–800 ml
    D. 800–900 ml

32. **What is the formula for calculating cerebral perfusion pressure (CPP)?**
    A. CPP = SBP + MAP and ICP
    B. CPP = MAP − ICP
    C. CPP = ICP − MAP
    D. CPP = MAP − CVP and ICP

33. **The goal for CPP is a pressure of**
    A. 50–80 mmHg
    B. 20–40 mmHg
    C. 10–20 mmHg
    D. 40–60 mmHg

34. **Spinal shock is defined as a(n)**
    A. Areflexia at or below the spinal cord injury
    B. Hyperreflexia and spasticity after a spinal cord injury
    C. Areflexia that rises above the site of injury
    D. Spasticity below the injury site

35. **Neurogenic shock differs from spinal shock in which of the following ways?**
    A. Neurogenic shock is a less severe form of shock with spinal cord injury that causes a brief decrease in blood pressure
    B. Neurogenic shock is a more severe form of shock that causes cardiovascular collapse in patients with a spinal cord injury above T6
    C. Neurogenic shock is a more severe shock that increases paralysis and death
    D. Neurogenic shock is a more severe form of shock that occurs within hours after a spinal cord injury and causes increased sympathetic outflow

36. **What is the effect of Cushing's syndrome in a patient with increased intracranial pressure?**
    A. Increased systolic blood pressure, widening pulse pressure, bradycardia
    B. Elevated blood pressure, narrow pulse pressure, tachycardia
    C. Bradycardia, low blood pressure, narrow pulse pressure
    D. Tachycardia, increased systolic blood pressure, widening pulse pressure

37. **What is the proper technique for eliciting a Babinski response?**
    A. Stroke the sole of the foot from side to side
    B. Stroke the sole of the foot along the lateral sole from the heel up toward the toes and across the ball of the foot
    C. Strike the heel and the ball of the foot
    D. Strike the Achilles tendon with a reflex hammer

38. **You are caring for a patient with increased intracranial pressure (ICP) caused by a traumatic brain injury. Which of the following clinical manifestations would indicate that the patient is experiencing increased brain compression causing brainstem damage?**
    A. Hyperthermia
    B. Tachycardia
    C. Hypertension
    D. Bradypnea

39. **The ED trauma educator is precepting a nurse new to the ED when a patient with a T2 spinal cord injury is admitted. The patient is soon exhibiting manifestations of neurogenic shock. What symptoms would the educator teach the new nurse to monitor this patient for?**
    A. Increased cardiac markers
    B. Hypotension
    C. Tachycardia
    D. Excessive sweating

40. **A patient with a spinal cord injury has a nursing diagnosis of altered mobility. The altered mobility increases the risk of deep vein thrombosis (DVT) in this patient. Which of the following would be included as an appropriate nursing intervention to prevent a DVT from occurring?**
    A. Placing the patient on a fluid restriction
    B. Applying thigh-high elastic stockings
    C. Administering an antifibrinolytic agent
    D. Assisting the patient with PROM exercises

41. **Your patient will be admitted to the Neuro ICU with a spinal cord injury with resultant paralysis. As a trauma nurse, you know the prevention of contractures is extremely important in the care of this patient. Measures to prevent contractures in a paralyzed patient include**
    A. Repositioning the patient every 2 hours
    B. Initiating range-of-motion exercises 1 week following the injury
    C. Initiating range-of-motion exercises 48 hours after the injury
    D. Performing range-of-motion exercises once a day

42. **A patient is admitted to the ED following an automobile accident. The patient has sustained a spinal cord injury. When re-assessing the patient, the nurse notes there is a sudden depression of reflex activity in the spinal cord below the level of injury. The trauma nurse should suspect which of the following as the cause of the change in the patient's condition?**
    A. A secondary injury
    B. Hypertension
    C. Spinal shock
    D. Hypovolemia

43. **Your patient has sustained a facial injury from walking into a scaffold at a construction site. The patient has mild swelling noted in the maxillary area, no motor or sensory deficits, has a GCS of 15, moderate pain at the injury site, and a fractured left upper incisor. On further assessment, it is noted that the maxilla moves independently from the rest of the face and malocclusion is present. This patient is probably suffering from**
    A. An ethmoid bone fracture
    B. A zygomatic arch fracture
    C. A LeFort I fracture
    D. A nasal bone fracture

44. **Your patient was struck in the left eye by a paintball. There is swelling around the orbit with crepitus. The patient states he has numbness in the upper lip and teeth. When the patient gazes upward, he has diplopia. As a trauma nurse, you know this patient probably has sustained a**
    A. LeFort III fracture
    B. A blowout fracture
    C. A middle fossa fracture
    D. A nasal ethmoidal fracture

45. **A patient is admitted to the ED with a suspected diffuse axonal injury. What would be the primary neuroimaging diagnostic tool used on this patient to evaluate the brain structure?**
    A. MRI
    B. PET scan
    C. X-ray
    D. Ultrasound

46. **The knee jerk, also known as the patellar reflex, is an example of**
    A. Functional upper motor neurons
    B. Nonfunctional lower motor neurons
    C. Nonfunctional upper motor neurons
    D. Functional lower motor neurons

47. A patient is brought to the emergency department after being involved in a motorcycle accident. He is found to have a T1 spinal cord injury. This patient is at increased risk for development of which of the following conditions because of his injury?

    A. Pulmonary edema
    B. Pulmonary emboli
    C. Decreased $PaCO_2$
    D. Increased vital capacity

48. A patient with a suspected head injury following an assault is being transported to the emergency department. What diagnostic test would the trauma nurse expect the physician to order to help determine treatment for preventing secondary injury?

    A. PET
    B. CBC
    C. ABG
    D. MRI

49. A sustained, rapid, and moderately deep hyperpnea is known as

    A. Cheyne-Stokes respirations
    B. Ataxic respirations
    C. An apneustic respiratory pattern
    D. Central neurogenic hyperventilation

50. While jumping on a trampoline, your new patient missed his landing, was catapulted off, and fell to the ground. The patient is being admitted to the ED with a C4 spinal cord injury. What nursing diagnoses could you document as a priority for this patient?

    A. Risk for impaired skin integrity related to immobility and sensory loss
    B. Impaired physical mobility related to loss of motor function
    C. Ineffective breathing patterns related to weakness of the intercostal muscles
    D. Urinary retention related to inability to void spontaneously

51. A nurse in the trauma bay is mentoring a new graduate working on the unit. Today they are talking about autonomic dysreflexia. What would the mentoring nurse tell the new graduate are the objectives of the care provided a patient experiencing autonomic dysreflexia?

    A. Improving mobility
    B. Improving sensory perception
    C. Empty the bladder completely
    D. Remove the triggering stimulus

52. The cranial nerve responsible for movement of the eyeball and innervation of the lateral rectus muscle is

    A. CN III
    B. CN VIII
    C. CN II
    D. CN VI

53. The three main branches of the trigeminal nerve are the

    A. Facial, abducens, and trochlear
    B. Supraorbital, supratrochlear, and infratrochlear
    C. Ophthalmic, maxillary, and mandibular
    D. Zygomatic, buccal, and cervical

54. **Your patient was kicked in the face while practicing Taekwondo 2 days ago. She awoke this morning with a headache and flashes of light in her peripheral vision. She also states she has floaters in her eyes and that her vision is "murky" in some areas. Your priority for treatment is to**
    A. Turn on all the lights
    B. Shield the eyes
    C. Check the ocular pH
    D. Arrange an ophthalmology consult

55. **Your patient was playing volleyball and was struck in the face by the ball when it was spiked. Two of your patient's teeth were avulsed. Which of the following is the best medium for transporting the patient's teeth?**
    A. Diet Coke
    B. Water
    C. Hank's solution
    D. Milk

56. **The gold standard for airway management in the patient with maxillofacial injuries is via**
    A. Nasotracheal intubation
    B. Tracheostomy
    C. Oral intubation
    D. A King airway

57. **Your patient was playing paintball when he removed his goggles to clean them. At that moment he was struck near the left eye by a paintball. He presented to the ED with complaints of burning in the eye. The physician elects to irrigate the eye to try and remove the paint. The best solution for irrigation is**
    A. Lactated Ringer's
    B. D_5 Isolyte M
    C. D_5W
    D. Sterile water

58. **While assessing a patient with a basilar skull fracture, the nurse notices a stain on the patient's pillow. The stain is a small amount of blood encircled by a pale yellow stain. This stain is called**
    A. A Halo sign
    B. Battle's sign
    C. Grey-Turner's sign
    D. Ludwig's sign

59. **Which of the cranial nerves (CN) are affected by a basilar skull fracture and leads to a loss of sense of smell?**
    A. I
    B. II
    C. VIII
    D. III

60. **Your patient was admitted with midface trauma and will require an otoscope for an intranasal examination. The physician will be assessing for**
    A. A LeFort II fracture
    B. Avulsed teeth
    C. Ocular injuries
    D. A septal hematoma

61. A patient with a closed head injury, has a Foley catheter. In 1 hour, her urine output increased from 30 ml/hour to 1000 ml of very pale, clear urine. The trauma nurse knows the increase in urine output is probably due to
    A. A volume shift from the third space
    B. Syndrome of inappropriate antidiuretic hormone
    C. Diabetes insipidus
    D. Diuresis from steroids

62. As a trauma nurse, you know the treatment of diabetes insipidus includes which of the following interventions?
    A. Fluid restriction
    B. Intravenous replacement to cover the increased urine output
    C. Diuretics
    D. Demeclocycline

63. In what manner could the spinothalamic tract be tested by the trauma nurse?
    A. Deep tendon reflexes
    B. Babinski reflex
    C. Pinprick or monofilament testing
    D. Patellar tendon reflex

64. Death from status epilepticus is usually caused by which of the following mechanisms?
    A. Airway blockage leading to severe cerebral hypoxia
    B. A hypermetabolic state within the brain
    C. Fall from a seizure causing head trauma
    D. Aspiration pneumonia

65. Your new patient has been diagnosed with sudden onset grand mal seizures. While transferring the patient to the gurney, you witness a seizure. What is the first action you should take to protect this patient?
    A. Hold the patient down to prevent injury
    B. Roll the patient to the right side and protect the airway
    C. Insert an oral airway and call for help
    D. Hit the Code Blue button

66. An example of a mnemonic commonly used to assess a patient's level of consciousness is
    A. TIPPS
    B. PQRST
    C. RRST
    D. AVPU

67. One of the most common causes for the symptoms of hyponatremia is
    A. An adrenal gland tumor
    B. An impaired thirst impulse
    C. Lung muscle paralysis
    D. Brain swelling

68. Which of the following statements is true regarding alveolar fractures?
    A. Alveolar fractures are usually secondary to a high-energy mechanism that results in injury to the upper, mid, and lower face
    B. Alveolar fractures must be composed of three of four facial units
    C. Alveolar fractures can occur in multiple locations secondary to the weak condylar neck
    D. Alveolar fractures may occur in isolation from a source of low-energy force

69. While moving your patient to a gurney for transport for a CT scan, the patient undergoes a tonic-clonic seizure. As a trauma nurse, your priority is to
    A. Immediately raise the head of the gurney
    B. Place a padded tongue blade between the teeth
    C. Administer oxygen by mask
    D. Establish and maintain a patent airway

70. Which of the following statements is false regarding the etiology of facial injuries?
    A. High-impact and low-impact forces are defined as greater or less than 20 times the force of gravity
    B. A high-impact force is all that is required to damage the mandible, maxilla, supraorbital rim, and frontal bones
    C. The nasal bone and zygoma may be injured by a low-impact force
    D. More than 30% of frontal bone fractures are likely to suffer an intracranial injury

71. About a week ago, an elderly patient was visiting a deli when a car drove through the front window, knocking the patient into a display cabinet. The patient only received a bruise over the left forehead and offered no other complaints. The patient denied treatment at that time. Over the past week, the patient has become confused to time and location. The family brought the patient to the ED for evaluation. As a trauma nurse, you suspect the patient may likely be suffering from
    A. An epidural hematoma
    B. A lacunar stroke
    C. Dementia
    D. A subdural hematoma

72. While assessing your patient's pupils, you note that the pupil has a teardrop shape. This finding is most likely indicative of
    A. A tumor on the optic nerve
    B. A detached retina
    C. A globe rupture
    D. A problem with CN VI

73. While performing a slit lamp procedure, you note the physician is using a cycloplegic agent. The purpose of this medication is to
    A. Block parasympathetic stimulus
    B. Stimulate the dilator muscle of the iris
    C. Act as a topical anesthetic
    D. Constrict the iris

74. Your new patient was admitted to the ED after being kicked in the eye during a martial arts demonstration. The patient was photophobic and complained of severe pain and nausea. The patient also suffered from blurred vision and blood in the anterior chamber of the eye. This patient is suffering from
    A. A globe rupture
    B. A retrobulbar hematoma
    C. Severe photophobia
    D. A hyphema

75. Two women fought over a latte at a local coffeehouse. One of the women is now a patient in your ED. The patient has pain in the left jaw, is unable to fully close her mouth or open her mouth. As a trauma nurse, you suspect this patient is suffering from
    A. A LeFort II fracture
    B. An orbital fracture
    C. A mandibular fracture
    D. A basilar fracture

76. Your patient has been diagnosed with acute angle glaucoma. The physician orders Diamox to be administered. As a trauma nurse, you know it is important to monitor serum levels for
    A. Hypercalcemia
    B. Hypokalemia
    C. Hypernatremia
    D. Hypoglycemia

77. Your patient is a middle-aged man who stated he was struck on the right side of his face with a fist during an attempted robbery. He had negative LOC, is alert and oriented four times. He has cervical tenderness, periorbital ecchymosis with tactile crepitus with facial swelling, and mild dysphagia. His chest X-ray showed mediastinal air. This finding is indicative of
    A. A pneumomediastinum
    B. A pneumothorax
    C. Cardiac tamponade
    D. A pleural effusion

78. Your patient was playing paintball when he removed his goggles to clean them. At that moment, he was struck near the left eye by a paintball. He presented to the ED with complaints of burning in the eye. The physician elects to irrigate the eye to try and remove the paint. The best solution for irrigation is
    A. Lactated Ringer's
    B. D$_5$ Isolyte M
    C. D$_5$W
    D. Sterile water

79. Your new patient was involved in a MVC. The patient states she had a backache and was distracted. Fortunately, the patient has no major injuries, but is complaining about bilateral eye pain, conjunctival erythema, and swollen eyelids. The patient also states that when she blinks, her eyes feel as if they have sand in them. She also states the symptoms started while driving home after she completed a session in a tanning bed this morning. As a trauma nurse, you suspect this patient suffers from
    A. Cataracts
    B. A corneal abrasion
    C. Photokeratitis
    D. A detached retina

80. Snow blindness can occur under which of the following circumstances?
    A. Arc welding, tanning beds, highly reflective snow fields
    B. Tanning booths, any snowy day, bright headlights at night
    C. Arc welding, headlights, flashlights
    D. Flashlights, headlights, any snowy day

81. Which of the following statements is false regarding injuries to the neck?
    A. The neck is considered a low vascular region except for the carotid arteries
    B. The internal jugular vein and carotid arteries are the most common vessels injured
    C. The esophagus and pharynx are more protected because they are bordered by the spine and airway
    D. Because they are located anteriorly, injuries to the pharynx and esophagus are less common than injuries to the trachea and pharynx

82. In the neck, zone I encompasses the area that
    A. Has a low morbidity of exploration
    B. Extends from the angle of the mandible of the jaw to the base of the skull
    C. Extends from the base of the neck (thoracic inlet inferiorly and the cricoid cartilage superiorly)
    D. Has a high rate of multiple vascular injury

83. **In the neck, zone III**
    A. Extends from the angle of the mandible of the jaw to the base of the skull
    B. Does not need angiography to delineate the site of injury
    C. Requires cranial nerve exploration
    D. Allows for simple distal vessel control

84. **Which of the following structures are found in zone I in the neck?**
    A. Carotid arteries and trachea
    B. Cranial nerves IX–XII and jugular veins
    C. Salivary and parotid glands
    D. Subclavian vessels and aortic arch

85. **Structures found in zone II in the neck include**
    A. Lung apices and larynx
    B. Vertebral bodies and cranial nerve roots
    C. Jugular veins and trachea
    D. Lung apices

86. **Which of the following statements is true regarding assessment of a patient with a neck injury?**
    A. In zone I injuries, exploration and repair do not require angiography
    B. Zone I injuries rarely require surgery and have the lowest mortality
    C. The exam is apparent in zone II and injuries have the highest mortality
    D. Minor blunt or penetrating trauma can lead to airway compromise

87. **When assessing the neck, it is imperative to determine if an emergency intervention is necessary. Hard signs are those kinds of signs. A soft sign provides necessary information, but allows time to perform diagnostics. Which of the findings listed below is an example of a soft sign?**
    A. Extensive subcutaneous emphysema
    B. A wide mediastinum
    C. Pulsatile bleeding
    D. An expanding hematoma

88. **Control of bleeding in a neck injured patient should best be performed by application of**
    A. Pressure dressings
    B. Blind clamp placement
    C. Gentle wound probing
    D. Local pressure only

89. **While assessing the neck and head of your patient, you note that the right pupil is consistently small. This condition is known as**
    A. Anisocoria
    B. Ptosis
    C. Anhidrosis
    D. Horner's syndrome

90. **Which of the following statements is accurate with regard to the phrenic nerve?**
    A. The phrenic nerve contains sympathetic nerve fibers
    B. Phrenic nerves only provide sensory supply to the diaphragm
    C. The phrenic nerve, when injured, cannot total paralyze the diaphragm
    D. Each phrenic nerve supplies only the mediastinum

91. **Which of the following nerves is the motor nerve to the larynx?**
    A. The stellate ganglia
    B. The recurrent laryngeal verve
    C. The superior cricoid nerve
    D. The recurrent pharyngeal nerve

92. **The brachial plexus supplies muscular and cutaneous innervation to an entire upper limb with the exception of the**
    A. Radial nerve
    B. Musculocutaneous nerve
    C. Axillary nerve
    D. Intercostobrachial nerve

93. **Regardless of the mechanism of injury, vascular injuries of the neck must be carefully evaluated. As a trauma nurse, you know**
    A. The right external carotid artery is the vessel likely to be damaged
    B. Angiography is a favored treatment for injuries to zones I and III
    C. Surgical stabilization is mandated for zone II injuries
    D. Endovascular stents are to be used for vertebral artery injuries

94. **Any impairment to the voice is known as**
    A. Dysphonia
    B. A laryngeal fracture
    C. Laryngo malacia
    D. Laryngeal compression

95. **When assessing laryngotracheal injuries, a common finding would not include**
    A. Tenderness over the trachea
    B. A thyroid fracture
    C. Dystonia
    D. Posterior neck subcutaneous emphysema

96. **Signs of esophageal injury would not likely include**
    A. Tracheal deviation
    B. Odynophagia
    C. A fluid leak into the left pleural space
    D. Excessive drooling

97. **What Glasgow Coma Scale score indicates coma?**
    A. 8–10
    B. 6–7
    C. 5–6
    D. 4–5

98. **Your patient has an old injury to C5. He has a blood pressure of 215/129 and his pulse is 175. What is the likely cause of his symptoms?**
    A. Autonomic dysreflexia
    B. Hypertension
    C. Spinal shock
    D. Neurogenic shock

99. **Your head-injured patient has developed nystagmus. Nystagmus may be defined as**
    A. Eyes deviated to the side of the injury
    B. A convergent gaze
    C. Rhythmic tremor or shaking of the eyes
    D. Divergent gaze

100. **Your patient had a grand mal seizure lasting 65 seconds. As soon as the seizure passed, the patient was fully awake and asking for food. Given the patient's reaction to his seizure, you should**
    A. Tell the patient you know he faked the seizure
    B. Feed the patient
    C. Notify the attending physician and anticipate a psychological evaluation
    D. Give Dilantin 1 gram slowly

101. **Your patient was injured while skateboarding and has a T8 spinal cord injury. He has been diagnosed with spinal shock. The ED nurse knows the symptoms of spinal shock include**
    A. Areflexia, autonomic dysfunction, loss of sensation, eliminatory dysfunction
    B. Areflexia, peripheral vasodilatation, decreased SVR, loss of sensation
    C. Areflexia, heightened sensation, cardiovascular shock
    D. Areflexia, bowel and bladder dysfunction, bradycardia

102. **The most accurate method of measuring intracranial pressure is**
    A. A subarachnoid bolt
    B. Intraventriculostomy
    C. An epidural catheter
    D. A subdural catheter

103. **Where should the transducer for any type of intracranial pressure monitoring system be placed?**
    A. Foramen ovale
    B. Aqueduct of Sylvius
    C. Foramen of Monroe
    D. Fourth ventricle

104. **When performing a neurologic examination, the six cardinal eye directions for eye movement are controlled by which of the following cranial nerves?**
    A. CN II, III, IV
    B. CN III, IV, VI
    C. CN II, V, VII
    D. CN V, VI, VII

105. **Your patient was admitted to the ED for seizure activity. As a trauma nurse, you should anticipate orders for which of the following laboratory tests?**
    A. CBC, lipid panel, toxicology screen
    B. CBC, toxicology screen, LFTs
    C. CBC, CMP, lipid panel
    D. CBC, CMP, sedimentation rate, CRP, RPR, toxicology screen

106. **Your patient is very depressed. The patient stated, "I don't want to die like my mother did with ALS." This patient is exhibiting behavior consistent with which Kübler-Ross stage of grief?**
    A. Denial
    B. Bargaining
    C. Anger
    D. Acceptance

107. **Your patient has been diagnosed with a basilar skull fracture after running into the pole holding the net at a basketball game. The patient suffers from facial palsy and deafness and blood is noted in the ear. The type of basilar skull fracture this patient has incurred is known as a(n)**
    A. Middle fossa fracture basilar skull fracture
    B. Anterior fossa basilar skull fracture
    C. Middle fossa basilar skull fracture
    D. Interrupted basilar skull fracture

108. **Your head injured patient has the best prognosis if exhibiting which of the following symptoms:**
    A. A grasp reflex
    B. Decerebrate posturing
    C. Flaccidity
    D. Decorticate posturing

109. **Your patient was a passenger in the front seat of a car that was rear-ended. During assessment, you note a "seat belt sign" on the upper abdomen and guarding in the periumbilical area. The patient states he cannot feel his legs., but demonstrates some spontaneous movement. The physician tries a tuning fork and the patient is unable to feel vibrations, but is able to feel pain on the lower leg. This patient appears to be suffering from**
    A. Brown-Sequard syndrome
    B. Posterior cord syndrome
    C. Cauda equina syndrome
    D. Central cord syndrome

110. **Your patient has suffered a cervical injury involving the right side of the sympathetic chain. The patient demonstrates ipsilateral pupil constriction, ptosis, and anhydrosis. This triad of symptoms is known as**
    A. The Superficial syndrome
    B. Trager's syndrome
    C. Rowe syndrome
    D. Horner's syndrome

111. **Pain that radiates along a dermatone is known as**
    A. Neurogenic pain
    B. Referred pain
    C. Ulnic pain
    D. Radicular pain

112. **Your patient was involved in a fight at a soccer game. Although two teeth were not avulsed, they have fractured through the enamel and dentin of the teeth. This type of injury is known as**
    A. A LeFort I fracture
    B. An Ellis II fracture
    C. A dental arch fracture
    D. A Hank's fracture

113. **A group of high school students began fighting at school. Your patient was struck in the side of the face by a heavy backpack. The patient complains of great difficulty opening and closing her mouth. She has significant periorbital ecchymosis, diplopia, and periorbital displacement. As a trauma nurse, you know this patient is probably suffering from**
    A. An orbital fracture
    B. A LeFort II fracture
    C. A zygomatic fracture
    D. A LeFort I fracture

114. **A completely irregular breathing pattern with deep and shallow breaths is known as**
    A. Cheyne-Stokes respirations
    B. Ataxic respirations
    C. An apneustic respiratory pattern
    D. Pyrogenic respiration

115. **Which of the following treatments is most likely to be used for a patient suffering from neurogenic shock?**
    A. Packed red blood cells
    B. Poikilothermy
    C. Phenylephrine
    D. Bladder irrigations

116. **As a trauma nurse, you know the type of fracture commonly associated with axial loading where C1 splits into several sections is known as a(n)**
    A. Upper cervical fracture
    B. Jeffersonian ring fracture
    C. Atlanto-occipital fracture
    D. Hangman's fracture

SECTION 4: ANSWERS

1. **Correct answer: C**
   A patient requiring definitive airway management would have a GCS score of 8. Intubation should be anticipated and supplemental oxygen should be given to keep the SaO_2 greater than 98%.

2. **Correct answer: B**
   An epidural catheter is the type of ICP monitoring device that is inserted below the skull and above the dura mater.

3. **Correct answer: C**
   If a patient is suffering from acute neurological deterioration, the patient will require a limited use of hyperventilation to prevent herniation. However, if the patient is ventilated, maintain the PCO_2 at approximately 35 mmHg.

4. **Correct answer: B**
   The Glasgow Coma Scale measures eye opening, motor response, and verbal response. It rates each with a total scale from 3 to 15, with 15 being a fully responsive patient. A score of 6–7 is comatose level. The longer that the patient remains in the lower score ranges, the worse the projected outcome.

   Glasgow Coma Scale (Adult)

Best Eye Response	Best Verbal Response	Best Motor Response
No eye opening (1)	No verbal response (1)	No motor response (1)
Eye opening to pain (2)	Incomprehensible sounds (2)	Extension to pain (2)
Eye opening to verbal command (3)	Inappropriate words (3)	Flexion to pain (3)
Eyes open spontaneously (4)	Confused (4)	Withdrawal from pain (4)
	Oriented (5)	Localizing pain (5)
		Obeys commands (6)

5. **Correct answer: D**
   High doses of methylprednisolone sodium succinate (Solu-Medrol) for the treatment of spinal cord injuries is no longer a recommended treatment. Because the immune system and wound healing is comprised, Solu-Medrol may cause wound infections, sepsis, pneumonia, GI hemorrhage, and pulmonary emboli.

6. **Correct answer: B**
   The normal range for intracranial pressure is 4–15 mmHg.

7. **Correct answer: C**
   Cerebrospinal fluid absorbed at an increased rate decreases intracranial pressure. CO_2 retention, PaO_2 less than 50 mmHg, and increased metabolic activity contribute to increased intracranial pressure.

8. **Correct answer: B**
   Autonomic hyperreflexia is a potentially life-threatening response to a minor stimuli seen after a spinal cord injury at T6 or higher. It occurs after the initial spinal shock has resolved. Symptoms can include severe hypertension, dysrhythmias, severe headache, and photophobia.

9. **Correct answer: D**
   Brown-Sequard causes ipsilateral (same side) motor paralysis and contralateral (opposite side) loss of pain and temperature sensation. This syndrome occurs because of the way the pyramidal tracts cross in the spinal column.

10. **Correct answer: C**

Decerebrate posturing displays as both arms fully extended and internally rotated, legs fully extended with toes pointed. Decerebrate posturing demonstrates the effect of pressure on the midbrain and pons. It is a very poor neurologic sign, especially if it continues for more than 4 hours.

11. **Correct answer: B**

Ipsilateral, or same side, pupil dilation is the symptom seen with uncal herniation across the tentorium. The tentorium is a fold of dura mater that supports the temporal and occipital lobes. This herniation puts pressure directly on CN III, causing pupil dilation. CN III also controls movement of the eyeball, dilates and constricts the pupil, and could result in ptosis. Size and shape of the pupil may be altered if the nerve is damaged.

12. **Correct answer: A**

Damage to Cranial nerve II results in a loss of vision and disruptions of the visual fields. CN III controls movement of the eyeball, the eyelid, and dilation and constriction of the pupil. The equality, size, and shape of the pupil may be altered and ptosis may occur if damaged.

13. **Correct answer: B**

With a normal doll's eyes or oculocephalic reflex, the eyes appear to move to the opposite direction from the head turn. For example, if the head is turned quickly to the patient's left, the eyes normally appear to move to the far right side. If the reflex is absent, the eyes appear fixed and do not move. This is a poor neurologic sign. It represents pontine and midbrain damage. It may be used in determining brain death.

14. **Correct answer: B**

Cerebrospinal fluid is formed by the choroid plexus of the third ventricle. The arachnoid villi, projections from the subarachnoid space, reabsorb the cerebrospinal fluid.

15. **Correct answer: C**

The cerebrospinal fluid should be clear and colorless with a protein count of 16–45 mg/dl, WBCs 0–5 cells/mm^3, and the glucose level should be approximately 80% of the serum glucose level.

16. **Correct answer: B**

Panic attacks, transient ischemic attacks, cardiac arrhythmias, hypertension, electrolyte disorders, hyperthermia, disease processes, trauma, and syncope are some causes of seizures. Psychological illness is not a medical diagnosis.

17. **Correct answer: C**

An abnormal response when testing for pronator drift indicates that the patient may have an upper motor neuron disease or weakness in the shoulder girdle. To elicit this response, have the patient stand for 20–30 seconds with both arms outstretched forward, palms up, and eyes closed. Tell the patient to hold that position while you tap the hands vigorously downward. The patient will not be able to maintain extension and supination and will drift into pronation.

18. **Correct answer: B**

The patient with a high cervical transection of the spinal cord can present with the following: sensation of the occiput, face, and ears; there is no diaphragmatic movement; no voluntary movement below the injury; and there is loss of bowel and bladder function. Patients with this level of injury often die due to pneumonia.

19. **Correct answer: C**

At C5-6 there is enough diaphragmatic movement to allow for adequate respiratory function. Injuries above C5-6 require some level of mechanical ventilation.

20. **Correct answer: D**

A motorcyclist skidded on the road, lost control of the motorcycle, then hit a curb. EMS reported that the patient lost consciousness for approximately three minutes and had been wearing a helmet at the time of the accident. The patient regained consciousness while being placed in the ambulance. At that time the patient was alert and oriented with a GCS of 15 and had no motor or sensory defects. About 20 minutes after arrival in the ED, the patient's GCS was only 10. The patient was confused, opened his eyes to painful stimuli, and demonstrated flexion withdrawal to pain. This patient is probably suffering from an epidural hematoma.

An epidural hematoma results from an arterial bleed, usually from a laceration to the middle meningeal artery. Classically, the patient loses consciousness for a brief period of time, then regains consciousness and is alert and oriented. Blood collects between the skull and dura mater, causing an increase in intracranial pressure, leading to a degradation in neurological status. Patients often have severe headache and may suffer from an ipsilateral pupil on the side of the injury and possible hemiparesis.

21. **Correct answer D**
The first step in conducting a neurological assessment is to determine the patient's level of consciousness. A patient who is obtunded will demonstrate the following symptoms:

- Drowsiness, follows simple directions with minimal external stimuli, indifferent to surroundings
- A lethargic patient is drowsy, but awakened easily with sluggish mental, verbal, and motor responses.
- A stuporous patient is aroused only by vigorous, continuous external stimuli, verbal responses may be incomprehensible. Motor responses may be quite minimal
- A comatose patient exhibits no verbal response, minimal withdrawal to pain, no voluntary neural response with vigorous stimulation—awareness and arousal absent

22. **Correct answer: A**
Trauma affecting the lower half of the face tends to occur more often between the C1 and C4, causing higher cervical fractures.

23. **Correct answer: C**
Your patient slipped down a flight of stairs, landing on the buttocks. The patient suffered a fractured coccyx and a severe shoulder sprain. As a trauma nurse, you know the patient is also likely to suffer from Cauda equina syndrome. Injury to the lower spinal cord results in possible motor and sensory loss in the lower body. Sometimes, bowel and bladder function is impaired.

24. **Correct answer: B**
The posterior cord contains the ascending sensory neurons for light touch, proprioception, and vibration. Sensations about the position of the body and limbs in addition to vibration sense and the ability to finely discriminate touch sensations are carried here. Pain and temperature sensation are preserved below the level of involvement.

25. **Correct answer: B**
The appropriate bandage used as a temporary treatment for a mandibular fracture would be a Barton bandage.

26. **Correct answer: D**
The fifth thoracic spinal nerve innervates at the nipple line. The dermatome innervates not only the skin but the organs, muscles, and tendons along the same path. It is important to know the dermatomes when dealing with spinal injuries because they help locate the level of the injury.

27. **Correct answer: B**
Today you are precepting a nursing student and demonstrating an assessment of pupillary function on your patient. The true statement about pupillary function is that parasympathetic control of the pupil is via innervation of the ocular motor nerve (CN III).

28. **Correct answer: C**
Personality changes and poor short-term memory are expected symptoms in a patient with left frontal lobe injury. The frontal lobe is responsible for personality, memory, motor function, Broca's area, and critical thinking skills.

29. **Correct answer: B**
One way to check for low calcium is to tap over a branch of the facial nerve. If the patient is hypocalcemic, the upper lip on the same side (ipsilateral) will twitch. This is known as Chvostek's sign. Trousseau's sign utilizes a BP cuff to elicit a carpopedal spasm indicative of hypocalcemia. Grey-Turner's sign is ecchymosis around the umbilicus, indicating abdominal issues, and Homan's sign is no longer used to assess for DVT.

30. **Correct answer: C**
A positive Babinski or plantar reflex is a sign of an upper motor neuron lesion. A positive Babinski reflex can be seen with spinal cord compression, head injury, and stroke. It is a pathologic sign.

31. **Correct answer: C**
About 400–800 ml of cerebrospinal fluid is produced daily by the average adult by the choroid plexus in the third ventricle. There is approximately 125–150 ml circulating in the ventricular system and spinal column at one time.

32. **Correct answer: B**
Mean arterial pressure minus intracranial pressures equals cerebral perfusion pressure. Cerebral perfusion pressure is a calculated measurement of the pressure gradient that allows blood to flow to the brain. The CPP may also be calculated using the CVP instead of the ICP because it is a measure of vascular resistance.

33. **Correct answer: A**
As cerebral perfusion pressure is a calculated measurement of the pressure gradient that allows blood to flow to the brain, the goal is a CPP of at least 50–70 mmHg. The normal CPP is 60—100 mmHg.

34. **Correct answer: A**
Spinal shock is defined as an areflexia at or below the spinal cord injury. Spinal shock can occur hours to weeks after an injury to the spinal cord. The patient develops flaccidity, loss of sensation, and loss of bowel and bladder function. Hyperreflexia and spasticity occurs after spinal shock resolves.

35. **Correct answer: B**
Neurogenic shock is a much more severe form of shock that may occur with spinal cord injuries at or above T6. The autonomic dysfunction causes increased vagal tone, which results in severe bradycardia, decreased cardiac output, peripheral dilatation, and decreased SVR.

36. **Correct answer: A**
The effect of Cushing's syndrome in a patient with increased intracranial pressure is increased systolic blood pressure, widening pulse pressure, and bradycardia. Cushing's syndrome is also known as the triad of symptoms. These are late indicators of a serious deterioration of neurologic status. This patient is at very high risk for herniation and death.

37. **Correct answer: B**
The proper technique for eliciting a Babinski response is stroking the lateral sole of the foot from the heel up to and across the ball of the foot. It should be done in one motion with a relatively sharp instrument like the end of a reflex hammer.

38. **Correct answer: A**
Signs of increasing ICP include slowing of the heart rate (bradycardia), increasing systolic blood pressure, and widening pulse pressure. As brain compression increases, respirations become rapid, blood pressure may decrease, and the pulse slows further. A rapid rise in body temperature is regarded as unfavorable. Hyperthermia increases the metabolic demands of the brain and may indicate brainstem damage.

39. **Correct answer: B**
Manifestations of neurogenic shock include decreased blood pressure and heart rate. Cardiac markers would be expected to rise in cardiogenic shock. Patients do not perspire on the paralyzed portions of their body due to blockage of sympathetic activity.

40. **Correct answer: B**

It is important to promote venous return to the heart and prevent venous stasis in a patient with altered mobility, especially if the patient has suffered a spinal cord injury. Applying elastic stockings will aid in the prevention of a DVT. The patient should not be placed on fluid restriction because a dehydrated state will increase the risk of clotting throughout the body. Antifibrinolytic agents cause the blood to clot, which is absolutely contraindicated in this situation.

41. **Correct answer: C**

Your patient will be admitted to the Neuro ICU with a spinal cord injury with resultant paralysis. As a trauma nurse, you know the prevention of contractures is extremely important in the care of this patient. Measures to prevent contractures in a paralyzed patient include initiating range-of-motion exercises 48 hours after the injury. Contractures develop rapidly with immobility and muscle paralysis. The exercises can be implemented within 48–72 hours after the injury. The exercises should ideally be performed multiple times a day. Repositioning alone will not prevent contractures.

42. **Correct answer: A**

A patient is admitted to the ED following an automobile accident. The patient has sustained a spinal cord injury. When re-assessing the patient, the nurse notes there is a sudden depression of reflex activity in the spinal cord below the level of injury. The trauma nurse should suspect this patient is suffering a secondary injury caused by swelling around the spinal cord.

43. **Correct answer: C**

Your patient suffered a facial fracture after walking into a scaffold. The patient suffered a LeFort I fracture. Hallmarks of this type of fracture include mild facial swelling, a maxilla that moves independently from the rest of the face, and malocclusion. Occasionally there may be fractured teeth or lip lacerations.

44. **Correct answer: B**

Eye injuries caused by small objects or a fist often cause orbital (blowout) fractures. Symptoms include periorbital edema, crepitus, diplopia when gazing upward, a step-off deformity of the periorbital rim, numbness of the upper lip and maxillary teeth due to damage to the infraorbital nerve. If surgery is indicated, it is likely delayed until edema resolves.

45. **Correct answer: A**

CT and MRI scans are the primary neuroimaging diagnostic tools and are useful in evaluating the brain structure. Ultrasound would not show the brain nor would an X-ray. A PET scan shows brain function, not brain structure.

46. **Correct answer: D**

The knee jerk, also known as the patellar reflex, is an example of a functional lower motor neuron. These reflexes are also known as deep tendon reflexes. The nerve impulse makes an arc from the tendon to the sensory portion of the spinal cord to the motor root and back to the patella, causing extension of the lower leg.

47. **Correct answer: A**

A patient is brought to the emergency department after being involved in a motorcycle accident.

He was found to have a T1 spinal cord injury. With injuries to the cervical and upper thoracic spinal cord, innervation to the major accessory muscles of respiration is lost and respiratory problems develop. These include decreased vital capacity, retention of secretions, increased $PaCO_2$ levels, decreased oxygen levels, respiratory failure, and pulmonary edema.

48. **Correct answer: C**

Treatments to prevent secondary injury include stabilization of cardiovascular and respiratory function to maintain adequate cerebral perfusion, control of hemorrhage and hypovolemia, and maintenance of optimal blood gas values. An ABG would give baseline blood values to have a foundation in the maintenance of optimal blood gas values. PET scans and an MRI would not aid in preventing secondary injury to this patient's brain.

49. **Correct answer: D**

   Sustained, rapid, and moderately deep hyperpnea is known as central neurogenic hyperventilation. It is unknown exactly how this mechanism functions.

50. **Correct answer: C**

   A C4 spinal cord injury will require ventilatory support, due to the diaphragm and intercostals being affected. The other nursing diagnosis could be used in a care plan but not designated as a higher priority than ineffective breathing patterns.

51. **Correct answer: D**

   Because this is an emergency situation, the objectives are to remove the triggering stimulus and to avoid the possibly serious complications. Improving mobility and improving sensory perception are nursing diagnoses for spinal cord patients. Emptying the bladder completely is the objective of having a catheter in place.

52. **Correct answer: D**

   The cranial nerve responsible for eyeball movement and innervation of the lateral rectus muscle is the abducens nerve, CN VI.

53. **Correct answer: C**

   The three main branches of the trigeminal nerve are the ophthalmic, maxillary, and mandibular.

54. **Correct answer: B**

   This patient is probably suffering from a detached retina. The eyes must be shielded immediately to prevent further injury. The patient is probably anxious because of the vision changes, so it is important to minimize external stimuli and eye movement. Arranging the ophthalmology consult is important but can be done after measures are taken to save the patient's vision.

55. **Correct answer: C**

   Hank's solution contains all the metabolites, such as Ca, PO_4, K^+, and glucose, necessary to maintain normal cell metabolism for several hours. Diet Coke is too acidic and will damage the teeth. Water is hypotonic and will cause the cells to lyse. Milk is occasionally used to transport teeth, but cells on knocked-out teeth roots in milk don't die immediately. However, they are unable to replicate (mitosis) and are less able to reform new cells when implanted.

56. **Correct answer: C**

   The gold standard for airway management in the patient with maxillofacial injuries is via oral intubation and is often performed with rapid sequence induction. Airway management modalities should be utilized based on the severity of the maxillofacial distortion, debris present, edema, and potential for compromise

57. **Correct answer: A**

   The best solution for irrigating the eye is lactated Ringer's solution because it has approximately the same pH (6–7.5) as tears (7.1). Paintball guns now are so advanced they shoot the paintball at the same velocities as pellet guns, but have 10 times the mass. The paintball is smaller than the orbit, so it has the potential for blowout fractures and complete disruption of the globe.

58. **Correct answer: A**

   The halo sign, a stain with a small amount of blood encircled by a pale yellow stain, is indicative of a basilar skull fracture. This can be a dangerous sign for the patient as meningitis can easily develop.

59. **Correct answer: A**

   CN I is the frequently affected cranial nerve in a basilar skull fracture and leads to a loss of sense of smell.

60. **Correct answer: D**

   Patients admitted with midface trauma should be assessed for septal hematoma with an otoscope for intranasal examination. A septal hematoma is blood collecting under the septum. If not treated it may deteriorate into an abscess or avascular necrosis. There is also the possibility that cerebrospinal fluid may be found, indicating an ethmoid bone fracture.

61. **Correct answer: C**

A sudden increase in urine output from 30 to 1000 ml/hour of pale, clear urine indicates diabetes insipidus. Diabetes insipidus (DI) is a serious decrease in antidiuretic hormone (ADH). The most common causes of neurogenic DI are closed head injury and posterior pituitary tumor removal. ADH is produced by the posterior pituitary gland. Closed head injury and cerebral edema lead to pressure on the pituitary gland, thus decreasing ADH. Other common causes of DI are lung cancer (small or oat cell carcinoma), leukemia, and lymphoma.

62. **Correct answer: B**

Treatment of diabetes insipidus includes intravenous replacement with D_5W ½ NS with 20 mEq of potassium is titrated to replace hourly urine output. Other therapies include DDAVP (desmopressin) nasal spray or a pitressin infusion. Strict I&O, monitoring electrolytes, and serum and urine osmolalities are also performed.

63. **Correct answer: C**

The spinothalamic tract may be tested by pinprick or monofilament testing. The spinothalamic tract carries impulses from the spine to the thalamus; thus, it is a sensory motor tract. The lateral spinothalamic senses pain and temperature, whereas the anterior tract senses light touch and pressure.

64. **Correct answer: B**

Death from status epilepticus is usually caused by a hypermetabolic state within the brain. Status epilepticus results in decreased oxygen and glucose levels in the brain, leading to the release of glutamate. The increased glutamate causes the influx of calcium into the neurons, destabilizing them electronically, which leads to cell injury and death.

65. **Correct answer: B**

The best action is to turn this patient to the right side and protect the airway. Because the seizure has already started, it would be impossible to safely insert an oral airway. Never try to restrain a patient having a seizure. Hitting the Code Blue button is certainly an option, but it doesn't help the patient immediately. Code buttons are not necessarily used in the ED as staff are present at all times. Precipitating events (if known), such as aura, onset, duration, nursing actions, and postictal state should be included in the nursing notes.

66. **Correct answer: D**

An example of a mnemonic used to assess a patient's level of consciousness is AVPU.
A: alert
V: responds to voice
P: responds to painful stimuli
U: unresponsive

67. **Correct answer: D**

Brain swelling causes most of the symptoms of hyponatremia. Sodium is found mostly in the body fluids outside the cells. When the amount of sodium in fluids outside the cells drops, water moves into the cells to balance the levels. This causes the cells to swell with too much water. Although most cells can handle this swelling, brain cells cannot because the skull is essentially a closed space. An impaired thirst impulse and lung muscle paralysis are symptoms of hypernatremia.

68. **Correct answer: D**

Alveolar fractures may occur in isolation from a source of low-energy force. They may also be the result of fracture line extension through the alveolar section of the mandible or maxilla. Panfacial fractures are usually secondary to a high-energy mechanism, which results in injury to the upper, mid, and lower face, and are composed of three of four facial units. Mandibular fractures can occur in multiple locations secondary to the weak condylar neck.

69. **Correct answer: D**

As a trauma nurse, it is imperative that you establish and maintain airway patency—it is always a priority intervention for a patient with tonic-clonic seizure activity. Using O_2 at this point will be ineffective because often patients do not breathe during seizure activity. Forcing a tongue blade between teeth may result in a human bite or broken teeth.

70. **Correct answer: A**

High-impact and low-impact forces are actually defined and greater or lesser than 50 times the force of gravity, not 20 times the force of gravity. So the statement is false.
The following statements are true:

- A high-impact force is all that is required to damage the mandible, maxilla, supraorbital rim, and frontal bones.
- The nasal bone and zygoma may be injured by a low-impact force.
- More than 30% of frontal bone fractures are likely to suffer an intracranial injury.

71. **Correct answer: D**

As a trauma nurse, you would probably suspect this patient is suffering from a subdural hematoma. The patient's history suggests this diagnosis. About a week ago, an elderly patient was visiting a deli when a car drove through the front window, knocking the patient into a display cabinet. The patient only received a bruise over the left forehead and offered no other complaints. The patient denied treatment at that time. Over the past week, the patient has become confused to time and location. There is no symptomology suggesting stroke or dementia. Epidural hematomas result in loss of consciousness (LOC) initially and tend to develop within 48 hours. This patient had no LOC.

Because of the previous mechanism of history, a subdural hematoma is likely. It is also important to note that elderly patients use anticoagulants and have friable veins and occasional coagulopathy issues.

72. **Correct answer: C**

While assessing your patient's pupils, you note that the pupil has a teardrop shape. This finding is likely indicative of a globe rupture, especially if the tip of the teardrop points to the rupture site.

73. **Correct answer: A**

While performing a slit lamp procedure, you note the physician is using a cycloplegic agent. The purpose of this medication is to block parasympathetic stimulus that constricts the iris by stopping the ciliary muscle from contracting.

74. **Correct answer: D**

This patient has a hyphema. The patient was admitted to the ED after being kicked in the eye during a martial arts demonstration. The patient was photophobic and complained of severe pain and nausea. The patient also suffered from blurred vision and blood in the anterior chamber of the eye. There are four grades of hyphema, determined by how much blood occupies the anterior chamber. Grade 1 means blood occupies less than 1/3 of the chamber, Grade 2 means 1/3 to 1/2 of the chamber contains blood. Grade 3 is occupation of 1/2 to less than the total space. Grade 4 means the entire chamber is occupied by blood.

75. **Correct answer: C**

Two women fought over a latte at a local coffeehouse. One of the women is now a patient in your ED. The patient has pain in the left jaw, is unable to fully close her mouth or open her mouth. As a trauma nurse, you suspect this patient is suffering from a mandibular fracture. The patient is also likely not to be able to hold a tongue depressor in the mouth, smile, or grimace. Always assess under the tongue for bruising. If the jaw was misaligned during the fight, injury may have occurred.

76. **Correct answer: B**

When Diamox is administered it is important to monitor potassium levels for hypokalemia. Hydrogen ion excretion in the renal tubules is inhibited and the low potassium levels may cause dysrhythmias.

77. **Correct answer: A**

This patient has a pneumomediastinum secondary to facial trauma that leads to subcutaneous cervicofacial emphysema and tracking of air into the mediastinum along lines of fascia. Granted this would be extremely rare, but it is important for the trauma nurse to consider even the remotest possibilities.

78. **Correct answer: A**
The best solution for irrigating the eye is lactated Ringer's solution because it has approximately the same pH (6–7.5) as tears (7.1). Paintball guns now are so advanced they shoot the paintball at the same velocities as pellet guns, but have 10 times the mass. The paintball is smaller than the orbit, so it has the potential for blowout fractures and complete disruption of the globe.

79. **Correct answer: C**
Bilateral eye pain, conjunctival erythema, swollen eyelids, and a feeling that something is in the eye is usually indicative of ultraviolet photokeratitis. Exposure to the ultraviolet light in the tanning booth may cause permanent injury such as cataracts.

80. **Correct answer: A**
Snow blindness, also known as radiation keratitis, can be caused by exposure to any UVB rays. Injury to the eyes caused by highly reflective snowy fields, especially in high altitudes, is where the term *snow blindness* originated. Today, exposure to UVB rays from welder's arcs, tanning booths, carbon arcs, photographic flood lamps, lightning, electric sparks, and halogen desk lamps are additional causes of this type of injury.

81. **Correct answer: A**
The statement that the neck is considered a low vascular region is false. It is considered a high vascular region.

82. **Correct answer: C**
In the neck, zone I encompasses the area that extends from the base of the neck (thoracic inlet (inferiorly) and the cricoid cartilage (superiorly).

83. **Correct answer: A**
In the neck, zone III extends from the angle of the mandible of the jaw to the base of the skull.

84. **Correct answer: D**
Structures found in zone I are subclavian vessels, brachiocephalic veins, common carotids, aortic arch, jugular veins, esophagus, lung apices, cranial nerve roots, and the c-spinal cord.

85. **Correct answer: C**
Structures found in zone II in the neck include the salivary and parotid glands, esophagus, trachea, carotid arteries, vertebral bodies, jugular veins, and cranial nerves IX–XII.

86. **Correct answer: D**
It is incumbent on the trauma nurse to try and ascertain if the patient is anticoagulated. Minor trauma to the neck, whether blunt or penetrating, may compromise the airway due to expanding hematomas. Also, make certain to check the area under a cervical collar or dressing to ascertain if there is a hidden injury.

87. **Correct answer: B**
Examples of soft signs include a wide mediastinum, hemoptysis, a voice change, dysphonia/dysphagia, and hematemesis.

88. **Correct answer: D**
Local pressure should be applied minimally and avoid compression of the ipsilateral carotid artery. Some patients do not have adequate collateral anterior cerebral circulation. Avoid pressure dressings, probing and clamps, and definitely no tourniquets.

89. **Correct answer: A**
A pupil that stays consistently small is known as anisocoria.

90. **Correct answer: A**
The phrenic nerve contains sympathetic nerve fibers. In the thorax, the phrenic nerve supplies not only to the mediastinal pleura, but the pericardium as well. Phrenic nerve injuries can paralyze the diaphragm.

91. Correct answer: D
The recurrent pharyngeal nerve is the motor nerve to the larynx. It supplies all the muscles except the cricothyroid muscle.

92. Correct answer: D
The brachial plexus supplies muscular and cutaneous innervation to an entire upper limb with the exception of an area of skin near the axilla innervated by the intercostobrachial nerve and the trapezius muscle.

93. Correct answer: B
Regardless of the mechanism of injury, vascular injuries of the neck must be carefully evaluated. As a trauma nurse, you know angiography is a favored treatment for injuries to zones I and III. On zone II, surgical stabilization may be useful for both stable and unstable patients. In addition, zone II injuries that are stable may be managed nonoperatively.

94. Correct answer: A
Any impairment to the voice is known as dystonia. Therefore, hoarseness is a form of dystonia.

95. Correct answer: D
When assessing laryngotracheal injuries, a common finding would not include posterior neck subcutaneous emphysema. The subcutaneous emphysema would be found anteriorly and often extends from the neck to the trunk. Thyroid fractures are common, the patient exhibits dystonia with hoarseness, hemoptysis, and tenderness over the trachea.

96. Correct answer: C
Signs of esophageal injury would not likely include a left pleural space fluid leak, but rather a leak into the right pleural space. Other signs of esophageal injury include excessive drooling, hyper salivation, odynophagia (extreme pain when swallowing), and dysphagia. Additional signs may include a sucking neck wound, subcutaneous emphysema, tracheal deviation, and pain when turning the neck.

97. Correct answer: B
A 6–7 is comatose level on the Glasgow Coma Scale. A score of 15 is a patient who is fully awake. A score of 3 means there is no eye, motor, or verbal response from the patient.

98. Correct answer: A
This patient has autonomic dysreflexia also known as autonomic hyperreflexia. This is a life-threatening exaggerated sympathetic response to minor stimuli. The stimuli may be a drafty room, a full bladder, or a bowel obstruction. Treating the cause will fix the problem. The symptoms include hypertension, severe headache, tachycardia or bradycardia, profuse sweating, or flushing.

99. Correct answer: C
Nystagmus, rhythmic tremor or shaking of the eyes, indicates pressure or damage to CN VIII (acoustic) in the vestibular portion. Shaking is usually stronger on one side and may occur in any of the cardinal eye directions.

100. Correct answer: C
Your patient had a grand mal seizure lasting 65 seconds. As soon as the seizure passed, the patient was fully awake and asking for food. Given the patient's reaction to his seizure, you should notify the attending physician and anticipate a psychological evaluation of this patient. If the patient had a genuine grand mal seizure, the postictal state is expected to last several hours and the patient would not be able to request food.

101. Correct answer: A
Symptoms of spinal shock include areflexia, autonomic dysfunction, loss of sensation, and eliminatory dysfunction. Spinal shock occurs hours to weeks after a cord injury, causing autonomic loss, and the severity of a spinal cord injury cannot be fully assessed until the shock has resolved.

102. **Correct answer: B**

The most accurate method of measuring intracranial pressure is intraventriculostomy. Because the catheter is inserted directly into one of the lateral ventricles, it is the most direct and accurate method of measuring intracranial pressure. The drain is inserted on the right side of the head. The ventriculostomy allows for not only drainage of excess CSF but also sampling of CSF to monitor for infection.

103. **Correct answer: C**

The transducer for any type of intracranial pressure monitoring system should be placed in the foramen of Monroe. The foramen of Monroe is the junction between the lateral ventricles and the third ventricle. It is located just above the ear.

104. **Correct answer: B**

The six cardinal eye movements test CN III (oculomotor), CN IV (trochlear), and CN VI (abducens). CN III is assessed by having the patient follow the examiner's finger or light up and out, up and in, down and out, and inward toward the nose. CN IV is assessed by having the patient follow the examiner's finger down and in toward the tip of the nose. CN VI is assessed by following the examiner's finger out toward the ear.

105. **Correct answer: D**

CBC, CMP, sedimentation rate, CRP, RPR, and a toxicology screen are the tests that need to be performed to help establish the cause of your patient's seizures. Seizures can be caused by illness, infection, overdose on drugs or alcohol, tertiary syphilis, dehydration, electrolyte imbalance, and cardiac arrhythmia.

106. **Correct answer: C**

Your patient is very depressed and stated, "I don't want to die like my mother did with ALS." Your patient is exhibiting behavior consistent with the Kübler-Ross anger stage of grief. The patient is angry at the diagnosis and afraid she will suffer the same fate as her mother. The five stages of grief identified by Kübler-Ross in 1969 are denial, anger, bargaining, depression, and acceptance. The patient can move through the stages in any order and can revisit a stage at any time. You should try to encourage the patient to express her feelings. The physician should also be notified, and the patient should receive counseling. Antidepressants may be considered.

107. **Correct answer: A**

Your patient has been diagnosed with a middle fossa basilar skull fracture after running into the pole holding the net at a basketball game. The patient suffers from facial palsy and deafness and blood is noted in the ear. Additional symptoms would include possible loss of lower facial sensation, a CSF leak, otorrhea, and tinnitus. Note that with any basilar skull fracture there is an increased potential for an intracranial infection.

108. **Correct answer: D**

If your patient demonstrates decorticate posturing, there is a likely better prognosis than available with the other levels of functioning noted above. Localization > withdrawal > decorticate posturing and positive Babinski > decerebrate posturing > grasp reflex, and finally, flaccidity.

109. **Correct answer: B**

This patient appears to be suffering from posterior cord syndrome. Your patient was a passenger in the front seat of a car that was rear-ended. During assessment, you note a "seat belt sign" on the upper abdomen and guarding in the periumbilical area. The patient states he cannot feel his legs, but demonstrates some spontaneous movement. The physician tries a tuning fork and the patient is unable to feel vibrations, but is able to feel pain on the lower leg.

The patient was rear-ended, so the head was thrown backward, a usual cause of this syndrome. The patient will also have intact temperature and crude touch and pressure sensation with loss of fine touch and pressure, along with proprioception.

110. **Correct answer: D**
Your patient has suffered a cervical injury involving the right side of the sympathetic chain. The patient demonstrates ipsilateral pupil constriction, ptosis, and anhydrosis. This triad of symptoms is known as Horner's syndrome.

111. **Correct answer: D**
Pain that radiates along a dermatome is known as radicular pain.

112. **Correct answer: B**
Your patient was involved in a fight at a soccer game. Although two teeth were not avulsed, they have fractured through the enamel and dentin of the teeth. This type of injury is known as an Ellis II fracture. As a trauma nurse, you know treatment should include application of calcium hydroxide. The calcium hydroxide helps protect the tooth by further exposure to saliva and air, which could result in pulpitis. Oral analgesia and referral to a dentist are necessary.

113. **Correct answer: C**
As a trauma nurse, you know this patient is probably suffering from a zygomatic fracture.

A group of high school students began fighting at school, and the patient was struck in the face by a heavy backpack. The patient complains of great difficulty opening and closing her mouth. She has significant periorbital ecchymosis, diplopia, and periorbital displacement. As a trauma nurse, you know this patient is probably suffering from a zygomatic fracture. This type of fracture is often caused by a blow to the side of the face. This patient would likely exhibit numbness in the medial cheek area, lower and upper lids. And some flattening of the cheek. There is usually a palpable defect over the arch.

114. **Correct answer: D**
Pyrogenic respirations are a completely irregular breathing pattern with deep and shallow breaths.

115. **Correct answer: C**
Patients suffering from neurogenic shock are likely to be treated with phenylephrine, an alpha-agonist. In neurogenic shock, the body undergoes vasodilation, cooling the core until the core temperature equals the ambient temperature (poikilothermy).

116. **Correct answer: B**
As a trauma nurse, you know the type of fracture commonly associated with axial loading where C1 splits into several sections is known as a Jeffersonian ring fracture. Patients are neurologically intact, but there is great danger because the pieces may migrate and cause instant death.

Clinical Practice: Trunk

- Abdominal
- Genitourinary
- Pulmonary Issues
- Thoracic

SECTION 5: QUESTIONS

1. **Which of the following structures is not located in the mediastinum?**
    A. The vagus and phrenic nerves
    B. Lymph nodes
    C. Esophagus
    D. Trachea

2. **Which statement below is false with regard to the thoracic duct?**
    A. The duct transports 60–70% of ingested fat into the blood stream
    B. The duct empties into the venous system at the junction of the subclavian and internal jugular veins
    C. The duct empties into the right jugular vein
    D. The duct is protected by the mediastinum anteriorly

3. **Advantages to the utilization of ultrasound when assessing thoracic injuries does not include**
    A. Ultrasound allows for rapid assessment
    B. Ultrasound does not require transport
    C. Ultrasound is noninvasive
    D. No expertise is needed to perform

4. **Immediate life-threatening injuries do not include which of the following situations**
    A. Cardiac tamponade
    B. A tension pneumothorax
    C. A flail chest
    D. An aortic rupture

5. **Which of the following situations is least likely to put a patient at risk for a tension pneumothorax?**
    A. Decreased intrapleural pressure
    B. Barotrauma
    C. Lung parenchyma injury
    D. A clamped chest tube

6. **The chest tube that was inserted in your patient for a pneumothorax became dislodged then fell to the floor. There will be a delay before a new chest tube can be inserted. As a trauma nurse, you know the appropriate emergency action to mitigate this problem is**
    A. Reuse the chest tube that fell to the floor after cleaning it with antiseptic
    B. Apply a three-sided sterile dressing to the wound
    C. Place a sterile, nonporous dressing on the wound
    D. Apply an occlusive dressing to the wound

7. **During the postcardiac arrest phase, titration of inspired oxygen to the lowest level to achieve an arterial oxygen saturation of _____ or greater is recommended.**
    A. 92%
    B. 94%
    C. 96%
    D. 99%

8. **Your patient has a confirmed flail chest. What alteration in acid–base balance would you expect this patient to have with this condition?**
    A. Metabolic alkalosis
    B. Metabolic acidosis
    C. Respiratory acidosis
    D. Respiratory alkalosis

9. Patients with uncontrolled asthma may receive steroids and neuromuscular blocking agents in an attempt to mitigate their symptoms. These patients are at increased risk for
   A. Hypertension
   B. Prolonged muscle weakness
   C. Renal failure
   D. Hepatic failure

10. When assessing the abdomen, it is generally divided into four quadrants. The right upper quadrant (RUQ) is assessed for injuries to the
    A. Stomach, spleen, splenic flexure of the colon
    B. Ascending colon, appendix, pancreas
    C. Liver, spleen, jejunum
    D. Liver, gall bladder, head of the pancreas

11. Which of the following statements is true when a patient has a pulmonary embolism?
    A. Respiratory acidosis occurs
    B. Heparin is used to dissolve clots
    C. Normal D-dimer results can rule out a pulmonary embolism
    D. Metabolic alkalosis develops

12. Pulmonary embolism is actually considered a complication of deep venous thrombosis. To assess for deep venous thrombosis, which of the following signs should be assessed?
    A. Moses's
    B. Davis's
    C. Corrigan's
    D. Hamman's

13. A middle-aged female was admitted to the ED after a fall from a tree. She now complains of stabbing substernal pain each time she changes her position. Her chest X-ray results were just relayed to you by the ED trauma attending. The patient has been diagnosed with a pneumomediastinum. A common significant finding in a patient with a pneumomediastinum is
    A. Cullen's sign
    B. Grey-Turner's sign
    C. Hamman's sign
    D. Handes's sign

14. Which of the following drugs is classified as a methylxanthine?
    A. Morphine
    B. Theophylline
    C. Prednisone
    D. Atropine

15. While ambulating your patient, he suddenly collapses. During your primary assessment, you discover the patient is in respiratory arrest but does have a perfusing rhythm. Prior to the arrival of additional ED staff, you obtain a bag-valve mask device. According to the 2015 American Heart Association guidelines for CPR and ECC, how often should you squeeze the bag to assist ventilations on this patient?
    A. Once every 4 seconds
    B. Once every 5–6 seconds
    C. 10–15 times/minute
    D. 12–15 times/minute

16. **Interpret the following arterial blood–gas values from a patient who was treated in your ED 4 days ago for a fractured ulna.**

    pH   7.43
    CO_2 37
    HCO_3 25

    A. Compensated respiratory acidosis
    B. Normal
    C. Compensated metabolic acidosis
    D. Compensated metabolic alkalosis

17. **Analyze the following arterial blood–gas values from a patient in acute kidney failure:**

    pH   7.11
    CO_2 67
    HCO_3 15

    A. Uncompensated respiratory acidosis
    B. Uncompensated metabolic alkalosis
    C. Compensated metabolic acidosis
    D. Uncompensated (mixed) respiratory/metabolic acidosis

18. **Analyze the following arterial blood–gas values for a patient who ingested methanol:**

    pH   7.39
    CO_2 24
    HCO_3 16

    A. Compensated respiratory alkalosis
    B. Compensated metabolic acidosis
    C. Uncompensated metabolic acidosis
    D. Uncompensated respiratory acidosis

19. **Which of the following statements about laryngeal mask airways (LMA) is true?**

    A. An LMA may be inserted by any nurse
    B. An LMA may cause hoarseness after removal
    C. The patient must have an absent gag reflex
    D. The LMA eliminates the risk of aspiration

20. **During a cardiac arrest, your patient aspirated gastric contents. Which of the following statements is true regarding this type of aspiration?**

    A. If the pH of the material is less than 2.5, necrosis will be minimal
    B. The patient always develops ARDS
    C. Onset of symptoms is gradual
    D. There is little danger of atelectasis

21. **Your patient was normally a very active skateboarder. Today he slipped and fell, causing several lacerations and a left Colles' fracture. During assessment, you ascertain the patient is dyspneic with a temperature of 101.4°F and some trouble swallowing. The patient was subsequently diagnosed with aspiration pneumonitis. As a trauma nurse, you know the most severe pulmonary reaction may occur from the aspiration of**

    A. A nonacidic liquid
    B. Salt water
    C. Gastric contents with a pH greater than 2.5
    D. Acidic food particles

22. **Pulse oximetry should never be used**
    A. To determine oxygen saturation values
    B. During a cardiac arrest
    C. As a determinant for predicting hemoglobin affinity for oxygen
    D. To help determine a patient's activity tolerance

23. **Which of the following statements is true regarding chest tube drainage systems?**
    A. Drainage of frank blood in amounts greater than 100 ml/hour is not significant
    B. Drainage tubing should be placed horizontally on the bed, then down to the collection chamber
    C. All drainage tubing should be dependent to the insertion site
    D. Chest tube drainage from a mediastinal tube should bubble in the water seal chamber

24. **Ecchymotic splotches sometimes seen on labia, scrotum, and perineum secondary to pelvic fractures are known as**
    A. Cullen's sign
    B. Coopernail sign
    C. Moses' sign
    D. Gray-Turner's sign

25. **Analyze the following blood-gas values from a patient who is suffering from asthma:**
    pH   7.47
    CO_2 29
    HCO_3 24
    A. Uncompensated respiratory alkalosis
    B. Compensated respiratory acidosis
    C. Compensated metabolic alkalosis
    D. Uncompensated metabolic acidosis

26. **Interpret the following arterial blood-gas values from a patient with atelectasis:**
    pH   7.46
    CO_2 29
    HCO_3 22
    A. Uncompensated metabolic alkalosis
    B. Uncompensated respiratory alkalosis
    C. Compensated respiratory alkalosis
    D. Compensated metabolic alkalosis

27. **Analyze the following arterial blood-gas values from a patient with restrictive lung disease:**
    pH   7.32
    CO_2 67
    HCO_3 25
    A. Uncompensated metabolic alkalosis
    B. Uncompensated respiratory acidosis
    C. Compensated metabolic acidosis
    D. Compensated respiratory acidosis

28. **Review the following arterial blood-gas values:**
    pH   7.37
    CO_2 36
    HCO_3 24
    A. Normal
    B. Compensated respiratory acidosis
    C. Compensated metabolic acidosis
    D. Compensated respiratory alkalosis

29. **One of the most effective ways to relieve bronchospasms is**
    A. To administer adrenalin
    B. To administer an antihistamine
    C. To administer prednisone
    D. To administer a B2 receptor agonist

30. **When the emergency department resident attempts to place a central line, air is accidentally introduced into the line when the IV tubing becomes disconnected. The best position in which to place this patient to minimize a venous air embolism is**
    A. Trendelenburg with left decubitus tilt
    B. Right side
    C. Reverse Trendelenburg
    D. Left side

31. **A risk factor for development of thrombotic emboli includes which of the following conditions?**
    A. A patient who is one week postpartum
    B. Carcinoma
    C. Long bone fractures
    D. Heparin administration

32. **Your patient was struck head-on by another car in a parking lot. The impact, though slow speed, caused the airbag to deploy. The powder from the airbag caused an acute exacerbation of reactive airway disease. The patient has a history of asthma. Which of the following signs indicates this patient is suffering from an acute episode of respiratory distress?**
    A. Expiratory wheezes
    B. Grunting
    C. Sternocleidomastoid retractions
    D. Inspiratory wheezes

33. **Your patient has ceased wheezing during his asthma attack. This change in his condition**
    A. Indicates the patient is improving
    B. Only means the nebulizer treatment is working
    C. Indicates the patient is in complete respiratory failure
    D. Means the patient's anxiety has decreased

34. **The American Heart Association has classified acute pulmonary embolisms into three categories: massive, submassive, or low risk. A submassive pulmonary embolism is characterized by**
    A. An acute PE with evidence of right ventricular dysfunction or myocardial dysfunction
    B. A patient without ventricular dysfunction
    C. An acute PE with sustained BP less than 90 mmHg for more than 15 minutes
    D. An acute PE with redistribution of ventilation to all lung fields

35. **Pulse oximetry readings are considered unreliable when oxygen saturation levels fall below**
    A. 55%
    B. 60%
    C. 80%
    D. 70%

36. **The nursing student assigned to you for the day asks you to explain the oxyhemoglobin dissociation curve. You reply that the oxyhemoglobin dissociation curve is**
    A. A relationship between dissolved oxygen and the affinity for oxygen by the hemoglobin molecule
    B. A graphic representation of carbon dioxide content versus oxygen content in arterial blood
    C. A measure of methemoglobin
    D. A way to calculate gas transport across the alveoli

37. **Your patient with COPD has been receiving 600 mg of theophylline daily in divided doses. Which of the following assessment findings should be reported to the physician immediately, as these findings represent potential theophylline toxicity?**
    A. The patient is lethargic
    B. Atrial tachycardia with occasional PVCs has developed
    C. The patient's blood glucose is 50
    D. The patient has a systolic blood pressure of 160 mmHg

38. **Which of the following actions should not be performed initially in the ED when a patient has sustained a pelvic fracture?**
    A. A FAST examination
    B. Placement of a urinary catheter
    C. Administration of analgesia
    D. Administration of a neuromuscular block

39. **A measurement of total oxygen consumption is**
    A. SvO_2
    B. $ETCO_2$
    C. $PtCO_2$
    D. SjO_2

40. **Your patient required endotracheal intubation. Which of the following statements is true regarding the use of capnography to verify endotracheal tube placement?**
    A. Placement of the device can be difficult to learn initially
    B. It is not necessary to auscultate lung sounds when this device is used
    C. $ETCO_2$ is a moderately reliable indicator of correct tube placement
    D. It is not a substitute for pulse oximetry

41. **Your patient had 1,420 ml of pleural effusion removed via thoracentesis and immediately began coughing and was dyspneic. You believe this patient has developed**
    A. Reexpansion pulmonary edema
    B. A pneumothorax
    C. A cardiac tamponade
    D. A hemothorax

42. **Three days ago, during a home renovation, your patient had several sheets of drywall fall on him. The result was two cracked ribs and multiple contusions. In the ED, the patient was placed on a 60% nonrebreather mask. The patient was sent home with supplemental oxygen at 2 L/minute via nasal cannula. The patient's family gathered personal belongings and the tubing used on the patient in the ED. At home, the patient was placed on the nonrebreather mask at 60% because the family thought it should be the same as what they saw in the hospital.**
    The patient returned to the ED today suffering substernal chest pain exacerbated when deep breathing. The patient also states his allergies are causing a dry cough, some nasal stuffiness, some pain in both ears, and a sore throat. The chest pain becomes more pronounced and pleuritic in nature. The patient is anxious because he thinks the pain was caused by his actions. This patient has been on a 60% nonrebreather mask for 2 days. It is likely this patient may be suffering from
    A. A pulmonary embolism
    B. Hypoxemia
    C. Hyperoxia
    D. Pneumothorax

43. **A student nurse asks you to explain the concept of hypoxemia. Hypoxemia is best defined as**
    A. A decrease in oxygen at the cellular level
    B. A decrease in oxygen at the alveolar level
    C. A decrease in oxygen levels in venous blood
    D. A decrease in oxygen levels in arterial blood

44. **Which of the following conditions is the most probable cause of the acid–base imbalance of uncompensated respiratory alkalosis?**
    A. Kidney failure
    B. A side effect of theophylline
    C. Hyperventilation
    D. Hypoventilation

45. **A renal transplant that results from humoral rejection or acute cellular rejection may be definitively diagnosed only via**
    A. Ultrasound
    B. Nuclear scan
    C. Doppler scan
    D. Renal biopsy

46. **Evaluate the following arterial blood-gas values from a patient who has been vomiting the past hour:**

pH	7.36
CO_2	27
HCO_3	19

    A. Compensated metabolic acidosis
    B. Compensated respiratory acidosis
    C. Uncompensated metabolic acidosis
    D. Uncompensated respiratory acidosis

47. **Analyze the following capillary blood-gas results for a patient on 21% oxygen who has been ambulating in the hallway:**

pH	7.44
CO_2	41
HCO_3	23

    A. Compensated respiratory acidosis
    B. Compensated respiratory alkalosis
    C. Normal
    D. Compensated metabolic acidosis

48. **Interpret the following arterial blood-gas results from a patient with a ventricular septal injury from a stab wound:**

pH	7.57
CO_2	22
HCO_3	32

    A. Uncompensated (mixed) respiratory/metabolic alkalosis
    B. Compensated respiratory acidosis
    C. Compensated metabolic alkalosis
    D. Uncompensated respiratory alkalosis

49. **Which of the following statements is true about agonal gasps?**
    A. Agonal gasps are an indication of an extra thoracic obstruction
    B. Gasping is a sign of cardiac arrest
    C. Gasping is an abnormal pattern, but one that will provide ventilation
    D. Agonal gasps indicate brain herniation

50. **The volume of gas remaining in the lungs at the end of one normal expiration is called**
    A. Residual volume
    B. Capacitance
    C. Total lung capacity
    D. Functional residual capacity

51. **The volume of gas left in the lungs following a maximal respiratory effort is known as the**
    A. Vital capacity
    B. Total lung capacity
    C. Residual volume
    D. Dead airspace

52. **The functional residual capacity is defined as**
    A. The amount of air in the lungs after normal expiration
    B. The amount of gas that can be forcefully exhaled after maximum inspiration
    C. The amount of gas normally exhaled after a maximum inhalation
    D. The amount of gas left in the lungs after a maximum exhalation

53. **Your patient was brought to the ED by ambulance from a rehabilitation center. The patient was evacuated because the kitchen area of the center caught fire. The patient has an indwelling catheter, is in a wheelchair, and has a temperature of 100.4°F. The respiratory therapist who has just drawn an ABG sample asks you if the patient has a fever. The possibility of fever will have what effect on the sample he just collected?**
    A. The PO_2 will be falsely elevated
    B. The pH will rise
    C. Fever has no effect
    D. The HCO_3 will be elevated

54. **The cells responsible for forming a barrier for alveoli are known as**
    A. Histiocytes
    B. Type II alveolar epithelial cells
    C. Macrophages
    D. Type I alveolar epithelial cells

55. **Analyze the following arterial blood–gas values obtained from a patient who is suffering from pneumonia:**
    pH   7.37
    CO_2 67
    HCO_3 36
    A. Uncompensated metabolic alkalosis
    B. Compensated respiratory acidosis
    C. Compensated metabolic acidosis
    D. Uncompensated respiratory acidosis

56. **Type II alveolar cells produce**
    A. Surfactant
    B. Phagocytes
    C. Macrocytes
    D. Carbon dioxide

57. **The FiO_2 for a nasal cannula set at a flow rate of 6 L/minute is**
    A. 21%
    B. 24%
    C. 30%
    D. 40%

58. **A diagnosis of asthma may be made by**
    A. A PEFR of 100–125
    B. A FiO_2 of 80%
    C. A decreased FEV_1
    D. Wheezing

59. **An absolute contraindication for use of rapid sequence intubation is**
    A. Total loss of facial and/or oropharyngeal landmarks, which requires a surgical airway
    B. An airway where intubation may not be successful
    C. A "crash" airway where the patient is in arrest
    D. There is no absolute contraindication for the use of rapid sequence intubation

60. **Which of the following situations is not an indication for the use of rapid sequence intubation?**
    A. Prolonged respiratory effort that results in fatigue or failure
    B. Uncooperative trauma patient with life-threatening injuries
    C. Stab wound to neck with expanding hematoma
    D. All cervical spine injuries

61. **During rapid sequence intubation (RSI), cricoid cartilage pressure is often used to help prevent vomiting and aspiration of gastric contents. The esophagus is obstructed by the pressure to the anterior neck. This maneuver is known as the**
    A. Hamman's maneuver
    B. King maneuver
    C. Sellick maneuver
    D. Pitt maneuver

62. **When performing CPR on a cardiac arrest patient, as a trauma nurse, you know the best, most reliable way to confirm placement of an endotracheal tube is**
    A. Auscultation of upper and lower lung fields
    B. Use of a CO_2 detector
    C. Continuous waveform capnography ($PetCO_2$)
    D. Pulse oximetry

63. **Interpret the following arterial blood–gas results from a victim of a gunshot wound to the chest:**
    pH   7.22
    CO_2 63
    HCO_3 23
    A. Compensated respiratory acidosis
    B. Uncompensated metabolic acidosis
    C. Uncompensated respiratory acidosis
    D. Normal

64. **One cause of decreased SvO_2 in a patient is**
    A. An increased metabolic rate
    B. Sedation
    C. A decreased metabolic rate
    D. Increased cardiac output

65. **Which of the following statements about diagnostic peritoneal lavage (DPL) is true?**
    A. The results of DPL are always accurate
    B. A Foley and gastric tube should be placed prior to the DPL
    C. If 3 ml of frank blood is readily drawn back, the unstable patient must go to the OR
    D. A DPL should be avoided in patients with spinal cord injuries

66. **Your patient has a hemothorax. What is the proper location of a chest tube for evacuation of a hemothorax?**
    A. Second intercostal space, midclavicular line
    B. Second intercostal space, midaxillary line
    C. Fifth intercostal space, midaxillary line
    D. Fifth intercostal space, midclavicular line

67. **Where does the hypoxemic drive to breathe originate?**
    A. The cerebellum
    B. The aortic and carotid arteries
    C. The hypothalamus
    D. The medulla

68. **Breathing high concentrations of oxygen may wash out nitrogen that is present in alveoli. The nitrogen helps keep the alveoli open. If oxygen replaces nitrogen in the alveoli, the alveoli will shrink and begin to collapse. This phenomenon is considered an adverse effect and is known as**
    A. Oxygen toxicity
    B. Absorption atelectasis
    C. A pulmonary dysplasia
    D. Pulmonary hypertension

69. **A patient recently admitted from the ED requires immediate intubation. The physician orders succinylcholine. Which of the following conditions is not a side effect of succinylcholine?**
    A. Malignant hyperthermia
    B. Increased intraocular pressure
    C. Hypotension
    D. Hypokalemia

70. **Patients who have sustained crush injuries are susceptible to**
    A. Hypokalemia
    B. Lowered CK levels
    C. Rhabdomyolysis
    D. Alkalized urine

71. **Soon after arriving for your shift, you assume the care of a patient with virtually no report given as to the patient's condition or diagnosis. The ED nurse who transferred your patient to you did report that your patient had been previously intubated by paramedics with a laryngeal mask airway (LMA). The patient is now conscious and is on a nasal cannula at 2 L/minute. Which of the following statements is true regarding the use of LMAs?**
    A. Nurses routinely insert these airways
    B. There is a low risk of aspiration
    C. It is a temporary airway
    D. The vocal cords must be visualized

72. **An action of nitric oxide includes which of the following effects?**
    A. Vascular smooth muscle relaxation
    B. To augment prostaglandin synthesis
    C. To release macrophages
    D. To increase pulmonary vascular resistance

73. **Which of the following statements is true regarding the administration of CPAP?**
    A. CPAP cannot be delivered via an endotracheal tube
    B. CPAP allows for a decrease in functional residual capacity
    C. CPAP provides decreased pressure to the posterior pharynx
    D. CPAP may be administered via nasal prongs

74. **An adverse effect of excessive CPAP is**
    A. Continuous need to increase oxygen over time
    B. A rise in intrathoracic pressure
    C. Intraventricular hemorrhage
    D. A sudden change in cerebral blood flow

75. **Your patient is suffering from acute liver failure. The arterial blood gas results from the sample drawn 1 hour ago show the patient has respiratory alkalosis. Which of the following arterial blood gas results would support that diagnosis?**
    A. pH 7.27, CO_2 24, HCO_3 24
    B. pH 7.47, CO_2 24, HCO_3 24
    C. pH 7.57, CO_2 44, HCO_3 32
    D. pH 7.37, CO_2 67, HCO_3 26

76. **In the ED, patients may be mechanically ventilated by a variety of ventilator modes. Which of the following ventilator modes allows the patient to breathe spontaneously?**
    A. HFV
    B. SIMV
    C. CMV
    D. Oscillator

77. **Your patient will require long-term ventilatory support via a tracheostomy. A disadvantage of using a tracheostomy tube is**
    A. Subcutaneous emphysema
    B. It increases airway resistance
    C. The airway is less stable
    D. It allows for right mainstem intubation

78. **Analyze the following arterial blood–gas values from a patient who has been taking large quantities of antacids:**

pH	7.53
CO_2	42
HCO_3	37

    A. Uncompensated metabolic alkalosis
    B. Compensated metabolic acidosis
    C. Uncompensated respiratory alkalosis
    D. Uncompensated mixed respiratory/metabolic alkalosis

79. **Your patient fell down a flight of stairs, breaking several ribs in two or more places and suffering internal injuries. Which of the following injuries would mandate the use of pain control?**
    A. Flail chest
    B. ARDS
    C. A splenectomy
    D. Hemothorax

80. **Your patient has sustained a stab wound to the area of the right anterior axillary line at the fifth intercostal space. The patient is hypotensive, tachypneic, tachycardic, and restless. O_2 at 100% via mask is provided. Two large bore IVs have been placed and crystalloids are infusing. As a trauma nurse, you would expect to prepare for**
    A. An autotransfusion
    B. Immediate surgery
    C. A paracentesis
    D. Placement of a chest tube

81. A blunt cardiac injury is most likely to affect which of the following chambers of the heart?
    A. Right ventricle
    B. Left ventricle
    C. Right atrium
    D. Left atrium

82. Your patient was resting quietly on the gurney, awaiting transport to X-ray to evaluate a possible fractured right tibia and patella. Suddenly the patient complains of right-sided chest pain, tachypnea at rate of 40, cyanosis, and JVD. No breath sounds are now audible over the right lung fields. The trachea is deviated to the left and heart tones are distant. This patient is most likely suffering from
    A. A pericardial effusion
    B. A tension pneumothorax
    C. A Ludwig's angina
    D. An inferior wall MI

83. If a projectile strikes the precordium during the vulnerable part of the cardiac cycle, this is known as
    A. Mechanical energy
    B. Kinetic force
    C. Blunt force
    D. Commotio cordis

84. The most common location of a sternal fracture is
    A. The xiphoid process
    B. The manubrium
    C. The sternal angle
    D. The sternoclavicular joint

85. Which of the following rib fractures are associated with high mortality?
    A. The first, second, and third ribs
    B. The right lower ribs
    C. The left lower ribs
    D. Fractures of ribs 4–9

86. Which of the following conditions is not considered a complication of a pulmonary contusion?
    A. ARDS
    B. Atelectasis
    C. Pneumonia
    D. Crackles

87. Your patient had a chest tube placed for a pneumothorax. The patient had his motorcycle fall on his chest, and was bruised and cracked rib 4 on the right. Your patient exhibits ST segment depression on his EKG along with moderate, substernal chest pain. These findings indicate a possible
    A. Anteroseptal MI
    B. Myocardial ischemia episode
    C. Lateral wall MI
    D. Pericardial tamponade

88. During inspiration your patient has a paradoxical rise in jugular venous pressure. This phenomenon is commonly associated with which of the following cardiac conditions?
    A. Mitral stenosis
    B. Right heart failure
    C. An anterior wall MI
    D. Increased ventricular compliance

89. Your patient came to the ED with severe abdominal pain following a blunt force injury suffered during an assault. It was determined that the patient is at extreme risk for peritonitis. The patient had a J-tube placed while waiting for an ICU bed. This patient is at great risk for which of the following electrolyte deficits?

    A. Sodium

    B. Magnesium

    C. Manganese

    D. Phosphorus

90. On an EKG, upright QRS in leads V_1 and V_2 indicate which of the following types of bundle branch block?

    A. Right

    B. Left

    C. Dual bundle branch block

    D. Only leads aVF and III diagnose bundle branch blocks

91. Structures located in the retroperitoneum include:

    A. Liver, spleen, sigmoid colon

    B. Adrenal glands, spleen, transverse colon

    C. Small intestine, liver, gall bladder

    D. Kidneys, adrenal glands, pancreas

92. Your patient suffered an episode of bradycardia that resulted in a heart rate decreasing to the 20s. The patient had just been deeply suctioned. The low heart rate was unresponsive to oxygen support and a dose of atropine, so assisted ventilation via a bag-valve mask was provided. The heart rate finally improved to prebradycardic levels. Which of the following potential complications of atropine administration may now occur?

    A. Diuresis

    B. Hypertension

    C. Rebound bradycardia

    D. Headache

93. A biomarker that is not cardiac specific but can be elevated by falls, cardiopulmonary resuscitation, and injections is

    A. C-reactive protein

    B. Myoglobin

    C. INR

    D. BNP

94. A sign of necrosis seen on an EKG would include

    A. Acute ST elevation

    B. A right BBB

    C. A left BBB

    D. A Q wave in Lead III

95. Your patient was observing practice at the local high school when she was struck by a player that overran the sidelines. The patient sustained a blunt chest injury and on assessment you auscultated a pericardial friction rub. A pericardial friction rub would be best heard at

    A. The 3rd intercostal space, on the left sternal border

    B. The 2nd intercostal space, right sternal border

    C. The 5th intercostal space, midclavicular line

    D. The 5th intercostal space, midclavicular line

96. **Increased production of urea may be due to**
    A. GI bleeding
    B. Low protein diet
    C. Congenital kidney disease
    D. Hypothermia

97. **You are assessing your patient's existing shunt prior to emergency hemodialysis. You note there is no thrill or bruit at the shunt site. Your next nursing action should be to**
    A. Call the surgeon to do a new graft
    B. Use a Doppler to determine graft patency
    C. Administer a bolus of heparin
    D. Continue with the hemodialysis, as there is nothing wrong

98. **Your patient sustained an injury to a kidney from a fall 2 days ago. resulting in hyperlipidemia, edema, low albumin in the blood, and proteinuria. These findings are indicative that the patient is suffering from**
    A. Nephrotic syndrome
    B. An abdominal infection
    C. A catheter-induced nephrotoxic injury
    D. Post-renal failure

99. **You suspect your patient is developing a pulmonary embolism. Signs and symptoms of a pulmonary embolus can include**
    A. Sinus bradycardia or a normal EKG
    B. Pleuritic chest pain, decreased cardiac output
    C. ABGs show respiratory acidosis, increased respiratory rate
    D. Decreased pulmonary artery systolic pressure

100. **Which of the following statements about a stable pelvic fracture is true?**
    A. A stable pelvic fracture results when the posterior elements of the ring are disrupted
    B. Stable pelvic fractures are only caused by direct trauma and crush injuries
    C. Stable fractures cause large amounts of bleeding
    D. Stable fractures do not transect the pelvic ring

101. **If a patient has truncal obesity and has sustained a pelvic fracture, it is possible to initially stabilize the fracture via**
    A. Internal rotation of lower extremities and taping the knees together
    B. Closing the fracture under fluoroscopy
    C. Surgery only
    D. Fluoroscopy

102. **The peritoneal cavity contains which of the following structures?**
    A. The small intestine, pancreas, adrenal glands
    B. The ascending and descending colon, aorta, vena cava
    C. The spleen, uterus, kidneys
    D. The liver, spleen, stomach

103. **Which of the following statements is true about an acute rotator cuff tear?**
    A. Symptoms appear slowly and result in moderate diffuse pain in the arm
    B. The patient is unable to adduct the arm and there is severe pain
    C. The patient experiences pain in the affected arm for about 6 hours
    D. The patient may feel a tearing sensation and exhibit point tenderness over the site

104. A 28-year-old male presents with peristernal pain that worsens on inspiration and movement. The patient states the pain began during multiple reps of weightlifting at a local gym. The patient could not maintain the weight and fell to the floor and wrenched his knee. The patient states no pain in the knee at this time, but the mid chest pain is worse. On inspection of the chest, no visual swelling, deformity, or ecchymosis is seen. On palpation, the skin temperature is noted to be normal and there is point tenderness over the area. It is likely this patient is suffering from
    A. Pericarditis
    B. A pleural effusion
    C. Costochondritis
    D. A fractured rib

105. Your patient was involved in a street fight and sustained multiple lacerations on the anterior chest, forearms and shoulders. The patient requires suturing and tetanus prophylaxis. The patient has a history of malignant hyperthermia. An appropriate local anesthetic agent for this patient is
    A. Lidocaine
    B. Procaine
    C. Mepivacaine
    D. Bupivacaine

106. Your patient was driving his car through an intersection when his vehicle was T-boned by another car. The patient suffered a fractured pelvis and left femur and was stabilized in the ED and is awaiting surgical fixation of the fractures. When auscultating lung sounds, you hear what you believe to be bowel sounds in the chest. The patient is experiencing moderate shoulder pain on the left side and he is mildly tachypneic. The probable diagnosis will be
    A. A fractured scapula
    B. A hemothorax
    C. Diaphragmatic rupture
    D. Bowel rupture

107. The anatomical borders of the abdomen include:
    A. The diaphragm, which forms the posterior border
    B. The anterior border, formed by the vertebral column
    C. The inferior border, which is formed by the pelvis
    D. The superior border, which is formed by the abdominal and iliac muscles

108. The type of vertebral fracture that results from the mechanism of injury known as hyperflexion is called a
    A. Wedge fracture
    B. Compression fracture
    C. Simple fracture
    D. Teardrop fracture

109. When palpating the abdomen under the right costal margin near the liver, you note the patient is unable to inhale deeply. This reaction is known as
    A. Kernig's sign
    B. Rovsing's sign
    C. Lentick's sign
    D. Murphy's sign

110. Which of the following organs is not located in the retroperitoneum:
    A. Spleen
    B. Pancreas
    C. Adrenal glands
    D. Ureters

111. Your patient has been on a nasal cannula and now requires a nonrebreather mask to maintain his oxygenation saturation at acceptable levels. A nonrebreather mask can deliver what percentage of oxygen when the O_2 flow rate is set at 10–15 L/minute?
    A. 24–40%
    B. 30–40%
    C. 50–60%
    D. 60–80%

112. You are attempting to draw an arterial blood–gas sample from an arterial line. The syringe requires a lot of force to move the cylinder. What effect will this high friction on the syringe have on blood–gas results, if any?
    A. It will put the artery into spasm
    B. The high friction will increase the $PaCO_2$
    C. The high friction will decrease the PaO_2
    D. There will be no effect on the results

113. One of the factors to be considered when assessing a patient for possible aspiration and chemical/aspiration pneumonitis is
    A. The possibility of using syrup of Ipecac
    B. The pH of the aspirate
    C. The type of infiltrates on CXR
    D. ABG results

114. An indication for surgical intervention with a patient who has a hemothorax and required chest tube placement would be
    A. An initial return of 900 ml of blood on initial chest tube placement
    B. Drainage of 200 ml an hour for 2 hours
    C. An initial return of 1,500 ml of blood on initial chest tube placement
    D. Drainage of 150 ml an hour for 4 hours

115. Which of the following statements about innervation of the heart is true?
    A. Beta-1 adrenergic receptors are located only in the atria
    B. Beta-2 receptors are located in both the atria and the ventricles
    C. Beta-1 receptors cause an increase in conductivity, heart rate, and contractility
    D. Alpha-1 adrenergic receptors affect the tone of the ventricular walls

116. The most sensitive cardiac marker is
    A. CK-MB
    B. Creatine kinase
    C. Troponin T
    D. Tropinin IIa

117. A biomarker that indicates an inflammation is present is
    A. C-reactive protein
    B. CK-MB isoenzyme
    C. White blood count
    D. Troponin 1

118. When auscultating the heart, a common area for hearing murmurs and ectopic beats is
    A. Erb's point
    B. Pulmonic area
    C. Aortic area
    D. Mitral area

119. **During insertion of a CVP catheter, your patient has a short run of V-tach and the EKG monitor shows unifocal PVCs. Your immediate response should be to**
    A. Administer lidocaine 1 mg/kg
    B. Hang an amiodarone drip
    C. Notify the physician who is inserting the catheter
    D. Immediately have the physician completely withdraw the catheter

120. **Which of the following statements would be inaccurate when describing classic seat belt injuries?**
    A. The "seat belt sign" corresponds with an intra-abdominal injury in about 80% of patients
    B. Impalement is considered a dirty wound and results in higher mortality rates
    C. Seat belt injuries include hollow viscus injuries and abdominal wall disruption
    D. Seat belt injuries may result in a flexion-distraction fracture of lumbar vertebrae (Chance fracture)

121. **Pelvic fractures are usually classified as stable or unstable. The definition of an unstable pelvic fracture is**
    A. A fracture where the pelvic ring is broken in one section and no rotational displacement exists
    B. A fracture with external rotation, vertical compression, and without shear
    C. The pelvic ring is fractured in more than one place with two displacements on the ring
    D. A fracture that involves moderate displacement of the ring

122. **While assessing a patient for possible splenic involvement and abdominal injury, the patient complains of a sharp pain in the left shoulder, slightly above the collarbone. This phenomenon is known as**
    A. A symptom indicating a left kidney injury
    B. A peritoneal sign
    C. Trousseau's sign
    D. Kehr's sign

123. **Your patient is about to undergo a diagnostic peritoneal lavage (DPL) to provide some information about a suspected hollow viscus injury. As a trauma nurse, you know if the test is performed too early, you may miss injuries on patients with**
    A. Previous laparotomies
    B. Injuries to the pancreas
    C. Obesity
    D. Third trimester pregnancies

124. **Your female patient has a fever, chills, pain on urination, moderate burning at the supra pubic area, and diarrhea. This patient is most likely suffering from**
    A. Acute renal failure
    B. A kidney infection
    C. A lower urinary tract infection
    D. An upper urinary tract infection

125. **Esophageal injuries are usually caused by penetrating trauma, rarely because of a rupture. There is a lack of a serosal layer, which may predispose a patient to a leak after surgical repair. Also, the esophagus narrows at primarily three locations, predisposing it to an injury. These three points of narrowing of the esophagus would not include**
    A. The arch of the aorta
    B. The cricoid cartilage
    C. The mediastinum
    D. The esophagogastric junction

126. Your patient was riding his bicycle carelessly and T-boned a car. The patient exhibited peritoneal guarding. Duodenal injury is suspected. Which of the following statements about duodenal injuries is true?
    A. Compression injuries are rare because the duodenum is protected by the liver
    B. The duodenum is primarily a retroperitoneal organ
    C. Most duodenal injuries do not have associated intra-abdominal injuries
    D. Vertebral column fractures are not associated with duodenal injuries

127. Pelvic fractures may result in significant blood loss. When soft tissues are injured, a systemic inflammatory response is initiated, resulting in the release of chemical mediators. These chemical mediators may result in a depletion of intravascular volume. These chemical mediators are called
    A. Histamines
    B. Free radicals
    C. Cytokines
    D. Addressins

128. An appropriate location for an IV in a patient suffering a major abdominal injury would be in which of the following vessels?
    A. Femoral
    B. Antecubital
    C. Tributary of superior vena cava
    D. External jugular

129. Contraindications for a pulmonary angiogram would include
    A. Perfusion deficits
    B. Vascular filling defects
    C. Pulmonary thromboembolism
    D. Pregnancy

130. Sudden anuria may be due to
    A. An embolic event
    B. Congestive heart failure
    C. Prostate enlargement
    D. Azotemia

131. The current definition of acute renal failure is
    A. Trauma to one or both kidneys
    B. Decrease in renal perfusion from shock or anaphylaxis
    C. A sudden or rapid decline in renal filtration function
    D. An obstruction to passage of urine

132. Post-renal AKI may be caused by
    A. Malignant hypertension
    B. Transplant rejection
    C. Neurogenic bladder
    D. Preeclampsia

133. Hypokalemia may cause significant changes in acid base balance. Which condition below is associated with hypokalemia?
    A. Respiratory alkalosis only
    B. Metabolic alkalosis only
    C. Both respiratory and metabolic alkalosis
    D. Metabolic acidosis only

134. **The primary site for urea synthesis is in the**
- A. Kidneys
- B. Liver
- C. Lungs
- D. Pancreas

SECTION 5: ANSWERS

1. **Correct answer: C**
   The esophagus is not located in the mediastinum. Structures in the mediastinum include the thymus, heart, trachea, thoracic duct, lymph nodes, vagus and phrenic nerves, and the sympathetic trunks.

2. **Correct answer: C**
   The thoracic duct empties into the left internal jugular vein, not the right. The duct does transport 60–70% of ingested fat into the bloodstream, and the duct is protected by the mediastinum anteriorly, and the spine posteriorly.

3. **Correct answer: D**
   Ultrasound does require training and expertise to perform well. Advantages of using ultrasound include that it is noninvasive, requires no transport, and is a rapid assessment tool to help diagnose thoracic and other injuries.

4. **Correct answer: D**
   An aortic rupture is considered a potentially life-threatening injury. Life-threatening injuries include airway obstructions, flail chest, cardiac tamponade, tension pneumothorax, open pneumothorax, and massive hemothorax.

5. **Correct answer: A**
   An increase in intrapleural pressure, not a decrease, is a result of a tension pneumothorax. Situations that place a patient at risk for a tension pneumothorax are rib fractures, barotrauma, clamped or clogged chest tubes, lung parenchyma injury, extension of a simple pneumothorax, and tracheobronchial tree injuries.

6. **Correct answer: B**
   The chest tube that was inserted in your patient for a pneumothorax became dislodged then fell to the floor. There will be a delay before a new chest tube can be inserted. As a trauma nurse, you know the appropriate emergency action to mitigate this problem is to apply a three-sided dressing to the wound. This would allow the untapped side to allow air to exit. This type of dressing helps prevent tension from developing.

7. **Correct answer: B**
   According to the 2015 American Heart Association guidelines for CPR and ECC, during the postcardiac arrest phase, titration of inspired oxygen to the lowest level to achieve an arterial oxygen saturation of 94% or greater is recommended when feasible. This may help avoid potential complications with oxygen toxicity.

8. **Correct answer: C**
   A flail chest is a very painful condition that limits respiratory effort because of the pain. Analgesia and sedation that may be required may also depress respiratory drive and excursion. The CO_2 will increase, PaO_2 will decrease, and the pH will be below 7.35. The patient will develop respiratory acidosis.

9. **Correct answer: B**
   Patients with uncontrolled asthma may receive steroids and neuromuscular blocking agents in an attempt to mitigate their symptoms. These patients are at increased risk for prolonged muscle weakness. Uncontrolled asthma symptoms during an attack may lead to prolonged and extensive muscle use to maintain independent respirations. Prolonged effort may result in respiratory failure due to respiratory muscle fatigue. Administration of a neuromuscular blocking agent further inhibits the smooth muscle retractions. Long-term steroid use has been linked to muscle wasting. Ventilatory weaning may be prolonged as respiratory muscles recover from both the disease process and pharmacologic intervention.

10. **Correct answer: D**
    When assessing the right upper quadrant of the abdomen, you are assessing injuries to the liver, gall bladder with the biliary tree, hepatic flexure of the colon, head of the pancreas, and duodenum. The left upper quadrant is assessed for injuries to the stomach, spleen, left lobe of the liver, left kidney and adrenal gland, the splenic flexure of the colon, and sections of the transverse and descending colon. Right lower quadrant assessment includes the ascending colon, appendix, secum, the right ovary and fallopian tube, and right ureter. The left lower quadrant assessment for injuries includes the descending and sigmoid colon, the left ovary and fallopian tube, and the left ureter.

11. **Correct answer: C**
    A normal D-dimer rules out a pulmonary embolism. If the D-dimer is elevated, it may be caused by multiple other conditions. Hyperventilation occurs subsequent to hypoxemia caused by the PE, so respiratory alkalosis will be present, not metabolic alkalosis. Heparin does not dissolve existing clots.

12. **Correct answer: A**
    Use Moses's sign to assess for deep venous thrombosis (DVT). Moses's sign is elicited by pressing the calf toward the tibia. This may also elicit pain. These results are not exclusive to DVT but may complement a diagnosis. Traditionally, we were taught to assess Homan's sign: dorsiflexion of the ankle while bending the knee. If that elicited pain, the patient had a problem with circulation and possibly DVT.

13. **Correct answer: C**
    A very common and significant finding in a patient with a pneumomediastinum is Hamman's sign. Hamman's sign is a "crunching" sound or a slight clicking sound with each heart sound auscultated over the apex of the heart.

14. **Correct answer: B**
    Methylxanthines are an important classification of drugs. In addition to theophylline, caffeine and theobromine are also methylxanthines. Methylxanthines can be found in coffee, tea, and cocoa. Low doses of drugs in this classification can stimulate cortical arousal and in higher doses cause insomnia. They can cause tachycardias and increase production of gastric acid and digestive enzymes. Methylxanthines also inhibit histamine release.

15. **Correct answer: B**
    While ambulating your patient, he suddenly collapses. During your primary assessment, you discover the patient is in respiratory arrest but does have a perfusing rhythm. Prior to the arrival of additional ED staff, you obtain a bag-valve mask device. According to the 2015 American Heart Association guidelines for CPR and ECC, you should squeeze the bag every 5–6 seconds to assist ventilations on this patient.

16. **Correct answer: B**
    The pH is between 7.35 and 7.45, the CO_2 is between 35 and 45 mmHg, and the HCO_3 is between 22 and 26 mEq/L. All the results are within normal ranges, so this ABG is considered normal. The distractor was the injury and there is a tendency to believe something must be wrong with a patient if information was included in the stem of a question.

17. **Correct answer: D**
    This is an uncompensated (mixed) respiratory/metabolic acidosis. The pH is less than 7.35, so the value is uncompensated acidosis. To determine whether the acidosis is respiratory or metabolic, find the value that represents acidosis. This would be both the HCO_3 less than 22 mEq/L and the CO_2 greater than 45 mmHg, meaning the cause of the acidosis is both respiratory and metabolic in nature.

18. **Correct answer: B**
    This blood–gas result indicates a compensated metabolic acidosis. The pH is between 7.35 and 7.45, so the gas is compensated, but the value is closer to acidosis, making the value compensated acidosis. Determine which respiratory or metabolic value is acidotic: in this case, the HCO_3 less than 22 mEq/L.

19. **Correct answer: C**
Prior to insertion of an LMA, the patient must have an absent gag reflex. The laryngeal mask airway cannot be inserted by nurses unless they have specialized training. The LMA does not usually cause hoarseness because it does not pass through the vocal cords. There is a high risk of aspiration with LMA usage.

20. **Correct answer: C**
Symptoms from aspirated gastric contents have a gradual onset. The patient may develop ARDS, but not always. If the pH is greater than 2.5, very little necrosis will occur. If the pH is less than 2.5, there is probability of pulmonary edema, necrosis, bleeding, and atelectasis.

21. **Correct answer: D**
The patient you are caring for was diagnosed with aspiration pneumonitis in addition to a Colles' fracture and various lacerations. As a trauma nurse, you know the most severe pulmonary reaction may occur from the aspiration of acidic food particles even if the particles are not obstructive. The pulmonary damage may be extensive. The patient will probably become hypercapnic, hypoxemic, and acidotic if not treated aggressively.

22. **Correct answer: B**
Pulse oximetry should never be used during a cardiac arrest. During resuscitation, blood pressure and blood flow may vary. The pharmacologic effects of medications such as vasoactive drugs used during resuscitation will compromise SpO_2 values.

23. **Correct answer: B**
Chest tube drainage tubing should be placed horizontally on the bed then down to the collection chamber. If a mediastinal chest tube is in place, bubbling in the water seal chamber may indicate a communication between the mediastinal space and the pleural space. The physician should be notified immediately. However, some sporadic bubbling will occur when suction is first turned on because fluid must displace air in the collection chamber. Chest tube tubing that is dependent or coiled will allow for the accumulation of drainage. This obstruction may increase pressure in the lung.

24. **Correct answer: B**
Ecchymotic splotches sometimes seen on labia, scrotum, and perineum secondary to pelvic fractures are known as Coopernail's sign.

25. **Correct answer: A**
This result signifies an uncompensated respiratory alkalosis. The pH is greater than 7.45, so the value is uncompensated alkalosis. To determine whether the alkalosis is respiratory or metabolic, find the value that represents alkalosis: in this case, the CO_2 less than 35 mmHg.

26. **Correct answer: C**
This result demonstrates a compensated respiratory alkalosis. The pH is between 7.35 and 7.45, so the value is compensated, but because it is closer to 7.45, the value is considered alkalotic. To determine whether the alkalosis is respiratory or metabolic, find the value that represents alkalosis: in this case, the CO_2 less than 35 mmHg.

27. **Correct answer: B**
This result is an uncompensated respiratory acidosis. The pH is less than 7.35, so the value is uncompensated. To determine whether the acidosis is respiratory or metabolic, find the value that represents acidosis: in this case, the CO_2 greater than 45 mmHg.

28. **Correct answer: A**
The pH (between 7.35 and 7.45), the CO_2 (between 35 and 45 mmHg), and the HCO_3 (22 and 26 mEq/L) are within normal ranges, so the ABG is considered normal. During exams, stress will often make a person look for detailed information and overlook the simplest explanation.

29. **Correct answer: D**
One of the most effective ways to relieve bronchospasms is to use a B_2 receptor agonist. The B_2 receptor agonists lower cellular calcium levels and relax bronchial smooth muscle. The selective B_2 receptor

agonists do not produce cardiac stimulation. The cardiac stimulation can result in tachycardia and reduced cardiac output.

30. **Correct answer: A**
When the ED resident attempts to place a central line, air is accidentally introduced into the line when the IV tubing becomes disconnected. The best position to place this patient to minimize the venous air embolism is Trendelenburg with left decubitus tilt. This position minimizes any air from migrating through the heart and into the lungs. Of course, everything depends on the patient's injuries and status.

31. **Correct answer: B**
Risk factors for thrombotic emboli include carcinoma. Neoplasms, obesity, trauma, dysrhythmias, congestive heart failure (CHF), and prolonged immobility are additional risk factors.

32. **Correct answer: C**
Your patient was struck head-on by another car in a parking lot. The impact, though slow speed, caused the airbag to deploy. The powder from the airbag caused an acute exacerbation of reactive airway disease. The patient has a history of asthma. As a trauma nurse, you know that sternocleidomastoid retractions indicate this patient is suffering from an acute episode of respiratory distress.

    Sternocleidomastoid retractions indicate that an asthmatic patient is using accessory muscles to facilitate ventilation. Air is trapped in the air passages, so the patient has to create a higher negative pleural pressure by elevating the rib cage.

33. **Correct answer: C**
Your patient ceased wheezing during his asthma attack. This change in his condition means respiratory failure and intubation are imminent. If the patient is wheezing, it means air is getting through a narrowed opening. Asthmatics undergo air trapping when the inspired air must exit through a narrowed air passage. If the patient stops wheezing, it means no air is able to enter or exit the air passages.

34. **Correct answer: A**
The American Heart Association has classified acute pulmonary embolisms into three categories: massive, submassive, or low risk. A submassive pulmonary embolism is characterized as an acute PE with evidence of right ventricular dysfunction or myocardial necrosis. A massive PE is defined as an acute PE with sustained BP less than 90 mmHg for more than 15 minutes, use of inotropes not the result of other causes, or signs of shock. A low-risk patient does not have any of the aforementioned conditions.

35. **Correct answer: D**
Pulse oximetry readings are considered unreliable when oxygen saturation levels fall below 70%. Pulse oximetry accuracy is impacted by patient motion, low perfusion, venous pulsation, light, poor probe positioning, edema, anemia, and carbon monoxide levels. It is important to compare pulse oximetry values against arterial blood gases to validate values below 70% on the pulse oximeter.

36. **Correct answer: A**
The oxyhemoglobin dissociation curve is a curve that reflects the relationship between dissolved oxygen and the affinity for oxygen by the hemoglobin molecule.

    The curve describes the relationship between available oxygen and the amount of oxygen carried by hemoglobin.

    - The horizontal axis is PaO_2, or the amount of oxygen available.
    - The vertical axis is SaO_2, or the amount of hemoglobin saturation with oxygen.
        » A PaO_2 of 60 or more is usually adequate.
        » At less than 60 mmHg, the curve is steep and small changes in PaO_2 greatly reduce SaO_2.
    - The term, *affinity* is used to describe oxygen's attraction to hemoglobin binding sites. Affinity changes with:
        » Variation in pH
        » Temperature

> » CO_2
> » 2,3 DPG levels
- In a left shift (alkalosis, hypothermia), oxygen will have a higher affinity for hemoglobin. Tissue hypoxia can result.
- In a right shift (acidosis, fever), oxygen has a lower affinity for hemoglobin. Blood will release oxygen more readily. More O_2 will be released to the cells, but less oxygen will be carried from the lungs.

37. **Correct answer: B**
Atrial tachycardia with occasional PVCs is an assessment finding that should be reported to the physician immediately as potential theophylline toxicity. Dosing at 600 mg/day is a high dose and places the patient at risk for toxicity. If diet and/or medications are taken that decrease normal theophylline excretion, the patient may quickly become toxic from the theophylline. Other symptoms to report include insomnia, anxiety, confusion, disorientation, headaches, hypotension, hyperglycemia, and abdominal pain with diarrhea, nausea, and vomiting. Diligently monitor electrolytes.

38. **Correct answer: B**
When a patient has sustained a pelvic fracture, a urinary catheter should not be placed immediately. Urethral injury should be ruled out either by examination or urethrography. If a urologist is unable to see the patient and a catheter must be placed, consider the use of a suprapubic catheter.
    If the nurse obtains vascular access, analgesia and fluids may be given. In addition to a FAST exam, a chest X-ray should be obtained to locate potential injuries and bleeding sites. If the patient is to receive a neuromuscular blockade, it is crucial to stabilize the pelvis first because the muscles may be the only thing maintaining pelvic stability.

39. **Correct answer: A**
SvO_2 is a measurement of total oxygen consumption.

40. **Correct answer: D**
The true statement is that capnography ($PetCO_2$) is not a substitute for pulse oximetry. Capnography monitors the concentration or partial pressure of carbon dioxide (CO_2) in the respiratory gases. A pulse oximeter measures the availability of sites on the hemoglobin molecule for oxygen transport versus how many sites are occupied.

41. **Correct answer: A**
Your patient had 1,420 ml of pleural effusion removed via thoracentesis and immediately began coughing and was dyspneic. This patient has developed reexpansion pulmonary edema. Removal of large amounts of pleural fluid increases negative intrapleural pressure. Edema occurs when the lung does not re-expand. The patient then develops a severe cough and dyspnea. If the symptoms occur during a thoracentesis, the procedure should be stopped.

42. **Correct answer: C**
Your patient is suffering substernal chest pain exacerbated when deep breathing. The patient also states his allergies are causing a dry cough, some nasal stuffiness, some pain in both ears, and a sore throat. The chest pain becomes more pronounced and pleuritic in nature. This patient has been on a 60% nonrebreather mask for two days. It is likely this patient may be suffering from hyperoxia. When patients receive high concentrations of oxygen for extended periods of time, very high amounts of oxygen free radicals are circulating. These radicals cause damage to the capillary–alveolar membrane. Enzymes are usually available to neutralize the radicals. When a patient suffers from oxygen toxicity, there are not enough enzymes to overcome the free radicals. If the oxygen level is not reduced, the damage to the vessels and parenchyma may lead to ARDS. It is to be noted that all the symptoms listed previously are probably the result of the hyperemic state, not an allergy. Symptoms usually resolve quickly once normal oxygen levels are restored.

43. **Correct answer: D**
Hypoxemia is a decreased oxygen level in the arterial blood or a PaO_2 less than 80 mmHg. Hypoxia is a decreased oxygen level at the cellular level.

44. **Correct answer: C**

Hyperventilating causes respiratory alkalosis because the patient is unable to get enough oxygen, often due to bronchial constriction. Hypoventilation causes a buildup of CO_2, causing respiratory acidosis, not respiratory alkalosis.

45. **Correct answer: A**

A renal transplant that results from humoral rejection or acute cellular rejection may be definitively diagnosed only via ultrasound. Ultrasound may be difficult to obtain or interpret due to ascites, obesity, or fluid in the retroperitoneal area. Doppler scans measure blood flow, and the flow is diminished due to prerenal and intrinsic AKI. Nuclear scans are of limited value because the excretion rates may be slowed by disease. The renal biopsy is the gold standard for diagnosing rejection.

46. **Correct answer: A**

This result is compensated metabolic acidosis. The pH is between 7.35 and 7.45, so the value is compensated, but because it is closer to 7.35, the value is considered acidotic. To determine whether the acidosis is respiratory or metabolic, find the value that represents acidosis: in this case, the HCO_3 at less than 19 mEq/L.

47. **Correct answer: C**

The pH is between 7.35 and 7.45, the CO_2 is between 35 and 45 mmHg, and the HCO_3 is between 22 and 26 mEq/L. All the results are within normal ranges, so this ABG is considered normal.

48. **Correct answer: A**

This result is an uncompensated (mixed) respiratory/metabolic alkalosis. The pH is greater than 7.45, so the value is uncompensated. To determine whether the acidosis is respiratory or metabolic, find the value that represents alkalosis. This would be both the HCO_3 at > 26 mEq/L and the CO_2 less than 35 mmHg, meaning the cause of the alkalosis is both respiratory and metabolic in nature.

49. **Correct answer: B**

According to the 2015 American Heart Association guidelines for CPR and ECC, gasping is in no way normal and is a sign of cardiac arrest.

50. **Correct answer: D**

Functional residual capacity is the volume of gas remaining in the lungs at the end of one normal expiration.

51. **Correct answer: C**

Residual volume is the volume of gas left in the lungs following a maximal respiratory effort.

52. **Correct answer: A**

The functional residual capacity is defined as the amount of air in the lungs after normal expiration. The formula for functional residual capacity is FRC = ERV (expired residual volume) + the RV (residual volume). The normal FRC in healthy lungs is about 2,000–3,000 ml.

53. **Correct answer: B**

Fever causes the pH to rise. Most ABG machines are calibrated to 37°C. If the patient has a fever, the oxyhemoglobin curve will be shifted to the right. More oxygen will be given off to the tissues, so the machine has to be calibrated to account for the temperature.

54. **Correct answer: D**

The cells that are responsible for forming a barrier for alveoli are type I epithelial cells. Type I cells line the outside of the alveoli and are easily inflamed by inhaled toxins or heated air. In addition, type I cells maintain the blood–gas interface. Type II cells produce surfactant.

55. **Correct answer: B**

This ABG result indicates a compensated respiratory acidosis. The pH is between 7.35 and 7.45, so the value is compensated, but because it is closer to 7.35 the value is considered acidotic. To determine whether the acidosis is respiratory or metabolic, find the value that represents acidosis: in this case, the CO_2 greater than 45 mmHg.

56. **Correct answer: A**

Type II alveolar cells produce surfactant. Surfactant is a lipoprotein and functions by increasing surface tension of alveoli and allowing alveoli to expand and contract. We should have some residual pressure in the alveoli at the end of respiration to keep the alveoli open (physiologic PEEP). If surfactant production is impaired, the alveoli's ability to exchange O_2 is compromised.

57. **Correct answer: D**

The FiO_2 for a nasal cannula set at a flow rate of 6 L/minute is 40%. The nasal cannula is generally considered a low-flow oxygen device unless connected to a high-flow system. If using a flow > 4 L/minute, the oxygen should be humidified to prevent drying the mucosal membranes.

58. **Correct answer: C**

A diagnosis of asthma may be made by a decreased FEV1. The forced expiratory volume (FEV) is how much air is exhaled during the first second of effort. This amount should be $\geq 75\%$ of the predicted normal value(s). In asthmatics, this value is decreased because of obstruction. The forced vital capacity (FVC) is the total amount of gas exhaled as forcefully and rapidly as possible after taking a maximal inspiration. The result should be above 80%.

59. **Correct answer: A**

An absolute contraindication for use of rapid sequence intubation (RSI) is a total loss of facial and/or oropharyngeal landmarks, which requires a surgical airway. Another absolute contraindication is a total upper airway obstruction that requires surgical intervention. Relative contraindications for RSI include an airway where intubation may not be successful or an arrest "crash" intubation when there is no time for pre-oxygenation, pretreatment, or induction and paralysis.

60. **Correct answer: D**

Rapid sequence intubation (RSI) is not necessary to use for all cervical spine-injured patients. It would be appropriate for use if there is edema and loss of airway patency. Prolonged respiratory effort that results in fatigue or failure, a stab wound to the neck with an expanding hematoma, and an uncooperative trauma patient with life-threatening injuries are indications for the use of RSI.

61. **Correct answer: C**

During rapid sequence intubation (RSI), cricoid cartilage pressure may be used to help prevent vomiting and aspiration of gastric contents. The esophagus is obstructed by the pressure to the anterior neck. This maneuver is known as the Sellick maneuver. The American Heart Association takes the position that the Sellick maneuver not be routinely used unless the person performing the maneuver is well trained and experienced.

62. **Correct answer: D**

When performing CPR on a cardiac arrest patient, as a trauma nurse you know the best, most reliable way to confirm placement of an endotracheal tube is continuous waveform capnography ($PetCO_2$).

63. **Correct answer: C**

This blood–gas result indicates an uncompensated respiratory acidosis. The pH is less than 7.35, so the value indicates an uncompensated acidosis. Next, determine which respiratory or metabolic value represents acidosis: in this case, the CO_2 greater than 45 mmHg.

64. **Correct answer: A**

One cause of decreased SvO_2 is an increased metabolic rate. An increased metabolic rate would increase the O_2 uptake by tissues, resulting in a lower value measured by venous blood gases. The other answers result in a lower tissue oxygen requirement, and thus higher values of oxygen remain in the bloodstream.

65. **Correct answer: B**

Prior to performing a DPL, a Foley and gastric tube should be placed. If 10 ml of frank blood is pulled back, an unstable patient must go to the OR. A DPL is indicated if a patient has a spinal cord injury, altered mental status, shock, decreased hematocrit, unexplained hypotension, or an unavailable CT or ultrasound.

66. **Correct answer: C**
    To evacuate a hemothorax, the tube is placed in the fifth intercostal space, midaxillary line. The chest tube will be low in the thoracic cavity and uses gravity to help clear the fluid. If a hemothorax is not completely removed, there is a possibility an infection will result, which can lead to empyema. When assessing a patient, it is a good idea to ask (if possible) the origin of any small scars on the thoracic area, as the patient may have had previous problems requiring a chest tube.

67. **Correct answer: B**
    The hypoxemic drive to breathe originates in the aortic and carotid arteries. In the bifurcation of the internal and external carotid arteries, carotid bodies and aortic bodies (in the carotid arch) are chemoreceptors. When the supply of oxygen decreases, stimulation of the aortic and/or carotid bodies occurs and, in turn, stimulates cortical activity. The result is adrenal gland secretions (epinephrine, norepinephrine), tachycardia, tachypnea, increased respiratory rate, and increased blood pressure.

68. **Correct answer: B**
    Breathing high concentrations of oxygen may wash out nitrogen that is present in alveoli. The nitrogen helps keep the alveoli open, resulting in residual volume. If oxygen replaces nitrogen in the alveoli, the alveoli will shrink and begin to collapse. Oxygen is absorbed into the bloodstream much faster than a replacement is available in the alveoli. The effect is very pronounced in areas of the lung only barely ventilated. This phenomenon is considered an adverse effect and is known as absorption atelectasis.

69. **Correct answer: D**
    Succinylcholine combines with acetylcholine to cause smooth muscle relaxation, not contraction. Prolonged use may cause a change in blocking action and result in potassium-regulated alterations in electrical activity. Side effects of succinylcholine include malignant hyperthermia and hypertension or hypotension, hyperkalemia, anaphylaxis, and increased intraocular pressure.

70. **Correct answer: C**
    Patients who have sustained crush injuries are susceptible to the development of rhabdomyolysis. Creatinine and myoglobin are released from damaged cells. Large amounts of myoglobin are toxic to kidney cells. Often, potassium is released from its normal intracellular compartmental to cause hyperkalemia. To help mitigate the rhabdomyolysis, crystalloids which have been alkalinized by sodium bicarbonate are used, along with the diuretic, mannitol. Use of mannitol increases urine output and helps reduce the excess potassium, and the bicarbonate helps mitigate acidosis.

71. **Correct answer: C**
    The laryngeal mask airway (LMA) was intended as a temporary airway. It requires minimal training to insert, but cannot be placed by RNs as a matter of course. The patient must be unconscious and/or without a gag reflex. The seal around the mask is a low pressure seal, so it cannot be used on patients with high peak ventilator pressures. The LMA has a significant risk of aspiration. Advantages with use of this airway are that it is simply blindly inserted into the hypopharynx, does not require visualization of the vocal cords, and does not traumatize the trachea. Patients will not have hoarseness or lose their voice altogether. At best, patients will complain of a mild sore throat.

72. **Correct answer: A**
    An action of nitric oxide is to cause vascular smooth muscle relaxation. Nitric oxide is the molecule released from the endothelium that enables smooth muscle relaxation. Nitric oxide inhibits platelet aggregation and adherence and is thought to alter vascular permeability. It may also participate in nonspecific immunity because it is generated when macrophages are activated.

73. **Correct answer: D**
    Continuous positive airway pressure (CPAP) may be delivered by nasal prongs, nasopharyngeal tubes, or endotracheal tubes. CPAP provides increased pressure to the posterior pharynx and increases transpulmonary pressure. It can prevent alveolar collapse and helps prevent obstructive apnea.

74. **Correct answer: B**

Excessive CPAP may increase intrathoracic pressure to the point of compressing the right atrium and vena cava. The preload will be decreased and cardiac output will be reduced.

75. **Correct answer: B**

The arterial blood gas results that support the diagnosis of respiratory alkalosis are pH 7.47, CO_2 24, HCO_3 24.

76. **Correct answer: B**

Synchronized intermittent mandatory ventilation (SIMV) still provides a set frequency of breaths and either volume or pressure. The patient is permitted to breathe spontaneously at his or her own volume between mandatory ventilations. If the spontaneous breath occurs at the same time as a mandatory breath, the ventilator will synchronize with the patient, thus preventing "stacked" breaths. The other modes of ventilation listed (CMV, HFV, and oscillation) represent full control of setting by an operator and not the patient's responses.

77. **Correct answer: A**

A disadvantage of using a tracheostomy tube is subcutaneous emphysema. There are a large number of potential complications with the use of a tracheostomy tube. Some of these complications include tracheal stenosis, tracheomalacia, aspiration, infection, hemorrhage, and pneumothorax.

78. **Correct answer: A**

This result is an uncompensated metabolic alkalosis. The pH is greater than 7.45, so the value is uncompensated. To determine whether the alkalosis is respiratory or metabolic, find the value that represents alkalosis: in this case, the HCO_3 at > 26 mEq/L.

79. **Correct answer: A**

A flail chest is a medical emergency and the patient must be intubated immediately. Pain control is absolutely necessary with a flail chest. A flail chest results when two or more adjacent ribs are broken in two or more places. The chest wall is unstable. Usually, during inspiration the chest wall moves outward with an increase in negative intrathoracic pressure. In cases of a flail chest, the opposite movement of the chest wall is seen. This is known as a "paradoxical" movement. Eventually, the result will be atelectasis and alveolar collapse, with possible development of ARDS. To adequately stabilize the fracture, sometimes neuromuscular blockade is used. The patient must be given pain medication and sedation. Also, pain is a priority because the work of breathing (WOB) needs to be reduced.

80. **Correct answer: D**

Your patient has sustained a stab wound to the area of the right anterior axillary line at the fifth intercostal space. The patient is hypotensive, tachypneic, tachycardic, and restless. O_2 at 100% via mask is provided. Two large bore IVs have been placed and crystalloids are infusing. As a trauma nurse, you would expect to prepare for placement of a chest tube.

The patient appears to have a patent airway, so intubation is not the priority intervention. The patient is, however, exhibiting signs of hypovolemic shock. The mechanism of injury is classic for a hemothorax. A chest tube will help relieve a hemothorax and allow for lung expansion, restore negative pressure, and evacuate the pleural cavity.

81. **Correct answer: A**

A blunt cardiac injury is most likely to affect the right ventricle because it usually suffers the force of blows to the chest. The right ventricle lies directly behind the sternum and close to the chest wall. The left ventricle is lateral to the sternum and less likely to be injured. Both atria are small and more protected as well.

82. **Correct answer: B**

The patient is suffering from a tension pneumothorax. This patient had been resting quietly on the gurney, awaiting transport to X-ray to evaluate a possible fractured right tibia and patella. Suddenly the patient complained of right-sided chest pain, tachypnea at a rate of 40, cyanosis, and JVD. No breath sounds are now audible over the right lung fields. The trachea is deviated and heart tones are distant.

83. **Correct answer: D**

    If a projectile strikes the precordium during the vulnerable part of her cardiac cycle, this is known as Commotio cordis. There may be a brief moment of consciousness or the patient will collapse immediately. Even with immediate attempts at resuscitation, survival is extremely rare.

84. **Correct answer: B**

    The most common location of a sternal fracture is the manubrium. Most fractures are caused by either direct or indirect blunt force trauma from contact sports, or assaults. Indirect fractures may occur as a result of deceleration injuries, stress fractures, or osteoporosis. Always look for and treat underlying trauma.

85. **Correct answer: A**

    Fractures of ribs 1–3 are associated with high mortality rates. A lot of force is required to fracture these ribs. Associated injuries may be to the brachial plexus, subclavian artery, cranial and thoracic areas. Other sequelae include, pneumothorax, pneumomediastinum, lacerations to brachiocephalic vessels, and laceration of the aorta.

86. **Correct answer: D**

    Crackles are not considered a complication of a pulmonary contusion. ARDS, atelectasis, pneumonia, and respiratory failure are complications of a pulmonary contusion.

87. **Correct answer: B**

    ST segment depression usually indicates myocardial ischemia. This patient also exhibited substernal chest pain, another finding seen with ischemia. The patient needs a 12-lead EKG immediately to determine if the ischemia is cardiac in origin.

88. **Correct answer: B**

    During inspiration, your patient has a paradoxical rise in jugular venous pressure. This phenomenon is commonly associated with right heart failure. Blood flow to the right ventricle is impaired because of a decrease in compliance or possibly fluid in the pericardial space. Blood backs up into the venous system, causing the increase in jugular venous pressure.

89. **Correct answer: A**

    This patient is at great risk for hyponatremia. Large amounts of extracellular fluids are in the peritoneal cavity. If sodium is lost in here, then the calcium is no longer available to be absorbed into the vasculature.

90. **Correct answer: A**

    Upright QRS in leads V_1 and V_2 show right bundle branch blocks. A simple way to remember which type of bundle branch block with a QRS wider than 0.12 seconds is to think of the turn signals on your car. For a right turn, you must push the lever up; for a left turn the lever must go down. So, looking at V_1 and V_2, if the QRS is upright, then there is a right bundle branch block. If V_1 and V_2 are downward in force, then it is a left bundle branch block.

91. **Correct answer: D**

    The structures found in the retroperitoneum include: kidneys, adrenal glands, pancreas, ascending and descending colon, small intestine, aorta, vena cava, a section of the duodenum, and major vessels.

92. **Correct answer: D**

    Atropine administration may result in headaches, dizziness, and coma. You should also observe for urinary retention and hypotension and tachycardia due to blocking of parasympathetic receptor sites.

93. **Correct answer: B**

A biomarker that is not cardiac specific but can be elevated by falls, cardiopulmonary resuscitation, and injections is myoglobin. Serum myoglobin is a test that measures the amount of myoglobin in the blood. Myoglobin is a protein in heart and skeletal muscles. Muscles use up available oxygen. Myoglobin has oxygen attached to it, so additional O_2 is available to muscles. If the muscle is damaged, myoglobin is released and excreted by the kidneys. In large amounts, kidney damage may occur. If the patient has suffered an infarct, myoglobin levels peak about 8 hours after infarct, rapidly returning to normal in about 18–24 hours.

94. **Correct answer: A**

Along with acute ST elevation, another indicator of necrosis would be an abnormal Q wave. If the Q wave appears within about 6 hours of a transmural MI, it is an ominous sign. If the Q wave is more than 0.04 seconds long, it is a sign of necrosis. In an inferior MI, the Q wave should not exceed 0.03 seconds or it is indicative of necrosis.

95. **Correct answer: A**

Your patient was observing practice at the local high school when she was struck by a player who overran the sidelines. The patient sustained a blunt chest injury and on assessment you auscultated a pericardial friction rub. A pericardial friction rub would be best heard at Erb's point, the third intercostal space, on the left sternal border.

96. **Correct answer: A**

Increased production of urea may be due to GI bleeding. Approximately 500 ml of whole blood equals 100 grams of protein. The extra protein must be converted to urea.

97. **Correct answer: B**

Lack of thrill and/or bruit may indicate that the graft has occluded and dialysis is not possible. It is best to use a Doppler to determine graft patency prior to any calls or administration of any medication. Although you may not hear or feel the thrill and bruit, the graft may still be patent. The surgeon should be notified if the Doppler study is negative. Heparin will not lyse an existing clot.

98. **Correct answer: A**

Your patient sustained an injury to a kidney from a fall two days ago, resulting in hyperlipidemia, edema, low albumin in the blood, and proteinuria. These findings are indicative that the patient is suffering from nephrotic syndrome. When glomeruli are damaged, proteins such as albumin leak into the bloodstream. In this disease, 3+ grams of protein may leak into the urine over 24 hours (20+ times normal). Hypoalbuminemia occurs because of the high levels of protein leaking via the kidneys. Low albumin causes fluid to move from blood to tissue, causing edema.

99. **Correct answer: B**

Signs and symptoms of a pulmonary embolus include pleuritic chest pain, tachypnea, anxiety, and tachycardia, and possible bloody frothy sputum.

100. **Correct answer: D**

Stable fractures do not transect the pelvic ring and usually do not cause excessive bleeding. A large percentage of patients with a pelvic injury also have trauma to other areas of the body.

101. **Correct answer: A**

If a patient has truncal obesity and has sustained a pelvic fracture, it is possible to initially stabilize the fracture via internal rotation of lower extremities and taping the knees together.

102. **Correct answer: D**

The following structures are located in the peritoneal cavity: liver, spleen, stomach, gall bladder, transverse and sigmoid colon, upper third of the rectum, uterus.

103. Correct answer: D
With an acute rotator cuff tear, the patient may feel a tearing sensation and exhibit point tenderness over the injury site. Pain is usually intense and will last a few days secondary to spasm and bleeding. The patient will not be able to abduct their arm without assistance.

104. Correct answer: C
Costochondritis is often found in persons who engage in repetitive activities such as tennis, in this case, weightlifting. This patient likely has costochondritis, but the trauma nurse should anticipate the patient being evaluated for possible cardiac pathology.

105. Correct answer: B
An appropriate local anesthetic agent for a patient with a history of malignant hyperthermia is procaine.

106. Correct answer: C
When auscultating lung sounds, you heard what you believe to be bowel sounds in the chest. The patient is experiencing moderate shoulder pain on the left side and he is mildly tachypneic. The probable diagnosis will be a diaphragmatic rupture
   This patient's abdominal contents have probably entered the thoracic cavity secondary to a diaphragmatic tear. If air also enters the thoracic cavity, it will increase intrathoracic pressure and help to transmit sound. It is usually the left side of the diaphragm that ruptures, and this patient was injured on the left. It is postulated that perhaps the liver, because it is large, protects the right side of the diaphragm. A fractured pelvis usually also results in almost a 50% increased probability of a ruptured diaphragm.

107. Correct answer: C
The inferior border, which is formed by the pelvis. The superior border is defined by the diaphragm, the anterior border by the abdominal and iliac muscles, and the posterior border is bordered by the vertebral column.

108. Correct answer: D
The type of vertebral fracture that results from the mechanism of injury known as hyperflexion is called a teardrop fracture. A small anterior edge of a vertebrae breaks and may impinge on the spinal cord. Sometimes the patient will also have a posterior malalignment of the vertebrae.

109. Correct answer: D
When palpating the abdomen under the right costal margin near the liver, you note the patient is unable to inhale deeply. This reaction is known as Murphy's sign. When the fingers are approximately over the location of the gallbladder, pain is usually most intense. The cause is likely injury from blunt trauma or underlying cholecystitis.

110. Correct answer: A
The spleen is not located in the retroperitoneum, but in the peritoneum. Other organs located in the peritoneum are the liver, diaphragm, stomach, some small bowel, and the transverse colon.

111. Correct answer: D
A nonrebreather mask can deliver 60–80% of oxygen when the O_2 flow rate is 10–15 L/minute. If both exhalation ports have one-way valves, then near 100% oxygen may be reached. To prevent suffocation in patients where the oxygen is disconnected, nonrebreathing masks now have only one one-way valve to prevent/limit inhalation of room air. This results in decreasing the highest concentration of actual inspired oxygen to 60–80%.

112. Correct answer: C
Using a vacutainer or a high friction syringe creates a vacuum. When that occurs, dissolved gases come out of solution, which decreases PaO_2 and $PaCO_2$. The increased effort to move the cylinder

may cause the artery to spasm and impede obtaining the sample but will not directly affect results.

113. **Correct answer: B**

The pH of the aspirate is very important. If the aspirate is acidic, there is an almost immediate creation of pulmonary edema. This is due to the collapse and breakdown of the alveoli, capillaries, and their interface. Atelectasis, possible intra-alveolar hemorrhage, and some interstitial edema lead to hypoxia. Alkalotic aspirate destroys surfactant, which causes alveolar collapse, leading to hypoxia. Other factors to identify are the type of material aspirated and the amount. Syrup of Ipecac is used for ingestions. ABGs would be considered more of a diagnostic tool.

114. **Correct answer: C**

An indication for surgical intervention with a patient who has a hemothorax and required chest tube placement would be more than 1,000 ml of blood during initial chest tube placement or more than 200 ml of blood for 2–4 hours.

115. **Correct answer: C**

Beta-1 receptors cause an increase in conductivity, heart rate, and contractility. They are an integral part of the sympathetic nervous system.

116. **Correct answer: C**

The most sensitive cardiac markers are troponin T and troponin I. These biomarkers show injury to myocytes, not just cell death. Troponin T can be elevated with skeletal muscle injury. Troponin I is diagnostic of an MI and can be falsely elevated in renal insufficiency.

117. **Correct answer: A**

A biomarker that indicates an inflammation is present is C-reactive protein. C-reactive protein is produced by the liver. Blood is mixed with an antiserum, which attaches to a specific protein. Levels of CRP may not be increased in people with rheumatoid arthritis and lupus. Some additional causes of elevated C-reactive protein levels are cancer, connective tissue disease, inflammatory bowel disease, rheumatic fever, tuberculosis, the last half of pregnancy or with the use of oral contraceptives, and possible uremia.

118. **Correct answer: A**

When auscultating the heart, a common area for hearing murmurs and ectopic beats is Erb's point. The location is the 3rd intercostal space, on the left sternal border.

119. **Correct answer: C**

If the CVP catheter is in the right ventricle and touches the myocardium, PVCs can result. Occasionally, the physician will insert the catheter a bit too far, causing PVCs. In this case, the catheter simply has to be withdrawn to a better position in the right atrium. This is a rare occurrence. If the patient's catheter was left in the right ventricle, the V-tach might continue and the patient might suffer cardiac arrest.

120. **Correct answer: A**

The "seat belt sign" corresponds with an intra-abdominal injury in about 80% of patients would be *inaccurate* when describing classic seat belt injuries.

121. **Correct answer: C**

The definition of an unstable pelvic fracture is when the pelvic ring is fractured in more than one place with two displacements on the ring. A rotational displacement is always present and bleeding is likely.

122. **Correct answer: D**

While assessing a patient for possible splenic involvement and abdominal injury, the patient complains of a sharp pain in the left shoulder, slightly above the collarbone. This phenomenon is known as Kehr's sign. When the spleen is ruptured, blood irritates the underside of the diaphragm and phrenic nerve. The pain is then referred to the area of the left shoulder.

123. **Correct answer: B**

Injuries to the pancreas and bowel may be missed if a diagnostic peritoneal lavage is performed too early. These injuries may not have had time to become evident. A DPL is difficult to perform on patients in their third trimester of pregnancy, patients who have had previous laparotomies, and patients who have suffered trauma and are obese.

124. **Correct answer: C**

This patient has fever, chills, pain on urination, moderate burning at the supra pubic area, and diarrhea. This patient is most likely suffering from a lower urinary tract infection. Females are more likely to have urinary tract infections than men because they have shorter urethras and bacteria can easily ascend the tract.

125. **Correct answer: C**

Three points of narrowing of the esophagus would not include the mediastinum. The esophagus narrows at primarily three locations, predisposing it to an injury. Those locations are the arch of the aorta, the cricoid cartilage, and the esophagogastric junction. In the event of leakage of gastric and esophageal contents into the mediastinum, the resulting necrotizing tissue damage and inflammation may cause sepsis, MODS, and death.

126. **Correct answer: B**

Your patient was riding his bicycle carelessly and T-boned a car. The patient exhibited peritoneal guarding. Duodenal injury is suspected. The duodenum is primarily a retroperitoneal organ. Compression fractures are associated with vertebral column fractures of the transverse processes and Chance fractures. Intra-abdominal injuries are almost always associated with duodenal injuries.

127. **Correct answer: C**

Pelvic fractures may result in significant blood loss. When soft tissues are injured, a systemic inflammatory response is initiated, resulting in the release of cytokines. These chemical mediators may result in a depletion of intravascular volume. Cytokines increase permeability of vascular endothelium, allowing shifting fluid from plasma to intravascular space.

128. **Correct answer: C**

An appropriate location for an IV in a patient suffering a major abdominal injury would be in a tributary of the superior vena cava as the inferior vena cava may be compromised.

129. **Correct answer: D**

Pulmonary angiograms require iodine-based radiographic contrast dye to be injected into the antecubital or femoral vein via catheter to the pulmonary artery. The pulmonary vasculature can then be visualized. The radioactive iodine crosses the blood–placental barrier, which is why this procedure is contraindicated in pregnancy. Other contraindications include allergy to shellfish, iodine, radiographic dye, and renal insufficiency.

130. **Correct answer: A**

Sudden anuria is usually due to post-renal AKI, such as from an embolic event. Mechanical obstruction of the urinary collection system is involved. The collection system is comprised of the renal pelvis, the ureters, the bladder, and the urethra.

131. **Correct answer: C**

The current definition of acute renal failure is a sudden or rapid decline in renal filtration function. Acute renal failure is now known as acute renal injury (AKI) and can be classified as prerenal, intrinsic, or post-renal. Because material covered on the TCRN exam reflects practice up to about 6 months ago, the new terminology should be added. Some item writers may use this new terminology on the exam.

132. **Correct answer: C**

Post-renal AKI may be caused by a neurogenic bladder. Other causes include tumor, tricyclic antidepressants, fibrosis, BPH, prostate CA, urethral obstruction, stone disease, and ligation during surgery. Malignant hypertension, transplant rejection, DIC, and preeclampsia are causes of intrinsic failure/injury.

133. **Correct answer: C**

Potassium and hydrogen move opposite of each other. When a patient is hypokalemic, hydrogen moves into the extracellular fluid, leading to both respiratory and metabolic alkalosis.

134. **Correct answer: B**

Over 99% of urea synthesis occurs in the liver. Dietary protein is converted into amino acids and peptides. About 90% of these molecules are absorbed and transferred to the liver. Any excess nitrogen is converted into urea.

Clinical Practice: Extremity and Wound

- Musculoskeletal Trauma
- Surface and Burn Trauma

SECTION 6: QUESTIONS

1. **A disadvantage of using negative pressure wound care (NPWC) devices is**
   A. A NPWC cannot be used on wounds associated with malignancies
   B. A NPWC removes interstitial fluid
   C. A NPWC promotes a moist healing environment
   D. A NPWC removes barriers to cell migration and proliferation

2. **A burn that involves muscle, fat, or bone is classified as a**
   A. First-degree partial thickness burn
   B. Second-degree partial thickness burn
   C. Third-degree full thickness burn
   D. Fourth-degree full thickness burn

3. **The area of a burn that has the closest contact with the heat source and sustains the most damage is the**
   A. Zone of stasis
   B. Zone of hyperemia
   C. Zone of erythema
   D. Zone of coagulation

4. **Which of the following substances contain large amounts of alkali?**
   A. Toilet bowl cleaners
   B. Swimming pool chemicals
   C. Oven cleaners
   D. Metal cleaners

5. **You are admitting a patient with a fractured femur, mild concussion, and multiple facial lacerations after a motor vehicle accident. The patient's blood-alcohol level was elevated despite his report of only drinking one standard-sized beer while with friends at a bar 3 hours prior to driving. His stated medical history includes OTC Pepcid use to treat GERD. What factor is most likely to have contributed to the patient's elevated blood-alcohol level?**
   A. The patient is not being honest and consumed more than one beer before driving
   B. The Pepcid increases the blood-alcohol level by delaying metabolism
   C. The patient consumed a larger than standard size beer
   D. The patient's report of waiting 3 hours prior to driving

6. **The inadvertent administration of a vesicant medication into surrounding tissue is known as**
   A. Compartment syndrome
   B. Extravasation
   C. Ischemic necrosis
   D. Infiltration

7. **Which of the following statements about superficial frostbite is true?**
   A. Use heavy blankets to help rewarm the entire patient
   B. The skin will be bright pink and feel cold to the touch
   C. Rewarm the affected part using warm water at 104–107.6°F
   D. Keep the affected part dependent

8. A 40 year old was admitted to your ED after a burn injury. He was helping his friend barbeque in the backyard and a sudden flame-up burned his chest, right shoulder, and chin. What finding would be indicative of probable smoke inhalation in this patient?

    A. PaO_2 81, met HgB level of 2%
    B. PaO_2 76, pCO_2 26
    C. Increased CO_2
    D. A carboxyhemoglobin of 18%, burned chin

9. The type of knee injury most likely to be caused by hyperextension trauma is

    A. A medial meniscus injury
    B. Severe muscle injury
    C. Anterior and posterior cruciate ligament injury
    D. A patellar dislocation

10. A fracture at the junction of the proximal and middle thirds of the ulna is known as

    A. A Volkmann's fracture
    B. A Monteggia's fracture
    C. An intercondylar fracture
    D. A Colles' fracture

11. A third-degree strain is distinguished by

    A. Point tenderness, localized pain
    B. Spasm
    C. Loss of muscle function
    D. Ecchymosis

12. A distinguishing characteristic of a patellar fracture is

    A. Patient inability to abduct the leg
    B. Patient inability to actively extend the knee
    C. The examiner's inability to adduct the leg
    D. The examiner's inability to aspirate fluid from the knee area

13. Your patient was running to first base during a baseball game. When he placed his foot on the bag he heard a loud sound and could not apply weight on that leg. He was assisted to a friend's car and transported to your facility. You note the patient is in moderate pain and cannot bear weight on the affected leg. As a trauma nurse, you suspect this patient is suffering from

    A. A patellar fracture
    B. A severe quadriceps tear
    C. An Achilles tendon rupture
    D. An anterior cruciate ligament tear

14. An example of a pathologic cause of a proximal humerus fracture is

    A. An automobile accident
    B. Bone cancer
    C. A fall
    D. Sports injuries

15. The type of amputation that has the greatest chance of reimplantation is

    A. Shearing
    B. Guillotine
    C. Avulsion
    D. Crush

16. **Which of the following statements about splints is not correct?**
    A. Splints are easier to apply than casts
    B. Splints are easily removed for inspection of an injured area
    C. Splints allow for swelling during the acute phase of an injury
    D. Splints are circumferential

17. **A closed wound that occurs when a blood vessel ruptures and bleeds into surrounding tissue is known as a(n)**
    A. Hematoma
    B. Contusion
    C. Abrasion
    D. Lacunar stroke

18. **Your patient has sustained a proximal humerus fracture and damage to the radial nerve. Which of the following observations validates this type of injury?**
    A. Swelling at the wrist
    B. Extension of the forefinger and middle finger
    C. Wrist drop
    D. The patient guarding his shoulder

19. **The ED physician is evaluating a patient for carpal tunnel syndrome. The physician will attempt to elicit Tinel's sign. Tinel's sign is considered positive when**
    A. Pain is felt in the ring finger of the affected arm
    B. Pain and paresthesia worsens when the medial nerve is tapped
    C. Numbness occurs when the backs of the hands are pressed together for 1 minute
    D. The thumb can be adducted

20. **While assisting a patient with fitting for a cane, the cane should be placed next to the heel on the _____ side and the elbow flexed at _____ degrees.**
    A. Injured; 45
    B. Uninjured; 20
    C. Injured; 15
    D. Uninjured; 30

21. **Your patient requires application of a long leg fiberglass splint. The patient should be positioned**
    A. Upright
    B. Supine
    C. Flat on the abdomen
    D. In semi-Fowler's

22. **If your patient is obese and has sustained a lower leg or unstable ankle fracture, which position would be inappropriate for splinting?**
    A. Upright
    B. Supine
    C. Prone
    D. Semi-Fowler's

23. **A necrotizing infection associated with animal bites is likely caused by which of the following organisms?**
    A. *Clostridium tetani*
    B. *Pasteurella multocida*
    C. *Staphylococcus*
    D. *Pseudomonas*

24. **When performing a peripheral nerve assessment for ulnar nerve impairment, normal findings include**
    A. The ability to fan the fingers and have feeling on top of the small finger
    B. Feeling on the dorsum of the thumb and the ability to extend the thumb
    C. The ability to oppose the thumb to the base of the small finger and to feel on the tip of the index finger
    D. Feeling on the palm and ability to clench the fist

25. **Which of the following actions must be performed when preparing a patient for fixed wing air transport?**
    A. Always use a pneumatic antishock garment (PASG)
    B. Bivalve a circumferential plaster cast
    C. Try to use air splints whenever possible
    D. Splint forearms with an anterior gutter splint

26. **Your patient was climbing a ladder in an attempt to hang Christmas lights. He slipped and fell on his outstretched arm. He sustained a fracture to the distal ends of the radius and ulna. This type of fracture is known as a**
    A. Colles' fracture
    B. Navicular fracture
    C. Scaphoid fracture
    D. Volkmann's fracture

27. **Which of the following medications is not appropriate for initial treatment of a patient with a pelvic fracture?**
    A. Hydrocodone bitartrate
    B. Oxycodone and acetaminophen
    C. Fentanyl
    D. NSAIDs

28. **Your patient has sustained an ulnar fracture. Which of the following types of splints would be appropriate for this type of injury?**
    A. A spade splint
    B. A gutter splint
    C. A spica splint
    D. A Hare splint

29. **The most common forearm fracture is a**
    A. Colles' fracture
    B. Homan's fracture
    C. Volkmann's fracture
    D. A distal radius fracture

30. **The nerve most commonly injured in a proximal humerus fracture is**
    A. The axillary nerve
    B. The radial nerve
    C. The suprascapular nerve
    D. The musculocutaneous nerve

31. **Which of the following muscles is not part of the rotator cuff?**
    A. Deltoid
    B. Supraspinatus
    C. Subscapularis
    D. Teres minor

32. **The most serious complication of casting and splinting is**
    A. Decreased circulation
    B. Paresthesia
    C. Pain
    D. Compartment syndrome

33. **At 5 to 7 days after a contusion is sustained, the periphery of the contusion changes color from the periphery to the inside and becomes**
    A. Reddish blue
    B. Yellow
    C. Brown
    D. Green

34. **If a patient presents with contusions that are yellow tinged, the contusion is probably about _____ days old.**
    A. 1–5
    B. 5–7
    C. 7–10
    D. 10–14

35. **Your patient was a restrained passenger in a rollover accident and sustained only multiple contusions on both legs. Appropriate patient teaching about RICE therapy includes**
    A. Keeping feet and legs dependent to increase the blood flow to the area
    B. Do not wrap or splint the extremities
    C. Do not take analgesics for 48 hours
    D. Apply cold packs × 20 minutes, four times a day for 48–72 hours

36. **A deformity of the distal portion of a joint that is angulated away from the midline of the body is called a**
    A. Sprain
    B. Valgus
    C. Varus
    D. Strain

37. **The type of fracture caused by an angulation force of direct trauma is known as**
    A. An oblique fracture
    B. A spiral fracture
    C. A transverse fracture
    D. A depressed fracture

38. **A posterior dislocation of the glenohumeral joint in the shoulder may be caused by**
    A. Falls from bicycles or motorcycles
    B. An athletic injury, usually a recurrent injury
    C. A direct blow to the point of the shoulder
    D. Seizures

39. **Which of the following statements is true regarding management of a severed part after a traumatic amputation?**
    A. Leave all foreign matter intact so it can be removed in the operating room
    B. Place the part in ice water for transport
    C. Scrub the severed part gently
    D. Rinse the part with a sterile isotonic solution

40. **Which statement does not represent a complication of air splinting?**
    A. Talcum powder or cornstarch cause breakdown of the skin
    B. Excessive pressure variations may exist
    C. Compression of nerves may occur
    D. Removal may be difficult

41. **When applying an air splint to an elderly patient, the trauma nurse should consider**
    A. Elevating the limb to aid blood flow to the heart
    B. Placing a thin layer of smooth padding under the splint
    C. Adducting the limb to ease stress
    D. Twisting the valve counterclockwise to even pressures and prevent skin breakdown

42. **The preferred splint for a femur fracture is**
    A. Kirschner wire
    B. A fiberglass spica splint
    C. A traction splint
    D. A posterior long leg splint

43. **Which of the following types of traction splints is classified as a unipolar traction splint?**
    A. Hare
    B. Fernotrac
    C. Kendrick
    D. Thomas

44. **Traction splints are used for**
    A. Distal fibula fractures
    B. Distal tibia fractures
    C. Upper extremity fractures
    D. Femur fractures

45. **You are assisting with the fitting of a patient for a walker. Your patient should have his or her elbow bent at**
    A. 20 degrees
    B. 30 degrees
    C. 40 degrees
    D. 45 degrees

46. **Your patient fractured his humerus in a car accident 3 weeks ago. Yesterday he developed a fever and now has a temperature of 101.7°F. He complains of pain in the upper arm, his capillary refill is 9 seconds, his distal pulses are moderate to poor, and his fingers are cold. There are small areas just distal of the cast that are swollen and look like bubbles. There is a foul odor emanating from the cast. As a trauma nurse, you suspect this patient is suffering from**
    A. Compartment syndrome
    B. *Clostridium tetani*
    C. Gangrene
    D. Tetany

47. **Your patient joined a parachuting club. On her first jump with the instructor their parachute failed to open completely, and they both forcefully struck the ground with their feet. The type of fractures this patient would probably incur would be**
    A. Calcaneus and thoracic
    B. Cervical and thoracic compression
    C. Lumbosacral compression and calcaneus
    D. Pelvic and thoracic

48. **A possible complication with the administration of a Thomas splint is**
    A. Flexion and outward rotation of the proximal femur
    B. Improvement of a muscle spasm
    C. Displacement of the distal third of the fractured femur
    D. Compression of the medial nerve

49. **When using a battery-powered ring cutter, it is important for the nurse to**
    A. Use the diamond disk for a gold ring
    B. Use the carbide blade for a steel ring
    C. Place the cutting guard over the ring
    D. Cover the area with a water-soluble lubricating jelly

50. **A complication that would not occur when removing an oral piercing is**
    A. Abscess formation at the piercing site
    B. Aspiration
    C. Tooth breakage
    D. Edema

51. **If a patient has sustained an unstable ankle fracture, which position would not be appropriate for splinting?**
    A. Supine
    B. Prone
    C. Upright
    D. Lateral

52. **A posterior short leg splint should be applied**
    A. From the metatarsal 1 inch below the popliteal area to 1 inch beyond the toes
    B. From 1.5 inches beyond the toes to 1.5 inches below the popliteal area
    C. From 2 inches below the popliteal area to 2 inches beyond the toes
    D. From 1 inch below the popliteal area to 2 inches beyond the toes

53. **Which of the following splints can be applied by one person?**
    A. Hare splint
    B. Thomas splint
    C. Kendrick splint
    D. Sager splint

54. **The _____ traction splint does not require anterior padding in the anterior groin area.**
    A. Kendrick
    B. Hare
    C. Sager
    D. Thomas

55. **Normal tissue pressure is approximately 10 mmHg. When a patient has compartment syndrome, a pressure exceeding _____ indicates the need for a fasciotomy.**
    A. 15–25 mmHg
    B. 20–30 mmHg
    C. 25–35 mmHg
    D. 30–40 mmHg

56. **When patients require wound cleansing, a solution that effectively kills Gram-negative and Gram-positive rods, viruses, and fungi is**
    A. Sterile water
    B. Hydrogen peroxide
    C. A povidone-iodine solution
    D. Tap water and soap

57. **Epinephrine is useful in the repair of which of the following types of injuries?**
    A. Patients with known peripheral vascular disease
    B. Lip lacerations that extend through the lip border
    C. The face and scalp to slow absorption
    D. Cartilaginous areas of the ear and nares

58. **All types of local anesthetics are vasodilators and cause relaxation of smooth muscles except**
    A. Cocaine
    B. Lidocaine
    C. Tetracaine
    D. Pramosone

59. **An example of an ester compound is**
    A. Procaine
    B. Lidocaine
    C. Mepivacaine
    D. Bupivacaine

60. **Your patient requires suturing of a laceration. The patient has a history of malignant hyperthermia. An appropriate local anesthetic agent for this patient is**
    A. Lidocaine
    B. Procaine
    C. Mepivacaine
    D. Bupivacaine

61. **Your patient is to undergo a digital block for a reduction of an interphalangeal joint dislocation. The anesthetic of choice is**
    A. Epinephrine
    B. Buffered lidocaine
    C. Prilocaine
    D. Benzocaine

62. **Your patient was admitted to the ED for multiple fractures and contusions after a motor vehicle accident this evening. She complains of dyspnea and petechiae are noted. Your patient is probably suffering from**
    A. A pulmonary embolus
    B. Thrombocytopenia
    C. A venous air emboli
    D. A fat embolus

63. **Your patient has sustained a laceration on the forehead. Which of the following statements is true about the treatment of wounds in this area?**
    A. Do not shave the eyebrows
    B. Only cleanse the skin with a mild antiseptic solution
    C. Observe for redness, swelling, heat, and discharge
    D. Use sunblock over the wound for at least 6 months

64. **What is the force of injury in gunshot wounds to the head after the bullet penetrates the skull?**
    A. The movement of the bullet through brain tissue
    B. Compression of the air around the bullet as it moves through the brain tissue
    C. The skull fragments as they penetrate the brain
    D. Tearing injuries as the bullet passes through the vessels in the brain

65. **Which of the following statements about abrasions is false?**
    A. Abrasions are full thickness denudations
    B. Dirt and debris must be removed from the face within 8 hours
    C. Avoid direct sunlight for at least 6 months
    D. Abrasions are quite painful

66. **If the full thickness of skin is peeled away from a digit, hand, foot, or limb resulting in devascularization of the skin, this type of injury is known as**
    A. An amputation
    B. A laceration
    C. A degloving injury
    D. A Petersen avulsion

67. **The patient you are caring for impaled his forearm on a wood fence. Which of the following statements about this type of injury is false?**
    A. Any remaining particles of wood may be difficult to visualize on an X-ray
    B. Vegetative foreign bodies are highly reactive and easily lead to infection
    C. Vegetative foreign bodies may require anesthetic for removal
    D. Soak the affected area for at least 30 minutes to facilitate removal

68. **Fibroblast activity maximizes about 1 week after a patient has sustained a laceration. The ED nurse knows the next probable step in the care of this patient is**
    A. Have the patient return to the ED and administer tetanus toxoid
    B. Continue observation of this wound for another week
    C. Culture the wound and obtain a WBC count
    D. Remove the sutures and use tape on the wound

69. **Which of the following wounds is at greatest risk of contamination from a *Pseudomonas* infection?**
    A. A laceration from a pocket knife
    B. A plantar puncture wound through a shoe
    C. A degloved finger
    D. A paper cut

70. **A necrotizing infection associated with animal bites is likely caused by which of the following organisms?**
    A. *Clostridium tetani*
    B. *Pasteurella multocida*
    C. *Staphylococcus*
    D. *Pseudomonas*

71. **The outermost area of burned tissue is known as**
    A. The zone of coagulation
    B. The zone of hyperemia
    C. The zone of stasis
    D. The zone of necrosis

72. **Use of 0.5% silver nitrate solution is a good treatment for burns because of its broad-spectrum antibacterial action. As a trauma nurse, you know a disadvantage of using this medication is**
    A. Metabolic acidosis
    B. Hypochloremia and hyponatremia
    C. Transient leucopenia
    D. Limited penetration of eschar

73. **If muscle is burned, what classification is this type of burn?**
    A. First degree
    B. Second-degree partial thickness
    C. Third-degree full thickness
    D. Fourth-degree full thickness

74. **Your patient has burns on the right arm that are circumferential (all the way around the arm). What is the highest immediate risk with this type of burn?**
    A. Infection into the bone
    B. Difficulty removing dead tissue
    C. Compartment syndrome
    D. Escharotomy

75. **Using the Parkland formula for burn resuscitation, calculate the fluid requirements (first 24 hours) for a patient who weighs 60 kg and is burned over 35% of his body.**
    A. 25,250 ml
    B. 8,400 ml
    C. 21,600 ml
    D. 11,000 ml

76. **When utilizing the Parkland formula to calculate fluid needs, the preferred fluid for burn resuscitation is**
    A. Normal saline
    B. D_5/Isolyte M
    C. Lactated Ringer's
    D. 45% dextrose

77. **Which of the following vasodilators should not be mixed with Ringer's lactate?**
    A. Nesiritide
    B. Captopril
    C. Cardene
    D. Epinephrine

78. **Humerus stress fractures are likely to occur from unconditioned or immature bones and muscles when engaged in**
    A. Playing ice hockey
    B. Catching a football
    C. Bowling
    D. Pitching a baseball overhand

79. **The retroperitoneal space may accumulate as much as _____ L of blood before venous tamponade occurs.**
    A. One
    B. Two
    C. Four
    D. Five

80. **Gas gangrene is most frequently associated with**
    A. *Staphylococcus aureus*
    B. Duck embryo vaccine
    C. *Clostridium perfringens*
    D. A virus

81. **Piercings and use of body jewelry is increasingly common. Which of the following statements is false regarding body jewelry?**
    A. Body jewelry should be removed prior to defibrillation
    B. Jewelry that is removed should be considered contaminated with body fluid
    C. Removal may allow healing and development of abscess formation
    D. Most jewelry is nonmagnetic and does not require removal for an MRI

82. **A boxer's fracture is a fracture involving the**
    A. Proximal second phalanx
    B. Distal fifth metacarpal
    C. Proximal third metacarpal
    D. Distal fourth phalanx

83. **Your patient was riding his motorcycle in traffic when he had to swerve suddenly to avoid a crash. The motorcycle went out from under the patient and he skidded on the pavement. The type of injury you would expect to see is**
    A. A laceration
    B. A fracture
    C. An avulsion
    D. Tattooing

84. **Your patient sustained a crush injury to his ankle about a week ago. He now is complaining of weakness, inability to sleep, difficulty speaking and swallowing, progressive muscle paralysis, and blurred vision. On examination you notice dilated, fixed pupils, and dry mucous membranes. Your patient is probably suffering from**
    A. Guillain-Barré syndrome
    B. Gas gangrene
    C. Hyperemia
    D. Wound botulism

85. **Your patient was removing weeds in his yard. As he reached toward the ground near his storage shed, he was bitten on the forearm twice. The wound bled moderately. The patient saw a raccoon running away from the scene and fearing possible rabies, sought treatment in your ED. Which of the following animal bites is most likely to result in the need for anti-rabies prophylaxis?**
    A. Dog
    B. Raccoon
    C. Rabbit
    D. Mouse

86. **Sutures placed in an upper or lower extremity and not over a joint should be removed within**
    A. 1–3 days
    B. 3–5 days
    C. 4–7 days
    D. 7–10 days

87. **What is a Bennett' fracture?**
    A. A fracture of the forefinger metacarpal
    B. A fracture plus dislocation of the metacarpal bone at the base of the thumb
    C. A comminuted intra-articular fracture of the thumb and CMC joint
    D. An open fracture of the middle finger

88. **Your patient fell from a 10-foot ladder. His hip is dislocated. How would you determine if the hip is anteriorly or posteriorly dislocated?**
    A. Anterior hip dislocations present with internal rotation
    B. Anterior hip dislocations present with adduction
    C. Posterior hip dislocations present without any rotation
    D. Posterior hip dislocations present with internal adduction

89. **The type of vertebral fracture that results from the mechanism of injury known as hyperflexion is called a**
    A. Wedge fracture
    B. Compression fracture
    C. Simple fracture
    D. Teardrop fracture

90. **Which of the following types of blast injury scenarios is most likely to cause the highest mortality and immediate death rates?**
    A. Bombings involving structural collapse
    B. Open-air detonations
    C. Enclosed space explosions
    D. Water explosions

91. **Which type of blast injury is caused solely by the direct effect of blast overpressure?**
    A. A quaternary blast injury
    B. A tertiary blast injury
    C. A primary blast injury
    D. A secondary blast injury

92. **The type of blast injury that is caused by objects that strike people is known as a**
    A. Tertiary blast injury
    B. A blast wave
    C. A tertiary blast injury
    D. A secondary blast injury

93. **A high-energy explosion that results in people flying through the air and striking other objects is known as a(n)**
    A. Tertiary blast injury
    B. Overpressure wave
    C. Primary blast injury
    D. Incidental blast injury

94. **Structural collapse injuries are least likely to be directly associated with**
    A. Rhabdomyolysis
    B. Radiological injuries
    C. Prolonged extrication
    D. Severe burns

95. **After a mass casualty event, care providers should**
    A. Admit 2nd and 3rd trimester pregnancies for monitoring
    B. Should provide verbal communication to all victims
    C. Provide follow-up for head injuries
    D. Base discharges on associated injuries

96. **A key concept of a blast injury would not include which of the following?**
    A. Injuries resulting in non-intact skin or mucous membrane exposure, hepatitis B immunization (within 7 days) and age-appropriate tetanus toxoid vaccine (if not current)
    B. All bomb events have the potential for radiological and/or chemical contamination
    C. Immediate primary closure for grossly contaminated wounds
    D. Primary blast injuries are more common in patients with skull fractures

97. **A compression of extremities or other parts of the body causing muscle swelling and possible neurological disruptions in the affected areas is the definition of**
    A. Compartment syndrome
    B. Rhabdomyolysis
    C. Myoglobinemia
    D. Crush syndrome

98. **In a hospital setting, the CDC recommends treating crush injuries aggressively to prevent further hypotension, metabolic abnormalities, and renal failure. Recommendations for the treatment of acidosis includes**
    A. Use of IV fluids and mannitol to diurese the patient at a rate of at least 100 ml/hour
    B. Treat open wounds with antibiotics, debride necrotic tissue, and use tetanus toxoid
    C. Administer sodium bicarbonate until urine pH reaches 6.5
    D. Use a short-term tourniquet on an affected limb until IV hydration is initiated

99. **Infected wounds without well approximated edges and which require formation of granulation tissue from the base of the wound upward require**
    A. Tertiary wound closure
    B. Secondary wound closure
    C. Primary wound closure
    D. Deep cleansing

100. **On occasion, wounds that are infected may be permitted to granulate with secondary intention. At that time, secondary sutures are used to approximate the edges. This type of wound closure is known as**
    A. Morrow's secondary closure
    B. Howard's wound refinement
    C. A tertiary wound closure
    D. A primary wound closure

101. **Which of the following statements is true regarding the care of frostbite on a patient's extremity?**
    A. Hemorrhagic blisters must have fluid extracted from them quickly
    B. Rub the extremity to assist the tissue to rewarm
    C. Once the tissue begins to rewarm, pain is minimized
    D. Rubbing the part increases friction and may damage tissue

102. **Pain relief for digital blocks on fingers and toes may involve the use of**
    A. Bupivacaine
    B. 5% Lidocaine
    C. Procaine
    D. Tetracaine

103. **The formation of edema after a burn injury is dependent on the mediators of inflammatory response to increase capillary permeability. Which of the following substrates would not be considered one of these mediators?**
    A. Thromboxane A2
    B. Bradykinin
    C. Prostaglandin
    D. Prostacyclin

104. **During the immediate post-burn period, which of the following fluids would be most beneficial?**
    A. Normal saline
    B. 0.45% normal saline
    C. Lactated Ringer's
    D. Albumin

105. **Your patient was burned over the anterior chest, right forearm, anterior neck, and the lateral aspect of the right leg. The burns on his right forearm have a white, leather-like appearance, and the patient has no sensation in that area. What classification of burn are these injuries to the right forearm?**
    A. First degree
    B. Second-degree partial thickness
    C. Third-degree full thickness
    D. Fourth-degree full thickness

106. **The burn on your patient's right arm is pink and blistered. When touched the patient screams with pain. This classification of burn is**
    A. First degree
    B. Second-degree partial thickness
    C. Third-degree full thickness
    D. Fourth-degree full thickness

107. **Initially, a burned area can be estimated by the Rule of Nines or using the palm as 1% of the body surface area. There are many ways to calculate the body surface area involved. If your patient was burned over 28% of his body and weighs 62 kg, calculate the total fluid requirements during the first 24 hours using the Parkland formula for burn resuscitation.**
    A. 2,131 ml
    B. 5,380 ml
    C. 9,452 ml
    D. 6,944 ml

108. **Your patient was a spectator at a soccer tournament when he was struck by lightning. He was thrown about 10 feet into a tree. He suffered a fractured left radius and ulna, a concussion, and burns on his left arm, chest, and right leg. He has been somewhat confused since the accident. Which of the following statements about lightning injuries is true?**
    A. Internal burns are common
    B. Barotrauma is rare
    C. Myoglobinuria is rarely seen
    D. DC current will most likely cause ventricular fibrillation

109. **If a patient sustains an injury from electromagnetic waves, such as those from an X-ray, the type of energy involved is**
    A. Mechanical
    B. Electrical
    C. Chemical
    D. Radiant

110. **When energy is transferred from a bullet to an individual, the type of energy transferred is called**
    A. Mechanical energy
    B. Kinematic energy
    C. Physical energy
    D. Thermal energy

111. **Your patient was driving and was rear-ended in a MVC. The patient was cleared but is suffering with pain from a sprained cervical area. There are no other injuries. The resident intends to write a medication order to help mitigate the pain. Your patient's physician order is for "Fentanyl 0.5 mg IM every 1–2 hours for pain." As a trauma nurse, you should**
    A. Administer as ordered via a rapid push
    B. Administer over 10 minutes to prevent apnea
    C. Notify the physician for clarification as the ordered frequency should be every 3–4 hours
    D. Notify the physician for clarification as the ordered amount should be 0.05 mg IM

112. **Which of the following patient populations is most at risk for an intravenous infiltration?**
    A. The elderly/children
    B. Patients having coronary bypass surgery
    C. Patients with central line IVs
    D. Patients with a history of IV drug abuse

113. **A possible adverse effect with the use of fentanyl is**
    A. Neutropenia
    B. Chest wall rigidity
    C. Hyperthyroidism
    D. Tachypnea

114. **Fentanyl administered intravenously is incompatible with**
    A. Piperacillin
    B. Phenytoin
    C. Esmolol
    D. Morphine

115. **Your patient was admitted directly to the ED with deep frostbite. Which of the following actions should not be performed immediately for this patient?**
    A. Remove the patient's wet clothing
    B. Administer warm, noncaffeinated fluids
    C. Administer narcotic analgesics
    D. Amputate tissue that is black in color

116. **A male patient was pumping gas when a spark ignited the fumes. He suffered full thickness burns of the right arm. During your initial assessment you note that eschar is present and the right radial pulse is not palpable. A Doppler pulse is also not discernible. Which of the following actions is appropriate at this time?**
    A. Move the arm away from the torso and elevate it on a pillow
    B. Escharotomy
    C. Morphine 4 mg IV
    D. Ice packs to reduce swelling

117. **Your patient was very anxious prior to a dislocated shoulder reduction. He received an IM injection of Versed. His blood pressure dropped from 142/80 to 88/56, and he became bradycardic. To counter this reaction, the patient should be given**
    A. Xanax
    B. Ativan
    C. Valium
    D. Romazicon

118. **The type of device made by combining radioactive materials and an explosive is known as a(n)**
    A. Improved nuclear device
    B. Radiologic dispersal device
    C. Simple radiological device
    D. Improved explosive device

119. **An example of a primary blast injury is**
    A. Hemorrhagic contusion
    B. Fractured femur
    C. An arm impaled by a stick
    D. Gunshot wound

120. **You have been designated to serve on your department's Policies and Procedures Committee. Best practice concerning hair removal prior to insertion of a peripheral IV would be to**
    A. Use a depilatory cream on fragile skin
    B. Use a pair of scissors
    C. Use a razor
    D. Leave the hair in place

SECTION 6: ANSWERS

1. **Correct answer: A**
   A disadvantage of using negative pressure wound care devices is NPWC cannot be used on wounds associated with malignancies. Advantages of NPWC include promotion of a moist healing environment, removal of barriers to cell migration and proliferation, and removal of interstitial fluid.

2. **Correct answer: D**
   A fourth-degree full thickness burn involves muscle, fat, fascia, or bone. This type of burn usually occurs as a result of deep thermal or electrical burns.

3. **Correct answer: C**
   The area of a burn that has the closest contact with the heat source and sustains the most damage is the zone of coagulation. This area is frequently necrotic. It is essential to debride the necrotic tissue because it cannot regenerate. Grafts may be used in this area.

4. **Correct answer: C**
   Oven cleaners contain large amounts of alkali. Additional alkaline substances include dishwasher detergent, laundry detergent, drain openers, and ammonia capsules.

5. **Correct answer: B**
   Pepcid (famotidine) has been found to increase blood-alcohol levels by delaying metabolism and may contribute to alcohol-related injuries. Patients have been known to underestimate the amount, frequency, and size of consumed alcoholic beverages, but some medications, such as Pepcid, can sustain blood-alcohol levels, contributing to risky behaviors. Risk of bleeding is amplified in patients who combine energy drinks containing ginseng or ginkgo biloba with alcohol.

6. **Correct answer: B**
   The inadvertent administration of a vesicant medication into surrounding tissue is known as extravasation. A vesicant is fluid or medication capable of causing necrosis, blistering, and tissue damage.

7. **Correct answer: C**
   When a patient is suffering from superficial frostbite, rewarm the affected part using warm water at 40–43.3°C (104–107.6°F). Keep the affected part elevated and do not place heavy blankets over the area. The skin will be a waxy, whitish color. The patient may also have numbness, tingling, or a burning sensation of the affected area. It is important to remember to only start rewarming if the area is not at risk for re-injury.

8. **Correct answer: D**
   A carboxyhemoglobin of 18% and a burned chin is suggestive of smoke inhalation in this patient. When a sudden flame-up comes near the face, the first instinct is to gasp. This inhalation of superheated air will cause swelling of the tissues in the air passages. This man was probably very near the flame as his chin was burned, and he is at great risk of a compromised airway and may need intubation.

9. **Correct answer: C**
   The type of knee injury most likely to be caused by hyperextension trauma is an anterior and posterior cruciate ligament injury.

10. **Correct answer: B**
    A fracture at the junction of the proximal and middle thirds of the ulna is known as a Monteggia's fracture. If the patient has sustained this type of fracture, there is often a dislocation of the radial head. Neurovascular function may be compromised. If the fracture is due to a direct blow, it is sometimes called a "nightstick fracture." Patients usually demonstrate swelling, pain on ROM, crepitus, and deformity.

11. **Correct answer: C**
    A third-degree strain is distinguished by loss of muscle function (at the time of the injury), discoloration, hematoma, swelling, and a "snapping" or "popping" noise at the time of the injury.

12. **Correct answer: B**

A distinguishing characteristic of a patellar fracture is the patient's inability to actively extend the knee. Patellar fractures are usually associated with trauma or indirectly from quadriceps contractions or severe pulls. The patient will be suffering with severe pain and exhibit hemarthrosis.

13. **Correct answer: C**

Your patient was running to first base during a baseball game. When he placed his foot on the bag he heard a loud sound and could not apply weight on that leg. He was assisted to a friend's car and transported to your facility. You note the patient is in moderate pain and cannot bear weight on the affected leg. As a trauma nurse, you suspect this patient is suffering from an Achilles tendon rupture. It is important to splint the foot in plantar flexion and apply a compression dressing and crutches. A walking cast may be ordered along with an orthopedic surgery consult.

14. **Correct answer: B**

A pathologic cause of a proximal humerus fracture is an existing condition such as bone cancer, bone cysts, osteoporosis, or Paget's disease.

15. **Correct answer: B**

The type of amputation that has the greatest chance of reimplantation is the guillotine. The edges are more easily approximated. Reimplantations of the upper extremities are more successful than those of the lower extremities.

16. **Correct answer: D**

Splints are not circumferential. Splints are not only noncircumferential but usually held in place by an elastic bandage. Splints allow for easy access to an injury site, are fast and easy to apply, and allow for swelling during the acute inflammatory phase of injury. Circumferential casts may cause pressure-related complications. These complications include skin breakdown, necrosis, compartment syndrome, and thermal injury.

17. **Correct answer: B**

A closed wound that occurs when a blood vessel ruptures and bleeds into surrounding tissue is known as a contusion. A hematoma may form secondary to a contusion. Patients need to be evaluated as to potential causes: abuse, anticoagulant use (including diet, use of power drinks), bleeding/clotting disorders, type of activity, medications (including vitamins as many now contain herbal anticoagulants).

18. **Correct answer: C**

A proximal humerus fracture with damage to the radial nerve results in wrist drop. The radial nerve innervates dorsal extrinsic muscles of the forearm. Damage to the nerve may be assessed by having the patient abduct and extend the thumb and attempt to extend the wrist. If the nerve is damaged, the fingers will be flexed at the MCP joints and the thumb will be adducted.

19. **Correct answer: B**

Tinel's sign is considered positive when pain and paresthesia worsen when the medial nerve is tapped along its course in the wrist.

20. **Correct answer: D**

While assisting a patient with fitting for a cane, the cane should be placed next to the heel on the uninjured side and the elbow flexed at 30 degrees

21. **Correct answer: B**

Your patient requires application of a long leg fiberglass splint. The patient should be positioned supine.

22. **Correct answer: C**

Obese patients placed in the prone position for splinting may have difficulty breathing.

23. **Correct answer: B**

A necrotizing infection associated with animal bites is likely caused by *Pasteurella multocida*. This infection may progress to cellulitis, osteomyelitis, and pleuritis. The disease itself is called pasteurellosis.

24. **Correct answer: A**

When performing a peripheral nerve assessment for ulnar nerve impairment, normal motor and sensory findings include the ability to fan the fingers and have feeling on top of the small finger. Feeling on the dorsum of the thumb and the ability to extend the thumb is an indication of normal motor and sensory function of the radial nerve. The ability to oppose the thumb to the base of the small finger and to feel on the tip of the index finger is the expected result when testing the medial nerve.

25. **Correct answer: B**

Prior to fixed wing air transport, it is necessary to bivalve a plaster cast if it is circumferential. Changes in atmospheric pressure will cause the extremity to expand. Air splints are dangerous because they may impede circulation due to gas expansion.

26. **Correct answer: A**

Fractures to the distal ends of the radius and ulna are known as Colles' or, occasionally, "silver fork" fractures. It is incumbent on the nurse to consider shoulder, humeral, or hand fractures as well. The lumbar area of the spine may have been injured and the patient may have a compression fracture and possible calcaneal fractures.

27. **Correct answer: D**

NSAIDs are not appropriate initial treatment for a patient with a pelvic fracture because of the high risk of bleeding. It is also a good idea to avoid NSAIDs until the patient has been ruled out for other injuries, hypertension, bleeding disorders, or if they are taking anticoagulants.

28. **Correct answer: B**

Your patient has sustained an ulnar fracture. An ulnar gutter splint is appropriate for this type of injury. This splint extends along the ulna, partially covering the forearm from below the elbow to the palm of the hand.

29. **Correct answer: D**

The most common forearm fracture is a distal radius fracture. This type of fracture is commonly caused by falls on an outstretched hand. This fracture may also be caused by direct injury. The nurse should observe and assess for radial shortening, ulnar nerve involvement, carpal tunnel syndrome, tendon rupture, and reflex sympathetic dystrophy.

30. **Correct answer: A**

The nerve most commonly injured in a proximal humerus fracture is the axillary nerve. The patient may suffer loss of sensation over the lateral deltoid area. Vascular injuries are rare, but the trauma nurse should carefully assess for neurovascular status because peripheral pulses may still be obtained because of collateral circulation around the scapula. The shoulder girdle may develop a mass that can be palpated and that may indicate an arterial rupture. An angiogram may be indicated.

31. **Correct answer: A**

The deltoid muscle is not considered to be a part of the rotator cuff. The four muscles considered part of the rotator cuff are the supraspinatus, teres minor, subscapularis, and the infraspinatus. The supraspinatus and the infraspinatus muscles are the most commonly injured muscles in the rotator cuff.

32. **Correct answer: D**

The most serious complication of casting and splinting is compartment syndrome. Compartment syndrome occurs when pressures in a closed space compromise blood flow and tissue perfusion. Ischemia results and potentially causes edema and impairment of vascular and neurological tissue.

Patients should be taught that increased pain, numbness, tingling, swelling, color change, or delayed capillary refill in the immobilized area is serious and requires an immediate visit to an ED or urgent care facility. The cast or splint will probably be removed.

33. **Correct answer: D**

At 5–6 days after a contusion is sustained, the periphery of the contusion changes color from the periphery to the inside and becomes green-tinged. The ED nurse needs to take color into consideration to help evaluate the history of the injury.

34. **Correct answer: C**
     If a patient presents with contusions that are yellow tinged, the contusion is probably about 7–10 days old. From 1 to 5 days the contusion is usually purple or reddish-blue, green from 5 to 7 days, yellow from 7 to 10 days, and brown at 10–14 days.

35. **Correct answer: D**
     Appropriate patient teaching about RICE therapy includes application of cold packs $\times$ 20 minutes, four times a day for 48–72 hours. Wrap the cold source to prevent thermal injury. Additional teaching should also include resting extremities and elevating as close to level of the heart as possible during the first 24 hours. Compression bandages with an elastic bandage should be used and analgesics taken as ordered.

36. **Correct answer: B**
     A deformity of the distal portion of a joint that is angulated away from the midline of the body is called a valgus. An example is a patient with "knock knees."

37. **Correct answer: C**
     The type of fracture caused by an angulation force of direct trauma is known as a transverse fracture. An oblique fracture is usually caused by a twisting force. A spiral fracture is often caused by a twisting force when the foot is firmly planted. A depressed fracture is caused by blunt force on a flat bone.

38. **Correct answer: D**
     A posterior dislocation of the glenohumeral joint in the shoulder may be caused by a tonic-clonic seizure. This type of rare injury occurs from an extended arm forcefully abducted and internally rotated.

39. **Correct answer: D**
     The amputated part should be rinsed with sterile normal saline or Lactated Ringer's. No tap water or other solutions should be used. The part should be placed in a plastic bag and then sealed shut. That bag should be placed in another container with ice and water or refrigerated to 4°C. The bag should be labeled with the patient's name, date, and time per hospital protocol.

40. **Correct answer: A**
     Talcum powder and cornstarch do not cause breakdown of the skin. Both talcum powder and cornstarch help prevent the air splint from adhering to skin and makes removal easier. Excessive pressure variations exist and pressure may cause compartment syndrome, nerve compression, and soft tissue damage. Loss of inflation may result in inadequate stabilization of the fracture.

41. **Correct answer: B**
     When applying an air splint to an elderly patient, the ED nurse should consider placing smooth padding under the splint. Adducting the limb may cause further injury and pain as would be elevating the limb. Turning the valve counterclockwise will open the valve and let air out.

42. **Correct answer: C**
     The preferred splint for a femur fracture is a traction splint.

43. **Correct answer: C**
     Kendrick splints are classified as unipolar splints. The Sager comes in both models. The unipolar splints use one metal rod to stabilize the leg. The bipolar splints—Hare, Thomas, and Fernotrac—have two metal rods, one for each side of the leg.

44. **Correct answer: D**
     Traction splints are specific for femur fractures. They cannot be used on foot, ankle, upper extremity, distal tibia, or distal fibula fractures.

45. **Correct answer: B**
     Your patient should have his or her elbow bent at 30 degrees while being fitted for a walker.

46. **Correct answer: C**
     This patient is suffering from gangrene. Your patient fractured his humerus in a car accident 3 weeks ago. Yesterday he developed a fever and now has a temperature of 101.7°F. He complains of pain in the upper arm, his capillary refill is 9 seconds, his distal pulses are moderate to poor, and his fingers are

cold. There are small areas just distal of the cast that are swollen and look like bubbles. There is a foul odor emanating from the cast.

47. **Correct answer: C**

Your patient joined a parachuting club. On her first jump with the instructor their parachute failed to open completely, and they both forcefully struck the ground with their feet. Since this patient landed on her feet, she most likely sustained calcaneus and lumbosacral compression fractures.

48. **Correct answer: A**

A possible complication with the administration of a Thomas splint is flexion and outward rotation of the proximal femur. A goal is to improve muscle spasm. Displacement would involve the proximal third of the fractured femur. The medial nerve is in the arm, so it would not be affected by the femur splint.

49. **Correct answer: D**

When using a battery-powered ring cutter, it is important for the nurse to cover the area with a water-soluble lubricating jelly to dissipate heat generated by the cutter. The patient can be easily burned during ring removal. It is also possible to place ice directly on the ring. Diamond disks are for cutting steel, iron, brass, and platinum. Carbide disks are for cutting gold, silver, copper, aluminum, and plastic.

50. **Correct answer: A**

A complication that would not occur when removing an oral piercing is abscess formation at the piercing site. The abscess may form after the removal, not during the removal.

51. **Correct answer: B**

Patients who have sustained unstable ankle fractures should not be placed in the prone position. The calf might be flexed and the splint may be improperly fitted, causing tissue damage or lack of support.

52. **Correct answer: C**

A posterior short leg splint should be applied from 2 inches below the popliteal area to 2 inches beyond the toes. The nurse should ensure the patient's foot is at 90 degrees to the leg and that circulation and knee flexion is not compromised.

53. **Correct answer: D**

The Sager splint may be applied by one person.

54. **Correct answer: C**

The Sager traction splint does not require anterior padding in the anterior groin area.

55. **Correct answer: D**

When a patient has compartment syndrome, a pressure exceeding 30–40 mmHg indicates the need for a fasciotomy.

56. **Correct answer: C**

Povidone-iodine solutions effectively kill Gram-negative and Gram-positive rods, viruses, and fungi. The nurse should always ask about patient sensitivity or allergies to iodine or shellfish prior to its use.

57. **Correct answer: C**

Epinephrine is useful in repairing injuries to the face and scalp by slowing absorption and lowering peak blood levels.

58. **Correct answer: A**

Cocaine is a vasoconstrictor. It is used frequently for patients with epistaxis. Cocaine should not be given to patients with a history of abuse or who are allergic to exogenous catecholamines.

59. **Correct answer: A**

An example of an ester compound is procaine. Esters are hydrolyzed by pseudocholinesterase in the serum. Cocaine is an ester but is excreted unchanged in urine. Esters usually cause more allergic reactions than other compounds.

60. **Correct answer: B**
An appropriate local anesthetic agent for a patient with a history of malignant hyperthermia is procaine.

61. **Correct answer: B**
For a reduction of an interphalangeal joint dislocation, the anesthetic of choice (from this selection) is buffered lidocaine. This procedure should be relatively short and the buffered lidocaine reduces pain from a digital block.

62. **Correct answer: D**
Fractures, usually long bone fractures, can release free fatty acids, which cause fatty emboli. Fat globules float around and obstruct the pulmonary vasculature.

63. **Correct answer: A**
Your patient has sustained a laceration on the forehead. Do not shave eyebrows because the eyebrows may not regrow normally and will look distorted.

64. **Correct answer: C**
The force of injury from a gunshot is compression of the air as the bullet passes through brain tissue. There are other factors that influence injury from bullets including caliber, proximity, and number of shots fired. For example, a 22-caliber bullet lacks the velocity to exit the skull but bounces off the hard surfaces inflicting great damage. A bullet from a large-caliber gun has a tendency to pass straight through the brain tissue and exit the skull on the opposite side.

65. **Correct answer: A**
Abrasions are partial thickness denudations of skin, not full thickness denudations. An abrasion may be quite painful because of exposed nerve endings. Avoid direct sunlight for at least 6 months because pigmentary changes may take place. Dirt and debris should be removed from the face within 8 hours and should be removed from extremities within 4–6 hours.

66. **Correct answer: C**
If the full thickness of skin is peeled away from a digit, hand, foot, or limb resulting in devascularization of the skin, this type of injury is known as a degloving injury.

67. **Correct answer: D**
Wounds that may have wood splinters should not be soaked because the wood absorbs liquid and swells, causing further pain and tissue damage. In addition, the wood may harbor bacteria and vegetative foreign bodies.

68. **Correct answer: D**
Fibroblast activity maximizes about 1 week after a patient has sustained a laceration. The wound may not have enough tensile strength to maintain the approximation of the wound, so using tape to maintain wound adhesion may be necessary.

69. **Correct answer: B**
The type of injury at greatest risk of contamination from a *Pseudomonas* infection is a plantar puncture wound through a shoe.

70. **Correct answer: B**
A necrotizing infection associated with animal bites is likely caused by *Pasteurella multocida*. This infection may progress to cellulitis, osteomyelitis, and pleuritis. The disease itself is called pasteurellosis.

71. **Correct answer: B**
The outermost area of burned tissue is known as the zone of hyperemia. Blood flow is increased because of the inflammatory process. fully reversible changes occur here, including tissue edema, hyperemia, anoxia, and exudate formation.

72. **Correct answer: B**

Hypochloremia and hyponatremia are disadvantages of using 0.5% silver nitrate solution for burn patients.

73. **Correct answer: D**

This is a fourth-degree burn. Not many people are familiar with this classification. This is a burn that not only involves muscle but it extends through muscle and bone.

74. **Correct answer: C**

The highest risk at this time is compartment syndrome. A circumferential burn may lead to compartment syndrome. Escharotomy is a procedure, not a direct risk. As a nurse you must constantly assess for quality of pulses. Edema may be so great as to completely cut off circulation in a limb and cause myoglobin-related renal failure. Elevating the limb may help drain fluid and mitigate further edema. If the pulse is lost, it still may not mean compartment syndrome is the cause. It could be due to not replacing lost volume secondary to the burn. Although infection is a risk, it is not the immediate risk.

75. **Correct answer: B**

The formula is $4 \times kg \times \%$ of burn. So, the calculation is for a 60 kg patient with a 35% burn surface area. $4 \times 60 = 240 \times 35 = 8,400$.

76. **Correct answer: C**

As mentioned previously, Lactated Ringer's (LR) is preferred for large volume resuscitation because LR contains 130 mEq/L of sodium compared with normal saline, which has 154 mEq/L. LR has a higher pH (6.5) compared to normal saline (5.0). The pH of the LR is close to a normal pH. The patient will be in metabolic acidosis, so the metabolized lactate will buffer the acidosis. LR is also an isotonic crystalloid.

77. **Correct answer: C**

Cardene cannot be mixed with Ringer's lactate or sodium bicarbonate infusions. According to studies, although the combination does not cause a precipitate, the Ringer's lactate inactivates 15–42% of the drug.

78. **Correct answer: D**

Stress fractures of the humerus are likely to occur from unconditioned or immature bones and muscles when engaged in pitching a baseball overhand. The rotator cuff, pectoralis major, and deltoid muscles may be weakened. An additional cause of this type of fracture is violent muscle contractions, such as those seen in seizures and electrical shock.

79. **Correct answer: D**

The retroperitoneal space may accumulate as much as 5 liters of blood before venous tamponade occurs. If the pubic symphysis diastasis is spread > 3 cm, venous tamponade may not occur until several units of blood have accumulated. If a posterior instability has occurred, it may result in a blood loss of more than 15 units.

80. **Correct answer: C**

Gas gangrene is most frequently associated with *Clostridium perfringens*. This pathogen is an anaerobic, Gram-positive, spore-forming bacillus. Other bacteria are also capable of producing gas, and non-clostridial organisms have been isolated in 60–85% of cases of gas gangrene. The most frequently identified aerobic Gram-negative bacteria were *Escherichia coli*, *Proteus* species, *Pseudomonas aeruginosa*, and *Klebsiella pneumoniae*.

81. **Correct answer: D**

Most jewelry is nonmagnetic and does not require removal for an MRI unless it covers the body part being examined. Body jewelry should be removed prior to defibrillation to prevent burns and arcing. Jewelry that is removed should be considered contaminated with body fluid. Removal of body jewelry may heal over the piercing site and promote development of an abscess.

82. **Correct answer: B**

A boxer's fracture is a fracture involving the distal fifth metacarpal. This type of fracture occasionally involves the head of the metacarpal but is known as a fracture of the fourth or fifth metacarpal neck.

83. **Correct answer: D**

The type of injury you would expect to see when a motorcycle rider skids on pavement is tattooing. This injury is caused by sideways (tangential) dermal and epidermal trauma. It is a form of abrasion. Nerve endings are exposed, and the wound is very painful. This wound requires meticulous care, debridement, and possible antibiotic prophylaxis.

84. **Correct answer: D**

Your patient is probably suffering from wound botulism. His symptoms of weakness, inability to sleep, difficulty speaking and swallowing, progressive muscle paralysis, and blurred vision with dilated, fixed pupils are classic for this condition. Botulinum toxin blocks motor nerves' ability to release acetylcholine, the neurotransmitter that relays nerve signals to the muscles. Eventually, the muscles of respiration will be affected and death will occur from respiratory failure.

85. **Correct answer: B**

Your patient was removing weeds in his yard. As he reached toward the ground near his storage shed, he was bitten on the forearm twice. The wound bled moderately. The patient saw a raccoon running away from the scene and fearing possible rabies, sought treatment in your ED.

Anti-rabies prophylaxis is administered as a matter of course to individuals who have been bitten by raccoons, bats, skunks, and foxes. Generally, patients bitten by rodents rarely require post-exposure anti-rabies prophylaxis.

86. **Correct answer: D**

Sutures placed in an upper or lower extremity and not over a joint should be removed within 7–10 days.

87. **Correct answer: B**

A Bennett' fracture is a fracture plus dislocation of the metacarpal bone at the base of the thumb. If the force of the injury is severe and the bone breaks into several pieces, it is known as a Rolando fracture.

88. **Correct answer: D**

If your patient fell from a 10-foot ladder and dislocated his hip, you would determine if the hip is anteriorly or posteriorly dislocated by the presentation. Posterior hip dislocations present with internal rotation and adduction. Anterior hip dislocations present with external rotation and abduction.

89. **Correct answer: D**

The type of vertebral fracture that results from the mechanism of injury known as hyperflexion is called a teardrop fracture. A small anterior edge of a vertebrae breaks and may impinge on the spinal cord. Sometimes the patient will also have a posterior malalignment of the vertebrae.

90. **Correct answer: A**

For the past several years, statistics show that bombings involving structural collapse are most likely to cause the highest mortality and immediate death rates (about 25%). Confined space bombings caused about 8% of immediate deaths and open-air detonations caused about 4% of immediate deaths.

91. **Correct answer: C**

Since air is easily compressible, where water is not, tissue damage affects air-filled structures like the lung, organs in the gastrointestinal tract, and tympanic membrane rupture.

92. **Correct answer: D**

The type of blast injury that is caused by objects (the airborne debris) that strike people is known as a secondary blast injury. The types of trauma associated with a secondary blast injury include bomb fragments, fragmentation injuries, and both penetrating and blunt injuries.

93. **Correct answer: A**

A high-energy explosion that results in people flying through the air and striking other objects is known as a tertiary blast injury. The blast wind can displace a victim, potentially causing blunt and penetrating injuries, traumatic amputations, and fractures.

94. **Correct answer: B**

Structural collapse is less likely to be associated with radiological injury. Associated injuries and causes that frequently occur are prolonged extrication, severe burns, rhabdomyolysis, compartment syndrome, renal failure, and possible inhaled toxins.

95. **Correct answer: A**

After a mass casualty event, providers should admit all 2nd and 3rd trimester pregnancies for observation, follow up on head injuries, wounds, eye, ear, and stress-related injuries. Because there will probably be multiple ear injuries, the victims may be deaf or have tinnitus, making oral communication virtually impossible. Communication in that case may have to be written.

96. **Correct answer: C**

Grossly contaminated wounds should have primary closure delayed. Other key concepts include non-intact skin injuries or mucous membrane exposure, need hepatitis B immunization (within 7 days). Additionally, victims should be given an age-appropriate tetanus toxoid vaccine if not current. Also, bombing casualties have the potential for radiological and/or chemical contamination. Another key fact from the CDC is that patients with skull fractures more commonly have primary blast injuries.

97. **Correct answer: D**

A compression of extremities or other parts of the body causing muscle swelling and possible neurological disruptions in the affected areas is the definition of crush syndrome. Local tissue injury may lead to multiple organ dysfunction, and metabolic issues such as hypocalcemia, hyperkalemia, and metabolic acidosis.

98. **Correct answer: C**

In a hospital setting, the CDC recommends treating crush injuries aggressively to prevent further hypotension, metabolic abnormalities, and renal failure. Recommendations for the treatment of acidosis include alkalinization of the urine. Administer sodium bicarbonate to bring the urine pH to 6.5. Uric acid deposition in the kidneys and myoglobin will be prevented.

The question asked for appropriate in-hospital care. The other answers dealt with pre-hospital care or provided wrong treatments.

99. **Correct answer: B**

Infected wounds without well approximated edges and which require formation of granulation tissue from the base of the wound upward require secondary wound closure. Sometimes a drain must be used and gauze packing is necessary.

100. **Correct answer: C**

On occasion, wounds that are infected may be permitted to granulate with secondary intention. At that time, secondary sutures are used to approximate the edges. This type of wound closure is known as a tertiary wound closure.

101. **Correct answer: D**

Rubbing frostbitten tissue increases friction and tissue damage. The rewarming process can be quite painful, so pain relief may be done by administration of NSAIDs or aspirin would be appropriate. Hemorrhagic blisters must be left alone. Clear blisters should have the fluid withdrawn.

102. **Correct answer: A**

Appropriate pain relief for digital blocks on fingers and toes may involve the use of bupivacaine (Marcaine). Procaine and tetracaine cause too many side effects and the dose of lidocaine is inappropriate.

103. **Correct answer: D**

The formation of edema after a burn injury is dependent on the mediators of inflammatory response to increase capillary permeability. Mediators active in the increased permeability of capillary membranes are bradykinin, prostaglandin, thromboxane A2, histamine, serotonin, blood products, and complement components.

Systemic capillary leak syndrome (SCLS) was first identified by Dr. Bayard Clarkson in 1960. SCLS is a rare syndrome that can have acute, severe, self-reversing, recurrent flares of leakage of large volumes of plasma into the interstitial space and body cavities. The cause is unknown but is often triggered by an upper respiratory infection or burns. There is no evidence of a genetic component to this syndrome.

Symptoms of SCLS are caused by the walls of the capillaries being triggered by injury or infection thereby losing their ability to maintain their stability allowing plasma to leak. Symptoms include swelling of various body parts, nausea, lightheadedness, hypotension leading to shock, organ failure, rhabdomyolysis, compartment syndrome, acute tubular necrosis and death if left untreated. The patient experiences hemoconcentration and hypoalbuminemia.

There are two phases of SCLS. The initial phase takes place over 1–3 days. During this period the patient may lose up to 70% of the plasma from circulation. Fluid resuscitation includes albumin, other colloidal solutions, and intravenous steroids. The second phase is the recruitment phase that occurs over the same time period as the initial phase. The major problem with this phase is the rapidity with which the extravasated fluid is reabsorbed. This can lead to pulmonary edema.

104. **Correct answer: C**
Lactated Ringer's (LR) is used for burn patients for a variety of reasons with many of the formulas for burn resuscitation. It is preferred for large volume resuscitation because LR contains 130 mEq/L of sodium compared with normal saline that has 154 mEq/L. LR has a higher pH (6.5) compared to normal saline (5.0). The pH of the LR is close to a normal pH. The patient will be in metabolic acidosis, so the metabolized lactate will buffer the acidosis. LR is also an isotonic crystalloid.

105. **Correct answer: C**
Third-degree full thickness burns destroy nerve endings because they extend into subcutaneous tissue. The tissue may have a whitish color and will be somewhat firm with a leather-like appearance. Sometimes you can see clotted vessels through the eschar.

106. **Correct answer: B**
This type of burn may be a superficial or a deep second-degree partial thickness burn. The nerve endings are still intact, and this burn is very painful. Sometimes burns can be deceptive. A reddened area that should be diagnosed as a first-degree burn may be overlooked when staff is calculating requirements for fluid and nutrient resuscitation. After a few hours these areas can develop blisters and are only then recognized as dermal burns. There is a new way of assessing burn levels by using a laser Doppler during the first week of treatment.

107. **Correct answer: D**
The Parkland formula was developed by Dr. Charles Baxter at Parkland Hospital in Dallas, Texas, in the 1960s and is still utilized today. It is used nationwide as a standard for fluid resuscitation. There are many other formulas in use, but this one is widely known and will probably be on the TCRN examination. The formula is 4 ml fluid × patient's weight (in kg) ×% of burn, so $4 \times 62 \times 28 = 6,944$ ml fluid requirement for the first 24 hours. Half the calculated volume is given in the first 8 hours, and then the remaining volume is given over the next 16 hours. Remember to calculate from the time the burn occurred.

108. **Correct answer: C**
Myoglobinuria is rarely seen with lightning burns. AC current usually causes ventricular fibrillation, and DC current usually causes asystole. In some cases, arrhythmias are delayed for up to 12 hours. The mechanism of lightning strikes is quite complex. There are several ways lightning can injure a person:

- A side splash from another object is probably the cause of this patient's injuries. The lightning hits something like a tree and then bounces off.
- A direct strike may also have occurred.
- Another type of strike can occur when the person is touching an object that is struck.

Ground current effect occurs when energy spreads out across the surface of the earth. Lightning has two strokes, upward and downward. If they do not meet, energy can be directed outward.

Internal burns are rare. Myoglobinuria rarely occurs. Generally, lightning causes cardiac and respiratory arrest, burns from metals touching the victim (watches, necklaces, earrings), and neurologic damage.

109. Correct answer: D

If a patient sustains an injury from electromagnetic waves such as those from an X-ray, the type of energy involved is radiant. Other sources of radiant energy are sunlight, sound waves, and radioactive emissions.

110. Correct answer: A

When energy is transferred from a bullet to an individual, the type of energy transferred is called mechanical energy. Energy is loaded onto the patient, and if the load overcomes the body's ability to tolerate it, injury to one or more of the body's tissues occurs.

111. Correct answer: D

An order for fentanyl 0.5 mg IM q 1–2 hours for pain should be questioned immediately as the dose is 10 times the normal dose. Transcription errors lead to potentially life-threatening reactions. Despite the use of electronic medication records, some facilities still must transcribe physician orders to the electronic record, leading to medication errors. Decimal placement can often be missed in scanning and faxing orders to the pharmacy. Order clarification by the nurse and pharmacy helps prevent such errors.

112. Correct answer: A

The elderly and children are at greatest risk for intravenous infiltration. The elderly have less elastic veins, and children have immature veins. Examples of other risk groups include patients who have had CVAs, diabetics, spinal injured patients, and severely debilitated patients.

113. Correct answer: B

Possible adverse effects of fentanyl include respiratory depression, chest wall rigidity, apnea, laryngospasm, abdominal distension, loss of bowel sounds, and generalized muscle rigidity.

114. Correct answer: B

Fentanyl administered intravenously is incompatible with phenytoin, azithromycin, and pentobarbital.

115. Correct answer: D

In patients with deep frostbite, amputations are not an emergency. An amputation may be performed days or weeks after the injury. Priorities are to remove wet clothing, rewarm the patient, administer warm, noncaffeinated fluids (if the patient has an intact gag reflex), administer analgesics, and consider tetanus prophylaxis.

116. Correct answer: B

A male patient was pumping gas when a spark ignited the fumes. He suffered full thickness burns of the right arm. During your initial assessment you note that eschar is present and the right radial pulse is not palpable. A Doppler pulse is also not discernible. As a trauma nurse, you know loss of the radial pulse indicates probable compartment syndrome; this is an emergency, and pressure must be relieved via an escharotomy, an incision through multiple layers of tissue. Any circumferential burn of the body may lead to impaired function and necessitate an escharotomy.

117. Correct answer: D

Romazicon is a benzodiazepine antagonist and should be given to counteract the effects of Versed. Xanax, Valium, and Ativan are also benzodiazepines.

118. Correct answer: B

The type of device made by combining radioactive materials and an explosive is known as a radiologic dispersal device.

119. Correct answer: A

Hemorrhagic contusion is an example of a primary blast injury. The blast injury occurs after an explosion that causes sudden changes in atmospheric pressure generating an overpressure that compresses tissue.

120. Correct answer: B

Best practice concerning hair removal prior to insertion of a peripheral IV would be to use a pair of scissors or disposable-head surgical clippers. Use of a razor might cause cuts or microabrasions, which increase the risk for infection. Depilatory creams should never be used as they might also provide a portal for bacterial entry.

Continuum of Care for Trauma

- End-of-Life
- Forensic Issues
- Injury Prevention
- Psychosocial
- Rehabilitation

SECTION 7: QUESTIONS

1. **Which of the following statements about the treatment of patient delirium in the emergency department is accurate?**
   A. No drug has been approved by the FDA to treat delirium
   B. Propofol is the best treatment when the cause of the delirium is unknown
   C. Benzodiazepines have the greatest efficacy in the treatment of delirium
   D. Delirium goes undetected in about 10% of patients

2. **Which of the following advanced directives does not exclude pain relief or comfort measures?**
   A. An out-of-hospital DNR
   B. A portable DNR
   C. A durable power of attorney for healthcare
   D. A do not attempt resuscitation order DNR

3. **Which of the following documents represent informed consent?**
   A. A Living Will
   B. An Allow Natural Death order
   C. An out-of-hospital DNR
   D. A physician statement

4. **Transplantable tissue would include**
   A. Pancreas
   B. Kidney
   C. Bone
   D. Liver

5. **Care of a patient who is scheduled for eye organ procurement should include**
   A. Instillation of artificial tears in the eyes
   B. Keeping the patient flat in bed
   C. Placing a warm cloth over the eyes
   D. Keeping the patient at ambient temperature

6. **Supporting and respecting the culture, beliefs, and values of the trauma patient is known as**
   A. Standard of care
   B. Moral agency
   C. Duty
   D. Advocacy

7. **An inappropriate action prior to preparing a critical patient for air transport would be**
   A. Place a gastric tube to prevent aspiration
   B. Continue the use of air splints
   C. Place chest tube
   D. Remove hanging weights if possible

8. **Protecting the viability of evidence for court purposes by removing doubt of tampering is known as**
   A. Evidence protection
   B. Legal forensic documentation
   C. Chain of custody
   D. Internal guardianship

9. **Your patient was found outside the ED entrance when dropped off by an unknown party. The patient sustained both stab wounds and gunshot wounds. Which of the following is an appropriate action while caring for this patient?**
   A. If the clothing is thick and difficult to cut, use one of the entry holes to begin cutting the material
   B. Do not wash the patient's hands, and cover the patient's hands with paper bags
   C. Use a felt marker to label the wounds for easier documentation
   D. Discard all contaminated clothing

10. **You are discussing organ donation with the family of a 24 year old who was in a car accident and not expected to live. The family states that their son has no living will or advanced directive. The bother states that during a party, the patient said that he would be a donor. The generally accepted legal next of kin order for the determination of patient wishes is**
    A. Agent, spouse, adult child, parent
    B. Spouse, parent, guardian, agent
    C. Parent, grandparent, guardian, adult who exhibits concern
    D. Adult child, parent, adult sibling, grandparent

11. **The definition of palliative care recognized in the United States is**
    A. Palliative care is care coordinated within one specific unit
    B. Patient and family hopes for peace and dignity are supported at the end of life
    C. Palliative and non-palliative caregivers must collaborate to provide family care needs
    D. Palliative care means patient and family-centered care that optimizes quality of life by anticipating, preventing, and treating suffering. Palliative care throughout the continuum of illness involves addressing physical, intellectual, emotional, social, and spiritual needs and to facilitate patient autonomy, access to information, or both

12. **You are caring for a patient with multiple sclerosis. The neurologist wants to start your patient on steroids for 5 days. Which of the following is true and should be considered by the palliative care team prior to beginning this medication?**
    A. What is the medical team's treatment goal?
    B. A pharmacist consultant is not necessary as the patient has been on this medication before
    C. Because the medication is only prescribed for 5 days, there is no need to monitor the patient's response
    D. Can any current medications be stopped prior to beginning this medication?

13. **Your patient with Stage IV esophageal cancer that has metastasized to the liver and bone is awaiting discharge home under hospice. During your assessment, the patient is short of breath with cough, has constipation, and vomits when eating solid foods. The patient complains that what bothers him most is he dislikes the vanilla-flavored shakes that come on his tray. What would be a high priority for this patient?**
    A. Ensure that respiratory administers his breathing treatments every 4 hours as ordered
    B. Call the physician to add a cough suppressant to the patient's medication list
    C. Call dietary to request a different flavored shake or if a flavor additive can be added
    D. Ensure that the patient has a stool softener added to the medication list

14. **Which of the following statements best defines palliative care?**
    A. Palliative care means medical and surgical care that optimizes quality of life by anticipating, preventing, and treating suffering
    B. Palliative care means medical and surgical care that optimizes quantity of life by anticipating, preventing, and treating conditions that are serious and life-threatening
    C. Palliative care means patient and family-centered care that optimizes quality of life by anticipating, preventing, and treating suffering
    D. Palliative care is the management of patients with medical conditions that can no longer be corrected with medical or surgical interventions

15. **Which statement below is false regarding intrahospital transfer of patients?**
    A. The responsibility of care for the patient rests on the receiving facility as soon as the patient leaves the sending facility
    B. Ensure properly trained personnel are available at both the sending and receiving facility
    C. Select the appropriate mode of transport
    D. Paperwork should include the transferring and accepting physician names

16. **Which of the following statements is untrue regarding responses to post-traumatic stress disorder?**
    A. Patients are less likely to socialize
    B. Patients may have decreased ability to complete home or work tasks
    C. Patients may become irritable and hostile
    D. Patients may exhibit regressive behaviors

17. **Which of the following statements is true about post-traumatic stress disorder (PTSD)?**
    A. Only war veterans experience PTSD
    B. PTSD is easy to diagnose
    C. Multiple traumatic events heighten the risk of PTSD
    D. Patients become less aggressive

18. **A teenager was involved in a climbing accident and was severely injured. The parents just arrived in your ED and their daughter died only minutes prior to their arrival. Initially, the parents stay a little while in the ED waiting room. Both parents have a glazed expression while at their daughter's bedside. As a trauma nurse, you recognize their response as**
    A. Adaptation to the environment
    B. The initial steps to coping
    C. The initial response to a crisis
    D. Normal and does not need to be addressed

19. **When a person makes a conscious or unconscious attempt to disavow the meaning or even the knowledge of an event to reduce anxiety or fear, it is known as**
    A. Regression
    B. Coping
    C. Powerlessness
    D. Ineffective denial

20. **The useful organization and incorporation of both new and old data, experience, and emotional capacities into the personality is called**
    A. Introspection
    B. Solidarity
    C. Introversion
    D. Integration

21. **Patients who have schizophrenia sometimes exhibit opposition or resistance, either covertly or overtly, to outside suggestions or advice. This behavior is known as**
    A. Projection
    B. Negativism
    C. Manipulation
    D. Antagonism

22. **"An acute change in consciousness that is accompanied by inattention and either a change in cognition or perceptual disturbance" is the definition of**
    A. Post-concussion syndrome
    B. Dementia
    C. Delirium
    D. Severe depression

23. **Your patient was admitted to the ED after a barroom brawl in which he suffered multiple minor stab wounds. He is angry and verbally assaults the staff. The goal of anger management for this patient would not include**
    A. Confronting the patient directly with whatever made him angry
    B. Discussing what in particular made the patient angry
    C. Discussing with the patient alternative and positive ways to express his feelings
    D. Developing positive ways for the patient to express his feelings when confronted with frustrating situations in the future

24. **Your patient sustained a guillotine amputation of his right foot and will be going to the OR in about 10 minutes. The patient's vital signs are stable and he is totally cognizant of his surroundings and condition. The patient's family is quite agitated and does not agree with the patient's advance directives. The family informs you that they want everything done for the patient and to ignore the patient's request for no resuscitative measures. Which of the following nursing interventions would be appropriate at this time?**
    A. Inform the family that the physician will meet with them to discuss treatment options
    B. Tell the patient about the family's concerns
    C. Notify the physician that all orders are to come from the family
    D. Inform the family that the patient is fully capable of making decisions

25. **Your patient suffered a concussion. She is currently unable to recognize familiar faces. This symptom is not explained by defective visual acuity or reduced consciousness or alertness. Her condition is not uncommon and is known as**
    A. Symbolization
    B. Thought insertion
    C. Transference
    D. Prosopagnosia

26. **Which of the following patients are most likely to exhibit signs of PTSD?**
    A. A 13 year old runaway boy
    B. A 24 year old female who witnessed a murder
    C. A 37 year old man arrested for his first DUI
    D. A 64 year old lady who experienced a 3.5 earthquake

27. **As a part of your assessment of a patient experiencing PTSD, which of the following symptoms are most likely to occur?**
    A. Denial that anything is wrong
    B. Total recall of the event
    C. Duration of symptoms longer than 1 week
    D. Calm speech and organized thought process

28. **Your patient inhaled a large amount of cocaine. He is now complaining of paresthesias and "something small like little pieces of rock crawling under my skin." This condition is a type of psychosis and is known as**
    A. Magnan's sign
    B. Drummond's sign
    C. Cullen's sign
    D. Wilder's sign

29. Your patient suffered multiple lacerations and contusions after running his car into a building. The police brought him to the ED and have arrested him for multiple violations including possible DUI. You believe the patient is undergoing alcohol withdrawal and exhibits diplopia, peripheral neuropathy, confusion, recent memory loss, and hyperexcitability. You suspect that this patient is suffering from
    A. Jorn's syndrome
    B. Leucine deficiency
    C. Increased carnitine levels
    D. Wernicke-Korsakoff syndrome

30. A fellow nurse was fine during day shift. She did mention that she wanted to attend a concert the next night but had to work. When you return to work the next day, you find the nurse called in sick. The nurse's behavior is probably an example of
    A. Mental fatigue
    B. Malingering
    C. Schizophrenic language
    D. Depersonalization

31. Today, you have been assigned to the triage area. A patient, who appeared quite docile initially, complained of a sprained ankle and difficulty urinating. The patient was assisted to a gurney and then moved to a holding area. The patient was evaluated and treated by ED staff. About an hour after he arrived at the triage area, you heard yelling and loud noises emanating from the treatment area. When you entered the ED, the patient was crawling over the bedrails, the bed linens were a mess, the Foley catheter was lying on the floor, and the patient was visibly upset and swearing. This behavior was unexpected and disruptive. As a trauma nurse, you suspect this patient may be suffering from
    A. Dementia
    B. Hyperactive delirium
    C. An allergic reaction
    D. Severe metabolic acidosis

32. If your patient is seeking freedom from a sense of worthlessness and loneliness, the patient is at the _____ level of Maslow's Hierarchy of Needs.
    A. Self-actualization
    B. Esteem and recognition
    C. Love and belonging
    D. Safety and security

33. Individuals who are driven toward unacceptable behaviors and who redirect their energy into more socially acceptable behaviors are using a psychological defense mechanism called
    A. Resolution
    B. Compensation
    C. Repression
    D. Sublimation

34. The false belief that something is wrong with one's body or body part is called
    A. Malingering
    B. Hypochondriasis
    C. Transference
    D. Somatic delusion

35. The fear of crowds is known as
    A. Acrophobia
    B. Agoraphobia
    C. Arachnophobia
    D. Aschizophobia

36. **Your patient is explaining his medical history to you when he simply stops speaking and looks around the room. His behavior is known as**
    A. Rude
    B. Affect
    C. Blocking
    D. Amnesia

37. **Simultaneous existence of contradictory or contrasting emotions toward a person or object is known as**
    A. Apathy
    B. Double bind
    C. Depersonalization
    D. Ambivalence

38. **Your patient cut his forearm and requires several stitches. He begins to hallucinate when the resident is only midway through the procedure. The patient is demanding, loud, and very insistent. His behavior worsens and disrupts the staff. You could categorize this patient's behavior as**
    A. Paranoid
    B. Self-absorbed
    C. Deteriorating
    D. Overanxious

39. **A young woman was admitted to the ED for observation after fighting at a friend's house. She has a right fractured humerus, a right Colles' fracture, mild concussion, and right orbital fracture. When paramedics arrived, she was found talking to herself, resisted medical care, and stated she could heal herself. During your assessment, you find the patient withdrawn, irritable, fatigued, and indecisive about what to do with her clothing. Your next action should be to**
    A. Request a drug screen
    B. Request a psychologist evaluation for schizophrenia
    C. Request a social worker to assess the patient's home life
    D. Evaluate the patient for feelings of suicide

40. **A false perception that is not grounded in reality and not accounted for by external stimuli is called**
    A. A fugue
    B. A hallucination
    C. An idea of reference
    D. Disorientation

41. **Your patient is a college student and was admitted to your unit after ingesting about 50 extra-strength acetaminophen tablets. Until now he has refused to say why he ingested the drug. About an hour after arrival, you find him crying. When you ask him why he is crying, he tells you he was sexually assaulted by an unknown male 3 weeks ago, and he is afraid this will brand him a homosexual. Which of the following responses is the most therapeutic?**
    A. "Don't worry, you'll get over this and be okay"
    B. "Let me get the psychologist to come talk with you tomorrow"
    C. "Why do you believe this will make you a homosexual?"
    D. "What is wrong with being a homosexual?"

42. **Binge eating, mutilation, obesity, drug abuse, and alcoholism are all examples of**
    A. Self-destructive behavior
    B. Psychotic behavior
    C. Neurosis
    D. A fugue

43. As the educator for your emergency department, you note an increased frequency of patients with underlying mental disorders being admitted. You overhear some negative comments regarding nursing assignments for these patients. You ask the nurses to complete a self-awareness survey regarding their beliefs and understanding of mental health issues. You should use this information to
    A. Determine which nurses should never care for patients with mental health issues
    B. Change nursing assignments immediately
    C. Determine which nurses should be written up and counseled
    D. Create an education program for the nurses to increase understanding of mental health issues and learn how to access resources

44. Depression often devastates families and often goes undiagnosed and misunderstood by families, the public, and the medical community. Which of the following statements is also true regarding depression?
    A. Depression is only seen in maltreated individuals
    B. Depression is easy to diagnose
    C. The elderly do not respond to antidepressant therapy
    D. Depression is recurrent and may increase in severity

45. Your patient was admitted to the ED for lower abdominal pain. The patient stated she fell when trying to get off her bicycle. After appendicitis and significant injuries are ruled out, the physician decides to admit the patient for observation. The patient continues grimacing and will not allow you to assess her abdomen. Suddenly, the patient becomes combative, pulls her IV out, tears off her IV dressing, and starts screaming at the staff. As a trauma nurse, your next action should be to
    A. Apply restraints by yourself as additional staff may scare the patient
    B. Wear personal protective equipment to enter her treatment area to apply restraints
    C. Call security to help subdue the patient
    D. Use a Posey restraint system to subdue the patient

46. A model of health and illness that suggests that links among the nervous system, the immune system, behavioral styles, cognitive processing, and environmental factors can put people at risk for illness is called a(n)
    A. Integration model
    B. Centration model
    C. Synergy model
    D. Biopsychosocial model

47. Your staff in the emergency department unit has just completed an unsuccessful code on a college age woman. Due to an unexpected cardiac event, the patient did not survive. Chaplain services are called in to assist with a nursing staff debriefing. Staff members experiencing which of the following emotions are at highest risk for psychological stress?
    A. Anger
    B. Fear
    C. Anxiety
    D. Denial

48. Your patient is a gang member and heavy alcohol abuser. During a fight almost 24 hours ago, the patient was shot in the leg and hand. His gang members left him at the entrance to the ED with a note explaining the injuries sustained the previous night. You observe the patient thrashing around on the gurney, and he is suddenly awake when you walk by. The patient is shaking, has vomited, and is tachycardic, hypertensive, and talking to people not in the room. You suspect this patient is
    A. Exhibiting signs of paranoid schizophrenia
    B. Experiencing delirium tremens
    C. Experiencing sepsis
    D. Experiencing drug withdrawal

49. **The stage between normal forgetfulness due to aging and the development of dementia is called**
    A. Loss of problem solving
    B. Mild cognitive impairment
    C. Pre-Alzheimer's
    D. Delirium

50. **Getting lost on familiar routes, having difficulty balancing a checkbook, and misplacing items may be signs of**
    A. Delirium
    B. Dementia
    C. Depression
    D. Confusion

51. **A mood state characterized by pessimistic thinking, lowered self-esteem, sadness, and guilt is called**
    A. Fugue
    B. Delirium
    C. Withdrawal
    D. Depression

52. **Patients with post-traumatic stress disorder may experience recurrence of a memory, feeling, or perceptual experience from the past. This condition is known as a**
    A. Disintegration
    B. Euthymia
    C. Flashback
    D. Fantasy

53. **A key to prevention of excess mortality and morbidity in patients at risk for alcohol withdrawal is the appropriate use of an instrument designed to assess the level of risk for alcohol withdrawal. An example of an instrument to assess risk of alcohol withdrawal is the**
    A. Bevington scale
    B. P.O.L.A.R.I. scale
    C. AWSS scale
    D. CIWA-AR scale

54. **During discharge teaching, you notice multiple bruises on the arms and reddened areas on the neck of your patient's cousin. You suspect she is being physically abused. What other indicator would support your assessment?**
    A. Extroverted behavior
    B. Denial of abuse when asked directly
    C. She volunteers information
    D. Hesitance to discuss home situation

55. **You are caring for a patient who was the driver in a motor vehicle accident in which a child was killed. The patient is combative and restless, hyperventilating, tachycardic, and has an elevated blood pressure. She states, "I've got to leave here . . . they'll arrest me . . . they'll lock me up . . . I can't believe this . . . there is no way out." As a trauma nurse, you know the best therapeutic response should be**
    A. "They should arrest you, you killed a child"
    B. "Calm down. It wasn't your fault"
    C. "Stop it. You are working yourself up. Look at me and focus on what I am telling you to do"
    D. "Just relax. They can't arrest you because you are a patient here"

56. Your patient is the lone survivor of a car crash that killed her parents and two siblings. She is recovering from a pneumothorax, hemothorax, and a left fractured tibia. She has been extremely depressed and withdrawn. You are discussing medications, psychiatric therapy, and the increased risk of suicide and suicidal behavior with the patient's distant relatives. The family members make each of the following statements. Which of the statements is false?

    A. "If she is considering suicide, she will make statements or give warnings of suicide"
    B. "We should trust our instincts if we feel she is in danger"
    C. "As she recovers from her depression, she is at greater risk of suicide"
    D. "If she talks about suicide or asks about pills, then she is just voicing the thought and will not attempt suicide"

57. Your patient is experiencing delirium tremens. Nursing interventions include keeping the room well lit and minimizing stimulation. Staff members continuously reorient the patient to time, place, and person. Haldol has been given as ordered, and the patient is in four-point restraints. Which of these nursing interventions should be discontinued?

    A. Reorientation
    B. Medication administration
    C. Restraints
    D. Controlling stimulation

58. Your patient is a young woman with diffuse abdominal pain and confusion. Just after admission, she had generalized seizures and bradycardia. Opioid overdose was suspected and she was given naloxone with only minimal effect. The patient is now lethargic, but does tell you she is a "body packer" to help pay for beauty school. She soon becomes hypotensive and bradycardic. Appropriate therapy includes

    A. Bowel irrigations, intubation, mechanical ventilation, anticonvulsants
    B. Sodium bicarbonate activated charcoal, hemodialysis
    C. Antiemetics, gastric lavage, bronchodilators
    D. Activated charcoal, sodium bicarbonate, vasopressors

59. Excessive motor activity that accompanies and is associated with a feeling of inner tension and is usually nonproductive and repetitious is called

    A. Displacement
    B. Idiosyncratic
    C. Lability
    D. Agitation

60. Your patient has dementia. The physician places a pen in the patient's hand while the patient has his/her eyes closed. The patient is unable to recognize the object as a pen. This failure to recognize objects despite intact sensory function is known as

    A. Cognition
    B. Conversion
    C. Displacement
    D. Agnosia

61. A patient undergoing an assessment for an ear injury becomes agitated because his friend was not allowed to accompany him to the treatment area. Despite reassurances that the exam will not take long, the patient throws a chair into the wall and begins disconnecting the suction and oxygen apparatus from the wall. Your first priority is to

    A. Call a code
    B. Be firm and establish clear limits on behavior
    C. Leave the room
    D. Sedate the patient

62. When a patient experiences a subjective human response to a perceived or actual threat, the range of response may vary from vague discomfort to panic and loss of control. This response is known as
    A. Transference
    B. Anxiety
    C. Internal loss of control
    D. A defense mechanism

63. The word used to describe observable behavior that represents the expression of a subjectively experienced feeling state (emotion) is known as
    A. Lability
    B. Affect
    C. Constricted
    D. Blunt

64. Patients with dementia often lose their ability to taste. An inability to taste is known as
    A. Dysgeusia
    B. Dysgnathia
    C. Micrognathia
    D. Macrognathia

65. The useful organization and incorporation of both new and old data, experience, and emotional capacities into the personality is called
    A. Introspection
    B. Solidarity
    C. Introversion
    D. Integration

66. Which of the following statements is true regarding physical collection of evidence during care of a sexually assaulted patient?
    A. Gloves should be changed when handling any new piece of evidence or with each new specimen collection
    B. The examiner may leave the room as often as needed to obtain supplies needed in assessment and care
    C. During vaginal assessment with a speculum, use water-based gel to prevent additional vaginal injury
    D. Only the examiner should remove patient clothing to preserve evidence

SECTION 7: ANSWERS

1. **Correct answer: A**

   No drug has been approved by the FDA to treat delirium. "An acute change in consciousness that is accompanied by inattention and either a change in cognition or perceptual disturbance" is the definition of delirium defined by the American Psychiatric Association.

   The Society of Critical Care Medicine (SCCM) believes that the first step in delirium management is to identify the causes of delirium. They have developed a mnemonic called THIINK to help determine the cause of delirium in a patient. The letter H in this mnemonic means hypoxemia. The mnemonic was designed for ICU patients but is applicable to the emergency department. This mnemonic will not be on the TCRN exam. Having said that, much emphasis is now placed on the identification and care of the patient with delirium. It is best to be over-prepared rather than underprepared.

   The THIINK mnemonic follows:

   Toxic situations: CHF, shock, dehydration deliriogenic meds (tight titration of sedatives).

   Hypoxemia

   Infection/sepsis (nosocomial)

   Immobilization

   New organ failure

   (e.g., liver, Kidney)

   Although there is no universally accepted core model of care for patients with delirium, The American Association of Critical Care Nurses (AACN) has adopted the ABCDE bundle. This core model is a mix of evidence-based practice strategies that can be incorporated into daily patient care. The purpose is to systematically reduce modifiable risk factors and improve patient outcomes. The letters A, B, C, D, and E mean Awakening and Breathing trial coordination, Choice of sedative, Delirium Detection, early progressive mobility, and Exercise

   If you read the research presented on the AACN website, it will be clear that although multiple studies have been done on patients, there is no clear consensus as to a medication regimen. It is believed that 65% of patients with delirium go undetected; the exact number of patients is unknown. The lack of detection is believed to be partly due to a lack of a standardized assessment tool. Two tools that have the highest degree of validity are the Confusion Assessment Method for the ICU (CAM-ICU) and the Intensive Care Delirium Screening Checklist (ICDSC). We suggest visiting the AACN website at *www.aacn.org/WD/practice/docs/practicealerts/delirium-practice-alert-2011.pdf* to read about delirium assessment and management.

2. **Correct answer: D**

   An advanced directive that does not exclude pain relief or comfort measures is an Allow Natural Death order or a DNR written with specific life-saving measures

3. **Correct answer: C**

   An out-of-hospital DNR represents informed consent. This type of consent requires a signature of the HCP as well as the patient/surrogate. This type of consent directs EMS to reserve cardiac/respiratory arrest resuscitation but may still provide assessment, assistance for choking, aggressive pain management, and grief counseling.

4. **Correct answer: C**

   Transplantable tissue would include bone, cornea, middle ear, heart valves, ligaments, tendons, bone marrow, and pancreatic islet cells. The other choices are organs, not tissue.

5. **Correct answer: A**

   If a patient will be an eye donor, use paper tape to keep eyes closed, instill artificial tears, keep the HOB elevated 20 degrees, try to prevent swelling with cool compresses over eyes, and attempt to refrigerate the patient when possible.

6. **Correct answer: D**

   Supporting and respecting the culture, beliefs, and values of the trauma patient is known as advocacy.

7. **Correct answer: B**

   Continuing the use of air splints is an inappropriate action prior to preparing a critical patient for air transport. With altitude change, the air expands leading to the rupture of the device, further injury, or compartment syndrome.

8. **Correct answer: C**

   Chain of custody is protecting the viability of evidence for court purposes by removing doubt of tampering. Other duties of the forensic nursing practice include evidence collection, as well as evidence preservation.

9. **Correct answer: B**

   When a patient's injuries are linked to a crime, it is important to not wash the patient's hands, and cover the patient's hands with paper bags. This preserves evidence for law enforcement. If clothing is thick and difficult to cut, do not use entry points to begin removal of clothing, and cut away from potential areas of evidence. Use diagrams and photos with measurement devices that lay near the wound for documentation instead of writing on the patient's skin as this will tamper with evidence. Any and all clothing, including scraps of material, should be handled as little as possible and placed in a secure container as part of the chain of custody.

10. **Correct answer: A**

    The generally accepted legal next of kin order for the determination of patient wishes is agent, spouse, adult child, then parent. Death and organ donation can be a very difficult conversation. For this scenario, the family states that their son has no living will or advanced directive. The brother states that during a party, the patient said that he would be a donor. Unfortunately, as a trauma nurse, you know that hearsay cannot be recognized as the legal granting of consent for organ donation.

11. **Correct answer: D**

    The definition of palliative care in the United States as described by both the US Department of Health and Human Services (HHS) Centers for Medicare and Medicaid Services (CMS) and the National Quality Forum (NQF) states, "Palliative care means patient and family-centered care that optimizes quality of life by anticipating, preventing, and treating suffering." Palliative care throughout the continuum of illness involves addressing physical, intellectual, emotional, social, and spiritual needs and to facilitate patient autonomy, access to information, or both.

12. **Correct Answer: D**

    When considering adding additional medications or treatments to the care of a patient receiving palliative care, it is important to assess the current medications for the ability to stop medication(s) prior to adding new medications or treatments. A current medication may be causing symptoms that are contributing to the patient's suffering. Halting a current medication or treatment may relieve the symptoms without the addition of new pharmacologic intervention. With any new medication, even if previously taken, the patient should always be monitored for reaction, adverse effects, and if the medication is acting as expected and there are no interactions with other medications or treatments. Involvement of a pharmacist as part of the palliative care team would be crucial for identifying medication interactions prior to administration and may be able to suggest alternates that would be a better choice to meet overall treatment goals. The overall goals of the treatment team, including patient wishes, should be taken into account prior to starting any new medications or treatments. Only evaluating the goals of one element of the palliative care team may exclude critical core goals and exceed patient threshold for intervention (Palliative Care Pocket Consultant, Ohio).

13. **Correct Answer: C**

    Although this patient has several disease-related complications that are causing him distress such as dyspnea, cough, constipation, and emesis, the patient focuses on a shake flavor as his major complaint. Our first instinct is to fix the disease processes, but by addressing the patient's priority, you may relieve unnecessary stress on the patient and provide a source of nutrition and hydration the patient may tolerate without emesis, which would relieve constipation symptoms. The patient's report of priority of symptoms should be considered the gold standard for prioritizing interventions with palliative and hospice care. Patient prioritization should supersede the healthcare provider's prioritization. Breathing treatments, cough suppressant, and stool softeners may aid in comforting the patient, but should be prioritized based on the overall treatment goals.

14. **Correct Answer: C**

The National Consensus Project for Quality Palliative Care states, "palliative care means patient and family-centered care that optimizes quality of life by anticipating, preventing, and treating suffering." Core values that support palliative care include collaboration and communication between patients, families, palliative and non-palliative healthcare providers, care is coordinated by an interdisciplinary team, care is concurrent or independent of curative or life-prolonging care, and patient peace and dignity are supported throughout the course of illness, during the dying process, and after death.

15. **Correct answer: A**

Responsibility of care for the patient when making an intrahospital transfer rests on the sending facility until the patient arrives at the receiving facility.

16. **Correct answer: B**

Patients with PTSD may have diminished concentration and are unable to concentrate on home or work tasks. Patients often regress, have increased anxiety, become aggressive, suffer panic attacks, avoid family, and reenact the event frequently. Patients with PTSD are more likely to attempt suicide than their peers without PTSD.

17. **Correct answer: C**

Post-traumatic stress disorder may result in many different symptoms. If the patient experiences multiple traumatic events, the risk for developing PTSD increases. Additional causes of PTSD can include physical or sexual abuse, neglect, harassment, death of a significant other, accidents, war, terrorist attacks, disasters, or life-threatening illnesses/injuries. PTSD may also be caused by witnessed domestic violence, suicide, or murder.

If the patient experiences multiple traumatic events, the risk for developing PTSD increases. Additional causes of PTSD can include physical or sexual abuse, neglect, harassment, death of a significant other, accidents, war, terrorist attacks, disasters, or life-threatening illnesses/injuries. PTSD may also be caused by witnessed domestic violence, suicide, or murder.

Patients with PTSD may have diminished concentration and are unable to concentrate on home or work tasks. Patients often regress, have increased anxiety, become aggressive, suffer panic attacks, avoid family, and reenact the event frequently. Patients with PTSD are more likely to attempt suicide than their peers without PTSD.

Denial is often seen in people with PTSD. Most people with PTSD will have trouble recalling the event and even omit significant details. Other symptoms include avoidance of people and places that remind them of the traumatic event; flattened affect, flashbacks, nightmares, and hallucinations may also occur. Symptoms must last more than a month to establish PTSD.

18. **Correct answer: C**

A teenager was involved in a climbing accident and was severely injured. The parents just arrived in your ED and their daughter died only minutes prior to their arrival. Initially, the parents stayed a little while in the ED waiting room. Both parents have a glazed expression while at their daughter's bedside. As a trauma nurse, you know the death of their daughter is causing the parents to experience the initial response to a crisis. The death was not expected and now involves environment and circumstances beyond the parents' experience or ability to cope. The crisis may last for weeks depending on available support systems, the healthcare team, parent education, culture, and spiritual intervention.

19. **Correct answer: D**

Ineffective denial is a nursing diagnosis accepted by the North American Nursing Diagnosis Association defined as denial that is detrimental to health when a person makes a conscious or unconscious attempt to disavow the meaning or even the knowledge of an event to reduce anxiety or fear.

20. **Correct answer: D**

The useful organization and incorporation of both new and old data, experience, and emotional capacities into the personality is called integration.

21. **Correct answer: B**

   Patients who have schizophrenia sometimes exhibit opposition or resistance, either covertly or overtly, to outside suggestions or advice. This behavior is known as negativism.

22. **Correct answer: C**

   "An acute change in consciousness that is accompanied by inattention and either a change in cognition or perceptual disturbance" is the definition of delirium defined by the American Psychiatric Association.

23. **Correct answer: A**

   Your patient was admitted to the ED after a barroom brawl in which he suffered multiple minor stab wounds. He is angry and verbally assaults the staff. As a trauma nurse, you know the goal of anger management for this patient would not include confronting the patient directly with whatever made him angry. Direct confrontation with the object of anger may further exacerbate the situation and limit the person's ability to deal positively with the situation. Instead, engage the person in a conversation regarding the stressor and assist him in identifying feelings and options.

24. **Correct answer: D**

   Sometimes family members do not have enough education to make proper decisions. In this case, the family needs to know that the patient is still capable of making decisions and that his wishes will be honored.

25. **Correct answer: D**

   Your patient suffered a concussion. She is currently unable to recognize familiar faces. This symptom is not explained by defective visual acuity or reduced consciousness or alertness. Her condition is called prosopagnosia and often resolves when the brain injury heals.

26. **Correct answer: B**

   The 24 year old female who witnessed a murder is at a high risk for development of PTSD. Any person who witnesses an intense event is at risk for PTSD. The symptoms may last months or even years. Other factors that influence how the person responds include their mental state at the time of the event, the intensity of the event, and any medical complications.

27. **Correct answer: A**

   Denial is often seen in people with post-traumatic stress disorder (PTSD). Most people with PTSD will have trouble recalling the event and even omit significant details. Other symptoms include avoidance of people and places that remind them of the traumatic event; flattened affect, flashbacks, nightmares, and hallucinations may also occur. Symptoms must last more than a month to establish PTSD.

28. **Correct answer: B**

   Your patient inhaled a large amount of cocaine. He is now complaining of paresthesias and "something small like little pieces of rock crawling under my skin." This condition is a type of psychosis and is known as Drummond's sign. As a trauma nurse, you know cocaine users have paresthesias, psychoses, and imagine they have a foreign body, in the shape of a powder or fine sand, under the skin that it is constantly changing its position.

29. **Correct answer: D**

   The patient undergoing alcohol withdrawal and who exhibits diplopia, peripheral neuropathy, confusion, recent memory loss, and hyperexcitability has exhibited symptoms of Wernicke-Korsakoff syndrome. Wernicke-Korsakoff syndrome is a thiamine deficiency and a metabolic encephalopathy.

30. **Correct answer: B**

   A fellow nurse was fine during day shift. She did mention that she wanted to attend a concert the next night but had to work. When you return to work the next day, you find the nurse called in sick. The nurse's behavior is probably an example of malingering. Claiming symptoms of illness or injury with intent to deceive in order to obtain a goal, for example, a claim of physical illness to avoid working, is known as malingering.

31. Correct answer: B

Today, you were assigned to the triage area. A patient, who appeared quite docile initially, complained of a sprained ankle and difficulty urinating. The patient was assisted to a gurney and then moved to a holding area. The patient was evaluated and treated by ED staff. About an hour after he arrived at the triage area, you heard yelling and loud noises emanating from the treatment area. When you entered the ED, the patient was crawling over the bedrails, the bed linens were a mess, the Foley catheter was lying on the floor, and the patient was visibly upset and swearing. As a trauma nurse, you suspect this patient is suffering from hyperactive delirium. This behavior is frequently associated with hyperactive delirium. Remember that a patient may also demonstrate hypoactive delirium (decreased responsiveness, a flat affect, withdrawal, lethargic, and apathetic).

32. Correct answer: B

If your patient is seeking freedom from a sense of worthlessness and loneliness, the patient is at the esteem and recognition level of Maslow's Hierarchy of Needs.

33. Correct answer: D

Individuals who are driven toward unacceptable behaviors and who redirect their energy into more socially acceptable behaviors are using a psychological defense mechanism called sublimation.

34. Correct answer: D

The false belief that something is wrong with one's body or body part is called somatic delusion. Malingering is the deliberate manufacturing of an illness to prolong treatment. Hypochondriasis is morbid concern with one's body or health in the absence of a physical cause.

35. Correct answer: B

The fear of crowds is known as agoraphobia. A phobia is a fear or dread of an act, an object, or a situation that is usually not realistically dangerous. However, the patient perceives that danger exists.

36. Correct answer: C

When a patient simply stops talking and there is a gap or interruption in speech that is related to absent thoughts or distractions, it is known as blocking.

37. Correct answer: D

Simultaneous existence of contradictory or contrasting emotions toward a person or object is known as ambivalence.

38. Correct answer: C

Because this patient's behavior is escalating, the correct categorization of the behavior is "deteriorating." The patient may be exhibiting some paranoid tendencies, but the cause of the hallucinations is unknown at this time.

39. Correct answer: D

You should first evaluate the patient's feelings, paying close attention to any statements indicating a risk for suicide or injury to staff. The patient is now exhibiting signs of depression after a manic episode. Patients with psychotic elements exhibited with mania, depression, or both may be misdiagnosed with schizophrenia, anxiety disorder, and/or drug abuse. Patients with bipolar disorder may swing between moods over minutes, hours, or days. Symptoms include hallucinations, delusions, and aggressive or violent behavior. Careful history may reveal a trend of manic and depressive episodes that would clarify the patient's true condition and lead to faster and correct treatment. A social worker should be involved, but ensuring immediate patient and staff safety is the primary concern.

40. Correct answer: B

A false perception that is not grounded in reality and not accounted for by external stimuli is called a hallucination.

41. Correct answer: C

This patient has opened up to you, and it is important to maintain the communication. Finding out why he feels homosexuality is bad gives insight to the suicide attempt. There are many other legal and ethical issues that must be addressed with this case. It is obvious the patient will need psychological counseling. After your conversation, you must follow your hospital's policy/procedure manual about reporting such incidents. "Don't worry, you'll get over this and be okay" and "Let me get the psychologist to come talk with you tomorrow" are not therapeutic, and they negate his feelings. Asking, "What is wrong with being a homosexual?" could be perceived as threatening.

42. **Correct answer: A**

Binge eating, mutilation, obesity, drug abuse, and alcoholism are all examples of self-destructive behavior. Self-destructive behaviors are those that over time will shorten or threaten length and quality of life.

43. **Correct answer: D**

You ask the nurses to complete a self-awareness survey regarding their beliefs and understanding of mental health issues. You should use this information to create an education program for the nurses to increase understanding of mental health issues and learn how to access resources. Surveys can be used to anonymously identify staff perceptions and determine educational opportunities. Mental health issues impact every person at some point in their lives. Whether due to a catastrophic event or ongoing psychological issues, it is important that nurses understand their own biases regarding mental health and be able to identify resources when caring for this population. If the nurses believe the survey will be used punitively, then data may be skewed to what the staff believe the surveyor is looking for, not the truth. Instead of changing assignments immediately, it is best to use the opportunity for education and professional growth.

44. **Correct answer: D**

Depression is recurrent and may increase in severity. Many cases report that after the first depressive episode, as many as 40% of individuals will experience another episode within 2 years. Often, these patients are diagnosed with multiple psychiatric disorders such as anxiety disorder, dysthymic disorders, disruptive behavior, or substance abuse. Depression may be seen in any patient, although environmental factors such as maltreatment can contribute to risk of depression. A patient with chronic illness, infection, or certain biochemical factors is also at risk for depression. Depression is difficult to diagnose unless there is an understanding of depression and risk factors. Unfortunately, depression can be just as severe in children and teens as in adults and is associated with approximately 80% of childhood and teen suicides. Undiagnosed and untreated depression can continue into adulthood impacting personal and professional relationships and the ability to function successfully in society.

45. **Correct answer: B**

When entering this patient's room or any patient's room to apply restraints, wear appropriate personal protective equipment to protect yourself against exposure to bodily fluids. The patient most likely has had a psychotic reaction and has exposed her IV site and removed her IV, resulting in a potential for exposure to bodily fluids. When attempting to place restraints on a combative patient, regardless of the age, at least four staff members should be present—one for each limb. The family should not be asked to participate in placement of the restraints as they are untrained and it may be seen as betraying the patient. Instead, family members should remain at a safe distance to avoid injury or interference with healthcare providers. A Posey is not the best choice because it leaves the patient's hands free to continue pulling on IV lines. Whenever restraints are in use, be vigilant to document continued need of restraints, type used, time placed, vital signs including airway, breathing, and circulation before and after restraints are placed, time of removal, and reassessments. Be sure to follow your facility's restraint protocols and policies. Patient and staff safety is paramount.

46. **Correct answer: D**

A model of health and illness that suggests that links among the nervous system, the immune system, behavioral styles, cognitive processing, and environmental factors can put people at risk for illness is called a biopsychosocial model.

47. **Correct answer: C**

Anger, fear, and denial are normal emotions in this situation, but staff members that feel anxiety are at the greatest risk. Anxiety is a common emotion found in psychological emergencies. Anxiety involves uncertainty of the unknown and may limit the person's ability to identify resources or initiate appropriate coping mechanisms. Debriefings after codes, both successful and unsuccessful, are therapeutic and allow staff to verbalize emotions in a safe and stable environment. As a team, the staff may identify ways to support families and each other during crisis and emergency situations.

48. **Correct answer: B**

Your patient is a gang member and heavy alcohol abuser. During a fight almost 24 hours ago, the patient was shot in the leg and hand. His gang members left him at the entrance to the ED with a note explaining the injuries sustained the previous night. You observe the patient thrashing around in the gurney, and he is suddenly awake when you walk by. He is shaking, has vomited, and is tachycardic, hypertensive, and talking to people not in the room. You suspect the patient is experiencing delirium tremens.

The timing of this patient's symptoms is consistent with alcohol withdrawal or delirium tremens (DTs). DTs usually are seen 12–24 hours after the last ingestion of alcohol as blood-alcohol levels drop. Effects may peak up to 15 days after DTs begin. Fluids, vitamins, nutrition, and short-term pharmacologic treatments are appropriate. The severity of symptoms is affected by the amount and duration of alcohol ingestion as well as underlying physical health, other drugs, and existing psychological status. There are no indications at this time that the patient is septic or has schizophrenia. There may be underlying drug withdrawal symptoms.

49. **Correct answer: B**

The stage between normal forgetfulness due to aging and the development of dementia is called mild cognitive impairment (MCI). People with MCI have mild problems with thinking and memory that do not interfere with everyday activities. They are often aware of the forgetfulness. Not everyone with MCI develops dementia.

Symptoms of MCI include:

- Difficulty performing more than one task at a time
- Difficulty solving problems or making decisions
- Forgetting recent events or conversations
- Taking longer to perform more difficult mental activities

50. **Correct answer: B**

Getting lost on familiar routes, having difficulty balancing a checkbook, and misplacing items may be signs of dementia. Additional early signs of dementia are inability to learn new information or routines, losing interest in things previously enjoyed, personality changes, and loss of social skills.

51. **Correct answer: D**

A mood state characterized by pessimistic thinking, lowered self-esteem, sadness, and guilt is called depression.

52. **Correct answer: C**

Patients with post-traumatic stress disorder may experience recurrence of a memory, feeling, or perceptual experience from the past. This condition is known as a flashback.

53. **Correct answer: D**

An example of an instrument to assess risk of alcohol withdrawal is the Clinical Institute Withdrawal Assessment of Alcohol Scale, Revised (CIWA-Ar). The CIWA-Ar measures 10 symptoms. Mild withdrawal is indicated by a score of less than 8. Autonomic arousal (moderate) withdrawal is indicated by a score between 8 and 15. Scores of 15 or more indicate impending delirium tremens. Appropriate use of this scale helps staff individualize and modify treatment regimens as needed. The CIWA-Ar categories and ranges are as follows:

- Agitation (0–7)
- Anxiety (0–7)
- Auditory disturbances (0–7)
- Clouding of sensorium (0–4)

- Headache (0–7)
- Nausea/Vomiting (0–7)
- Paroxysmal sweats (0–7)
- Tactile disturbances (0–7)
- Tremor (0–7)
- Visual disturbances (0–7)

54. **Correct answer: B**

Abuse may be suspected if the cousin denies abuse in the presence of bruising, injury to bones, and ecchymosis around the throat. Many abused women and children have stories of a positive home life and excuses to explain injuries due to clumsiness. Due to the likely introverted personalities of abused individuals, it is important to establish a safe zone and trust to encourage honest communication and to begin assistance to escape the abuse.

55. **Correct answer: C**

The goal at this point is to regulate the patient's breathing and stabilize vital signs. Using a firm and quiet voice with simple sentences can help the severely anxious patient focus and diffuse the anxiety. Severely anxious individuals are less able to see options and cope at this stage. Goals should include decreasing any unnecessary stress and remaining available to the patient for communication. The statement, "Calm down. It wasn't your fault" speaks to facts not known. Statements like, "They should arrest you, you killed a child" are judgmental.

56. **Correct answer: D**

"If she talks about suicide or asks about pills, then she is just voicing the thought and will not attempt suicide" is not an accurate statement. Careful consideration and observation should be given to any person voicing any thought or plan regarding suicide. Many individuals will provide warnings about their suicidal thoughts, thereby providing those in the family or in proximity the opportunity to intervene. Such warnings are often cries for help and intervention. Family members should pay close attention to any impression or instinct that the person is considering suicide. As individuals enter and exit depression, they are at greatest risk for suicide as they have sufficient mental focus to form a plan and energy or motivation to carry it out.

57. **Correct answer: C**

Restraints should only be used if alternative methods for behavioral correction are ineffective. There is no indication that the patient is violent or has caused any threat to staff or self. Restraints should only be used as a last resort to prevent injury to self and staff. Reorientation, medication, and controlling external stimulation are all effective methods for controlling behavior.

58. **Correct answer: A**

Body packer is a term used for people who transport narcotics in body cavities. In this case, it is probable that a packet may have ruptured. Bowel irrigations, intubation, mechanical ventilation, and anticonvulsants may be required as treatments for this patient. More doses of naloxone may be necessary, along with supportive treatment for opioid overdose. Be alert for bradycardia, hypotension, respiratory depression, and hypothermia.

59. **Correct answer: D**

Excessive motor activity that accompanies and is associated with a feeling of inner tension and is usually nonproductive and repetitious is called agitation. As nurses, we observe agitation frequently in patients who fidget, wring their hands, pull on clothes or bedding, and who are unable to lie or sit still.

60. **Correct answer: D**

The failure to recognize objects despite intact sensory function is known as agnosia and is often seen in patients with dementia.

61. **Correct answer: B**

This patient is acting out his frustration. It is important to act immediately to set firm clear goals and limits to behavior. It is crucial you remain with the patient until he calms down, then attempt to discuss his feelings. Obviously, if you believe you or the patient is in imminent danger, call for help.

62. **Correct answer: B**

When a patient experiences a subjective human response to a perceived or actual threat, the range of response may vary from vague discomfort to panic and loss of control. This response is known as anxiety. When anxiety levels increase, the patient feels the physiologic effects from sympathetic nervous system stimulation. After the initial excitement, patients often experience a decrease in coping skills and problem-solving ability, and a narrowed perceptual field.

63. **Correct answer: B**

The word is used to describe observable behavior that represents the expression of a subjectively experienced feeling state (emotion) is known as affect.

64. **Correct answer: A**

Patients with dementia often lose their ability to taste. An inability to taste is known as dysgeusia.

65. **Correct answer: D**

The useful organization and incorporation of both new and old data, experience, and emotional capacities into the personality is called integration.

66. **Correct answer: A**

When collecting physical evidence during care of a sexually assaulted patient, gloves should be changed when handling any new piece of evidence or with each new specimen collection to prevent cross-contamination. Before beginning the examination, ensure that all necessary equipment is available in the room because the examiner may not leave the room once the examination begins. If an examiner leaves the room, the chain of custody will be broken, impairing future litigation. The patient should be allowed to remove clothing as able. Use a clean sheet on the floor to recover any soil or debris dropped from clothing during removal. Photos should be taken before removal of clothing and serially when performing the assessment. During the vaginal assessment with a speculum, tap water, not gels or lubricants, should be used. Gels and lubricants may alter sperm and dilute specimen collection.

SECTION 8

Professional Issues

- Disaster Management
- Ethical Issues
- Regulations and Standards
- Trauma Quality Management

SECTION 8: QUESTIONS

1. **The ethical principle that guides nurses to "Do No Harm" means**
   A. Beneficence
   B. Justice
   C. Non-malfeasance
   D. Paternalism

2. **Taking a positive action with compassion to help a patient is an example of**
   A. Utilitarianism
   B. Paternalism
   C. Justice
   D. Beneficence

3. **Being truthful with patients as well as honest, fair, dedicated, and loyal to our patients is a definition of**
   A. Justice
   B. Fidelity
   C. Paternalism
   D. Utilitarianism

4. **As a trauma nurse, you are assisting at a train derailment with at least 40 victims. As you enter the triage area, you note four patients who have been marked with yellow tags. Patients with this designation**
   A. Do not require medical attention
   B. Need immediate intervention
   C. Are deceased
   D. Are considered walking wounded

5. **A disaster victim who requires immediate intervention and transport, treatment within minutes (up to 60), and has injuries compromising his or her respiratory status is classified by which of the following colors during triage?**
   A. Yellow
   B. Black
   C. Green
   D. Red

6. **The Centers for Disease Control and Prevention (CDC) has defined biologic agents that may be used as weapons based on ease of dissemination and ease of transmission. Which of the following statements is not a concept considered by the CDC as a threat for a biologic agent that may be used as a weapon.**
   A. The threat of high mortality and public health impact
   B. Potential for panic and social disruption
   C. Requirements for public health preparedness
   D. Disruption of the electrical grid

7. **A foundation of disaster management to reduce loss of life and property from natural or manmade disasters, limiting or avoiding potential impact, as well as incorporating lessons learned from previous events is the definition of**
   A. FEMA
   B. Mitigation
   C. Triage
   D. Incident management

8. **When performing a secondary performance improvement review,**
   A. Real-time patient care cannot be affected
   B. Outcomes are improved because immediate changes can occur in the plan of care
   C. Outcome data is not immediately available
   D. Feedback to providers is immediate

9. **The goal of disaster management is**
   A. To reduce the number of deaths within the first week following a disaster
   B. To do the most good for the greatest number of people
   C. Making certain supplies are always available and stored within ten miles of a potential event
   D. Development of disaster triage plans

10. **After a disaster, or any incident that creates stress for those involved, it is critical that time is allotted for care providers' psychological health. An eight-step formal process that takes place 1–14 days after the event is known as**
    A. Critical Incident Stress Management class
    B. Defusing
    C. Resolution
    D. Debriefing

11. **Many times nurses experience conflicts when asked to assist patients with decision making. The obligation to assist the patient in making a decision when the patient does not have sufficient data or expertise is called**
    A. Paternalism
    B. Moral agency
    C. Interdependence
    D. Assumptive thinking

12. **In healthcare, actions are right or wrong based on a set of rules and morals. This ethical approach is known as**
    A. Social contract theory
    B. Deontology
    C. Moral agency
    D. Natural law

13. **Evidence to the public that a nurse meets established standards of quality and patient safety is provided by**
    A. The Nurse Practice Act
    B. Institutional policies
    C. Innovation and clinical inquiry
    D. Certification

14. **Which of the following elements would not be necessary to establish in order to determine malpractice?**
    A. Injury
    B. Breach of duty
    C. Physician relation
    D. Duty of care

15. **An important element of evidence-based practice is the evaluation of research and application of findings. Research is conducted using the**
    A. Empiric method
    B. Standardized method
    C. Sample method
    D. T-test method

16. **A statistical variable**
    A. Represents the possible outcomes
    B. Is an estimate generated from a sample
    C. Is a measured characteristic of a population
    D. Is the manipulated or changing characteristic being measured

17. **The clinical nurse specialist is discussing types of data that is collected. Which of the following represents qualitative data?**
    A. Blood pressure
    B. Temperature
    C. Pain level
    D. Pulse rate

18. **Which of the following is a true statement regarding variables?**
    A. The independent variable is the fixed variable and cannot be manipulated
    B. The dependent variable is a fixed variable and cannot be changed
    C. The dependent variable is the measured outcome or effect
    D. The independent variable is the studied outcome

19. **A researcher is discussing the type of data that will be collected during a study in the trauma bay. Initially, the research team wants to focus on categorical data. You know that which of the following is an example of categorical data.**
    A. Ethnicity
    B. Age
    C. Height
    D. Weight

20. **Which of the following levels of measurement is the lowest level?**
    A. Interval
    B. Nominal
    C. Ordinal
    D. Ratio

21. **You are collecting data from parents regarding car seat use. You ask if the parents always use a car seat, yes or no. This is an example of**
    A. Interval data
    B. Quantitative data collection
    C. Dependent variable
    D. Nominal data

22. **Every state has its own nurse practice act that determines qualifications into professional nursing. Nurse practice acts were not originated to**
    A. Set standards for nursing
    B. Protect the public
    C. Allow for disciplinary action
    D. Allow for an unlimited practice of nursing

23. **According to the Health Insurance Portability and Accountability Act of 1996 (HIPAA), individuals are not entitled to**
    A. Devise policies and procedures that address privacy
    B. Authorize use of personal medical records
    C. Access personal medical records (with an option to amend the record)
    D. Object to or restrict the use of personal medical records

24. **The law that was instituted to prevent "dumping" of patients unable to pay for medical treatment is known as?**
    A. HIPAA
    B. TRIAGE
    C. EMTALA
    D. TALAEM

25. **Under EMTALA guidelines, any individual presenting to an ED requesting treatment must be provided appropriate, stabilizing treatment for medical conditions including active labor within the capability of the ED. If the hospital is in violation, it may be subject to fines, loss of Medicare provider status, and civil litigation. A potential violation would include**
    A. The transferring facility must arrange appropriate transportation, ensure trained personnel and life-support equipment is available
    B. Obtaining written informed consent from the patient or patient's representative prior to transport to another facility
    C. Verifying the receiving facility has available space and qualified personnel
    D. Failure of the sending facility to verify acceptance by the receiving physician prior to transport

26. **The type of consent that involves an oral or written agreement to treatment, assessment, evaluation, medications, X-ray films, and laboratory studies is known as**
    A. Expressed consent
    B. Implied consent
    C. Involuntary consent
    D. Informed consent

27. **A nurse in the bay next to yours is thrown back across the room after she attempted to plug in a piece of equipment. After providing emergency medical care for electrocution, the supervisor asks you to complete an incident report. Which of the following statements is true regarding documenting an incident report?**
    A. Never refer to the existence of an incident report in the treated nurse's chart
    B. Draw conclusions about the portions of the event you did not witness
    C. State liability clearly in the document
    D. Refer to multiple biomedical repair requests concerning the equipment involved

28. **Your town has just endured multiple tornado touchdowns and a large storm. Multiple patients begin arriving in your emergency department. Which approach to triage during this mass casualty event would be appropriate?**
    A. Comprehensive triage
    B. Adult initial assessment
    C. Level 5 triage
    D. Simple triage

29. **What is the incubation period for inhalation anthrax?**
    A. 7–10 days
    B. 5–7 days
    C. 7–60 days
    D. 20–30 days

30. **What are the initial symptoms for inhaled anthrax?**
    A. Mild, flu-like symptoms
    B. Severe dyspnea and productive cough
    C. High fever, cough, and stridor
    D. Cutaneous lesions, cough, and high fever

31. **Your hospital is put on an external disaster notice after a ricin poisoning incident at a local train station. Your ED prepares to accept casualties. What makes ricin so toxic to humans?**
    A. Ricin causes respiratory failure
    B. Ricin causes renal failure
    C. Ricin inhibits protein synthesis, leading to cell death
    D. Ricin destroys the mitochondria in the cell, causing cell death

32. **Your patient works at a fast-food restaurant. She found an envelope that was torn and had white powder falling out of the tear. She and her fellow employees were sent to the hospital and are being evaluated for possible inhalation anthrax. What is the treatment of choice for this patient?**
    A. Penicillin G 2 million units intravenously every 6 hours
    B. Ciprofloxacin 400 mg intravenously every 12 hours
    C. Doxycycline 500 mg intravenously every 12 hours
    D. Augmentin 875/125 mg intravenously every 12 hours

33. **What form of isolation should be used for the patient with inhalation anthrax?**
    A. Full isolation with laminar air flow
    B. Droplet precautions
    C. Standard contact precautions
    D. Reverse isolation

34. **EMTALA regulations require emergency treatment to be given for all of the following persons except**
    A. A pregnant woman in labor in her car outside the emergency room
    B. A gunshot victim found in the alley next to the hospital
    C. A visitor who suffers a heart attack in the deli next door to the emergency department
    D. A woman who exhibits stroke symptoms while attending a class in the education department

35. **Which of the following situations is a violation of EMTALA?**
    A. An apneic patient is intubated prior to transport to another facility for open heart surgery
    B. A woman has delivered a baby, but not the placenta, prior to transport to the obstetrical unit
    C. Dopamine and dobutamine have been started to maintain blood pressure prior to transport to an intensive care unit
    D. A gunshot victim with a nicked artery requires manual pressure while being transported to surgery

SECTION 8: ANSWERS

1. **Correct answer: C**
   The ethical principle that guides nurses to "Do No Harm" is the definition of non-malfeasance.

2. **Correct answer: D**
   Taking a positive action with compassion to help a patient is the meaning of beneficence and is the core of advocacy.

3. **Correct answer: B**
   Being truthful with patients as well as honest, fair, dedicated, and loyal is a definition of fidelity in nursing.

4. **Correct answer: B**
   As a trauma nurse, you are assisting at a train derailment with at least 40 victims. As you enter the triage area, you note four patients who have been marked with yellow tags. Patients with this designation require medical care and are unlikely to die without immediate intervention. Transport can be delayed as injuries, though possibly serious, will not deteriorate immediately.

5. **Correct answer: D**
   A disaster victim who requires immediate intervention and transport, treatment within minutes (up to 60), and has injuries compromising their respiratory status, is classified by the color red (immediate) during triage.

6. **Correct answer: D**
   The threat of high mortality and public health impact, potential for panic and social disruption, and requirements for public health preparedness are definitely concepts to be considered with a potential biologic threat.

7. **Correct answer: B**
   A foundation of disaster management to reduce loss of life and property from natural or manmade disasters, limiting or avoiding potential impact, as well as incorporating lessons learned from previous events is the definition of mitigation.

8. **Correct answer: C**
   When performing a secondary performance improvement review, outcome data is not immediately available as it is a retrospective review.

9. **Correct answer: B**
   The goal of disaster management is to do the most good for the greatest number of people.

10. **Correct answer: D**
    An eight-step formal process that takes place 1–14 days after a stressful incident is a debriefing. Defusing is a three-step program that should start immediately after an event and hopefully before the participant sleeps.

11. **Correct answer: A**
    The obligation to assist the patient in making a decision when the patient does not have sufficient data or expertise is called paternalism. The nurse has the duty to do no harm (non-malfeasance) and should not take away the patient's autonomy.

12. **Correct answer: B**
    In healthcare, actions are right or wrong based on a set of rules and morals. This ethical approach is known as deontology. Deontology emphasizes duty (obligation) to another human being.

13. **Correct answer: D**
    The public can be assured by evidence that a nurse meets established standards of quality, and patient safety is provided by certification.

14. **Correct answer: C**

    There are four necessary elements necessary to determine malpractice: Duty of care, breach of duty, injury, and causation. Physician relation is a nebulous statement and has no bearing on the question.

15. **Correct answer: A**

    Research is conducted using the empiric method, which is the systematic observation and experimentation to gather data that either confirms or refutes your expectations. A sample is a subset of the population you are studying. A t-test is a type of statistical test used to assess the difference in the mean value of interval or ratio level variable.

16. **Correct answer: D**

    A statistical variable is the manipulated or changing characteristic being measured. An example would be a patient's temperature or blood pressure. Probability represents the possible outcomes or the likeliness an outcome will occur. A statistic is an estimate generated from a sample. A parameter is a measured characteristic of a population.

17. **Correct answer: C**

    Pain is an example of qualitative data as the number assigned by the patient represents a non-numerical meaning. For example, 10 is the worst pain possible and 0 is no pain. Blood pressure, temperature, and pulse rate represent actual numbers and are considered quantitative.

18. **Correct answer: C**

    The dependent variable is the measured outcome or effect in a study. In the hospital, a common dependent variable example would be length of stay. The independent variable is the variable (intervention or action) that is measured or controlled in the experiment. An example could be the number of minutes that a patient ambulates in the hall. To summarize the example, the belief (hypothesis) is that patient ambulation (independent variable) impacts length of stay (dependent variable).

19. **Correct answer: A**

    Ethnicity is an example of categorical data. It has a finite number of classifications or groups that can be applied, which cannot be represented in fractions. Categorical data is typically qualitative. Other examples include: gender, religion, and sexual orientation. Age, height, weight, and so forth are examples of continuous variables and can be measured on a continuum, even in fractional form. Continuous variables are often quantitative in nature.

20. **Correct answer: B**

    Nominal data, such as gender (male, female), is the lowest level of measurement because it only offers two choices. Ordinal data is the next step up and represents data that can be ranked, i.e., worst to best. Interval data is the next step up for data measurement is exhaustive, exclusive, and has a rank order with numerically equal intervals, but no absolute end. Temperature is an example of an interval level of measurement. Ratio data represents the highest level of measurement. Ratio data is exhaustive, exclusive, ranked with equal intervals, and has an absolute zero. Blood pressure is a common ratio level data collected in research.

21. **Correct answer: D**

    Nominal data has two choices or answers, such as a yes or no response to car seat use. This data is qualitative in nature. An example of this question using ordinal data would be, "never, usually, always" use of a car seat. Interval or ration level would be number of days per week you use the car seat. When creating a research question, the highest level of data collection (ratio) is the best choice and will provide the largest number of options for data analysis.

22. **Correct answer: D**

    Nurse practice acts were **not** originated to allow for an unlimited practice of nursing. In addition to setting the standards for nursing, protecting the public, and guidelines allowing for disciplinary actions, Nurse Practice Acts provide scope of practice guidelines, and define and limit the practice of nursing.

23. **Correct answer: A**
    According to the Health Insurance Portability and Accountability Act of 1996 (HIPAA), individuals are *not* entitled to devise policies and procedures that address privacy, which is a hospital's responsibility. Individuals are entitled to authorize the use of personal medical records, who accesses that record and may restrict the use of the medical record.

24. **Correct answer: C**
    The Emergency Medical Treatment and Active Labor Act (EMTALA) is the law that was instituted to prevent "dumping" of patients unable to pay for medical treatment. This law affects all institutions with Medicare provider agreements in effect.

25. **Correct answer: D**
    Failure of the sending facility to verify acceptance by the receiving physician prior to transport is an EMTALA violation. If the hospital is in violation, it may be subject to fines, loss of Medicare provider status, and civil litigation.

26. **Correct answer: A**
    Expressed consent is the type of consent that involves an oral or written agreement to treatment, assessment, evaluation, medications, X-ray films, and laboratory studies.

27. **Correct answer: A**
    When filing an incident report, never refer to the existence of an incident report in the treated patient's chart, as this opens the facility to liability. Documentation should remain factual and included details of which the documenter has direct knowledge. Never assign blame to persons, facility, or equipment, just facts. If you have knowledge of defective equipment that remains in use and is involved in a patient or other person's injury, then liability may shift to you for not removing the equipment from use.

28. **Correct answer: D**
    In a mass casualty with victims spread over multiple areas, it is best to use simple triage. The victims may be decentralized as are the triage sites. The victims can be sorted into groups so those needing immediate treatment or have life-threatening injuries may receive immediate transport.

29. **Correct answer: C**
    Inhalation anthrax has an incubation period of 7 days to as long as 60 days after exposure. Symptoms are initially vague and flu-like such as malaise, low-grade fever, and nausea. These symptoms quickly progress to profound diaphoresis, chest discomfort, and rhonchi. The mild symptoms occur in the first 5 days of the illness followed by a brief rally. There is then an abrupt onset of high fever and severe respiratory distress. Death occurs as early as 24–36 hours after symptoms begin.

30. **Correct answer: A**
    Inhalation anthrax starts with mild, nonspecific symptoms such as malaise, low-grade fever, fatigue, and cough. Untreated, death occurs within 24–36 hours from respiratory failure.

31. **Correct answer: C**
    Ricin is made from castor beans and is one of the most toxic substances known. It interferes with protein synthesis and causes cell death. Chewing castor beans may cause some symptoms, but the most lethal form is inhaled. The toxin is not spread by casual contact. The most likely victims would be seen in enclosed areas such as subway trains, buses, or small rooms. It is usually aerosolized with some liquid like water or a weak acid.

32. **Correct answer: B**
    Ciprofloxacin, a fluoroquinolone antibiotic, is the drug of choice for inhalation anthrax. Doxycycline, a tetracycline derivative, may also be used, but the dosage is incorrect. Penicillin G is not an option as the bacteria, *Bacillus anthracis*, becomes beta-lactamase positive, making the penicillin ineffective. Augmentin is not used for this situation, and it is only given orally.

33. **Correct answer: C**
The CDC states that contact precautions are all that is required for inhalation anthrax. Standard precautions may include the use of a face mask if the patient is having a productive cough.

34. **Correct answer: C**
EMTALA regulations do not mandate the hospital provide emergency care to be given on property not belonging to the hospital. If an individual experiences a medical emergency anywhere on hospital grounds or within 250 yards, then the hospital is obligated to assess, stabilize, and treat as necessary. Exceptions to the rules include if the emergency occurs on property covered by another Medicare or other licensed facility such as an adjoining medical office building, surgicenter, or urgent care.

35. **Correct answer: B**
Transportation of a woman who has delivered a baby, but not the placenta, is a violation of EMTALA. Complications may occur if the placenta is expelled during transport; therefore, it is required that the mother be held in the emergency department until the placenta is delivered. Intubation, medication administration, and treatments that initiate stabilization must be completed prior to transport. Interventions are not expected to necessarily fix the problem but allow for safe transport without greater complications.

SECTION 9

Environmental and Pharmacology

- Pharmacological Issues
- Toxicological Issues

SECTION 9: QUESTIONS

1. After a patient ingests toxic levels of iron, there is a latent asymptomatic phase. This phase may cause caregivers to underestimate the continuing risk to the patient. This latent phase usually occurs _____ hours after ingestion.
   A. 1–4
   B. 2–12
   C. 8–16
   D. 16–24

2. The toxic ingredient in automobile antifreeze is
   A. Freon
   B. Ethanol
   C. Methanol
   D. Ethylene glycol

3. An acid that is absorbed even through intact skin, causing local and systemic effects, is
   A. Ethylene glycol
   B. Hydrofluoric acid
   C. Carbonic acid
   D. Acetic acid

4. Which statement is true regarding alkaline substances?
   A. The pH is lower than 2
   B. Vascular thrombosis may result
   C. Eschar forms over the burned area
   D. Alkalines dehydrate tissues

5. Which of the following substances contain large amounts of alkali?
   A. Toilet bowl cleaners
   B. Swimming pool chemicals
   C. Oven cleaners
   D. Metal cleaners

6. Symptoms of salicylate poisoning include
   A. Respiratory acidosis and bradycardia
   B. Lethargy and hypotension
   C. Abdominal cramping and hyperglycemia
   D. Tachycardia and hyperthermia

7. The antidote for iron poisoning is
   A. No antidote is available, treat symptoms only
   B. Chelation
   C. Deferoxamine
   D. Activated charcoal

8. Poisoning by arsenic may cause which of the following symptoms?
   A. Pneumonia, renal dysfunction
   B. Tachycardia, hypertension
   C. Paresthesia, cerebral edema
   D. Convulsions

9. **A middle-aged, retired school teacher presented initially to the ED for cocaine intoxication. After admission, he begins to complain of severe epigastric pain. The patient's lab results are as follows: WBC 17.5 with 76% neutrophils, hematocrit 41%, LDH 341, platelets 226, BUN 7, creatinine 1. Urine analysis shows trace of proteins, few RBCs, and + urine toxicology for cocaine. What is the likely cause of this patient's pain?**
   A. Peptic ulcer disease
   B. Renal infarction
   C. Gastroenteritis
   D. Infarcted mesenteric artery

10. **The acid–base imbalance likely to be seen with an iron overdose is**
    A. Respiratory acidosis
    B. Metabolic alkalosis
    C. Metabolic acidosis
    D. Respiratory alkalosis

11. **A possible side effect of cocaine is**
    A. Malignant hyperthermia
    B. Cherry red skin
    C. Paralytic ileus
    D. Constricted pupils

12. **Your patient has overdosed on metoprolol. As a trauma nurse you know an appropriate nursing action would be to**
    A. Prepare for cardioversion
    B. Administer activated charcoal
    C. Have a pacer at the bedside
    D. Prepare to administer beta-blockers

13. **Which of the following is not considered a direct source of energy that would lead to a patient's injury?**
    A. Electrical
    B. Oxygen deprivation
    C. Chemical
    D. Thermal

14. **Rocky Mountain spotted fever is caused by**
    A. A parasite
    B. Fleas
    C. Rotavirus
    D. Fungi

15. **The antidote for digoxin overdose is**
    A. Calcium gluconate
    B. Digoxin immune fab
    C. Glucagon
    D. Potassium chloride

16. **Which type of isolation is required for vancomycin-resistant enterococci (VRE) infections?**
    A. Standard or universal precautions
    B. Reverse isolation
    C. Contact isolation
    D. Droplet isolation

17. **Signs of vitamin D toxicity include**
    A. Seizures
    B. Increased susceptibility to respiratory diseases
    C. Azotemia
    D. Hypocalcemia

18. **Which of the following drugs should be held while your patient is receiving diltiazem hydrochloride?**
    A. Nitroglycerin
    B. Digoxin
    C. Insulin
    D. Rifampin

19. **Acetaminophen overdose may take as long as 2 weeks to resolve. From 72 to 96 hours after ingestion, the patient's symptoms will include**
    A. Pallor, lethargy, and metabolic acidosis
    B. Increased renal function
    C. Right upper quadrant pain and increased serum hepatic enzymes
    D. Jaundice, confusion, and coagulation disorders

20. **Which of the following statements about cocaine is false?**
    A. Cocaine use, even just one time, can cause rhabdomyolysis
    B. Cocaine and tobacco use are associated with spontaneous abortion
    C. Laboratory specimens should be kept on ice
    D. Cocaine causes placenta accreta

21. **Your patient has a history of cluster migraine headaches and has been treated with lithium. Today the patient slipped on a newly waxed floor and struck her head on a table. There was no LOC, but the patient received a deep laceration on the back of her head and fractured her ulna. Her lithium level on admission was 1.7 mmol/L. This value would correspond with which of the following symptoms?**
    A. Somnolence and coma
    B. Ataxia and diarrhea
    C. Seizures and flattened T wave
    D. Manic-depressive behavior

22. **What is the causative organism for Lyme disease?**
    A. *Escherichia coli*
    B. *Klebsiella pneumonia*
    C. *Serratia marcescens*
    D. *Borrelia burgdorferi*

23. **Which of the following is not an action of diltiazem (Cardizem)?**
    A. Blocks calcium channels
    B. Relaxes coronary vessels
    C. Increases peripheral vascular resistance
    D. Prolongs AV conduction

24. **Which of the following is not an action of octreotide acetate (Sandostatin)?**
    A. Increases gastrointestinal motility
    B. Inhibits serotonin secretion
    C. Decreases pancreatic secretion
    D. Decreases hepatic venous pressure

25. **Your patient received spinal Duramorph. As you are transferring the patient from the gurney to the bed, you note that the patient has periodic apnea and audible wheezing. What other adverse reactions should you anticipate in this situation?**
    A. Hypotension and decreased intracranial pressures
    B. Bradycardia and increased libido
    C. Palpitations and anemia
    D. Rapid capillary refill and bounding pulses

26. **What are the primary actions of milrinone?**
    A. Vasodilation and positive inotropy
    B. Vasodilation and positive chronotropy
    C. Positive chronotropy and vasodilation
    D. Beta and alpha receptor inhibitor

27. **Your patient with hyperthyroidism is being started on metoprolol for angina. What would happen if the patient suddenly stops taking this drug?**
    A. No effect
    B. Leukopenia
    C. Thyroid storm
    D. Bradycardia

28. **Metoprolol is prescribed for hypertension. If dosing exceeds 400 mg daily, the patient should be monitored closely for**
    A. Bronchospasms
    B. Agitation
    C. Increased HDL
    D. Flushing

29. **During your history and physical assessment of a middle-aged female admitted for chest pain, she reports a history of a shingles outbreak 3 months ago. You should question which of the following physician orders to obtain clarification?**
    A. Aspirin 160 mg daily
    B. Morphine 2 mg IV PRN
    C. Nitroglycerin 2 sprays every 3–5 minutes for chest pain
    D. Oxygen via nasal cannula PRN

30. **Your patient, a victim of a black widow spider bite, became obtunded, bradycardic, apneic, and hypotensive soon after arrival in the ED. Your first action should be to**
    A. Administer morphine 2 mg IV
    B. Administer antivenin
    C. Tie a tourniquet around the leg
    D. Prepare to intubate

31. **A college student was helping a friend clean out a garage yesterday. He developed a raised area that initially looked like a mosquito bite but is now red, pus-filled, and inflamed. He is admitted to the ED with a necrotizing wound. You suspect a brown recluse spider bite. This patient should not exhibit which of the following signs and symptoms?**
    A. Dyspnea
    B. Nausea and vomiting
    C. DIC
    D. Wet cough

32. **Cadmium accumulates in the lungs, liver, and kidneys following exposure to**
    A. Cigarette smoke
    B. Asbestos
    C. Lead paint
    D. Freshwater fish

33. **Which of the following considerations should the trauma nurse know prior to the administration of vancomycin?**
    A. Vancomycin is nephrotoxic
    B. Vancomycin must be administered intramuscularly
    C. Vancomycin should always be given with an aminoglycoside
    D. Vancomycin is specific for *Staphylococcus aureus*

34. **Which drug is known to cause nephrogenic diabetes insipidus?**
    A. Demeclocycline
    B. Morphine
    C. Lactulose
    D. Vasopressin

35. **Calcium channel blockers act primarily on**
    A. Serotonin uptake
    B. Arteriolar tissue
    C. Lung receptors only
    D. Reduction of cardiac output

36. **Your new patient was brought into the emergency room after collapsing at a party. Her cardiac and neurologic workup is negative. Her preliminary urine drug screen is also negative, so she was transferred to the ED. What do you suspect may have caused her collapse?**
    A. GHB
    B. Dehydration
    C. Ecstasy
    D. Metoprolol

37. **Which of the following statements is false regarding the use of activated charcoal for suspected or confirmed poisoning?**
    A. Activated charcoal adsorbs most poisons
    B. Activated charcoal adsorbs metals
    C. Activated charcoal cannot be mixed with ice cream
    D. Single doses of activated charcoal are indicated for serious poison exposures

38. **Your patient is preparing to go home after treatment with antivenin for a black widow spider bite. Which of the following discharge instructions is appropriate?**
    A. "You may experience muscle spasms for only a few days"
    B. "You may experience tingling and weakness for several years"
    C. "Call your doctor immediately if you have joint or abdominal pain or begin to have trouble breathing"
    D. "It is normal to have a rash or fever in the next 3 days"

39. **You are preparing to administer a loading dose of theophylline to your patient with COPD. For every 0.5 mg/kg given, you would expect a ___ increase in blood theophylline levels.**
    A. 0.25 mcg/ml
    B. 0.5 mg/ml
    C. 0.75 mg/ml
    D. 1 mcg/ml

40. **Which medication listed is both an analgesic and an amnestic?**
    A. Barbiturates
    B. Propofol
    C. Atropine
    D. Ketamine

41. **Multiple doses of activated charcoal should be used for ingestion of**
    A. Theophylline
    B. Gentamicin
    C. Aspirin
    D. Acetaminophen

42. **Which statement about plague is incorrect?**
    A. Plague is caused by *Yersinia pestis*
    B. Aerosol droplets may spread plague person to person
    C. Plague is usually transmitted by rats
    D. Plague may be used as a biological weapon

43. **Your patient lived in the country at a camp all summer and ate large quantities of deer and fish. He was admitted to the ED for respiratory distress, weight loss, vomiting, and numbness around the mouth. He is also suffering from mouth sores, and he drools constantly. His probable diagnosis is**
    A. Botulism
    B. Chlamydia infection
    C. Difficile infection
    D. Mercury poisoning

44. **Your patient lives on a ranch. Yesterday he complained of a stiff neck and was very lethargic. Last night he was found unconscious and had apparently vomited and possibly aspirated. He was immediately transported to your ED. After a preliminary evaluation, he was admitted to the ED. This patient probably has**
    A. Pneumonia
    B. West Nile virus
    C. Western equine encephalitis
    D. A brain tumor

45. **Which of the following choices is not a form of anthrax?**
    A. Nonspecific
    B. Cutaneous
    C. Pulmonary
    D. Gastrointestinal

46. **An ambulance brought in a patient from an incident at a bus station. The ED is full and the only available bed is yours in the holding area. The patient is irritable, confused, and has paresthesias around the mouth. He is having watery, rice-like diarrhea, nausea, and vomiting. These symptoms are indicative of**
    A. Arsenic poisoning
    B. Digoxin toxicity
    C. Methanol poisoning
    D. Insecticide poisoning

47. **Aspirin inhibits platelet aggregation by**
    A. Inhibiting thrombin
    B. Inhibiting fibrin
    C. Inhibiting thromboxane
    D. Inhibiting fibrinogen

48. **Your diabetic patient with chronic pain is being started on Duragesic patches. You would anticipate what changes to the patient's insulin dosing?**
   A. No change is anticipated
   B. The amount of insulin administered to this patient will increase
   C. The amount of insulin administration to this patient will decrease
   D. The amount of insulin administration will only decrease during the first 24 hours of administration of a Duragesic patch

49. **Your patient drove his truck into the short wall between his house and his neighbor. Your patient suffered two avulsed teeth, forehead and cheek lacerations, and bruised knees. You note the patient states he lost control of the truck because of incessant coughing that has continued for the past week. The patient has a fever, and demonstrates increased respiratory effort, so a blood culture was done. The blood culture revealed the presence of *E. coli*. Which of the following antibiotics would have the best effect on the bacteria?**
   A. Ganciclovir
   B. Gentamycin
   C. Cytarabine
   D. Cefoxitin

50. **Phosphodiesterase inhibitors are inotropes that can also cause vasodilation and are referred to as inodilators. Which of the following medications is classified as an inodilator?**
   A. Nitroglycerin
   B. Cardizem
   C. Milrinone
   D. Labetalol

51. **The normal range for a serum amiodarone is __ to ___ mcg/ml.**
   A. 2.5 to 3.5
   B. 1 to 2.5
   C. 1 to 3
   D. 1.5 to 3.5

52. **Calcium channel blockers act primarily on**
   A. Serotonin uptake
   B. Arteriolar tissue
   C. Lung receptors only
   D. Reduction of cardiac output

53. **Your patient with recurrent VT was started on intravenous amiodarone today. Which of the following signs should the ED nurse monitor closely during administration of the initial loading dose?**
   A. Urine output and parathyroid levels
   B. Urine output and liver function tests
   C. Thyroid levels and hypertonicity
   D. Observe for greenish discoloration of the skin and change in thyroid levels

54. **Your patient with an implanted cardiac defibrillator should have thresholds checked frequently during administration of which of the following drugs?**
   A. Amiodarone
   B. Nesiritide
   C. Nitroglycerin
   D. Anisindione

55. **Nesiritide is an appropriate drug to help treat which of the following heart conditions?**
    A. Constrictive pericarditis
    B. Acute decompensated congestive heart failure
    C. Chronic obstructive cardiomyopathy
    D. Pericardial tamponade

56. **To monitor the effectiveness of anticoagulant therapy, the international normalized ratio (INR) is frequently used. For a patient with atrial fibrillation, a therapeutic range for INR would be**
    A. 3.5–4.5
    B. 1.5–3
    C. 2–3
    D. 5–6.1

57. **While caring for your patient on nesiritide, you note a decrease in urine output. Which of the following lab results should you immediately report to the physician?**
    A. BUN/Creatinine ratio greater than 20
    B. Serum bicarbonate 25 mEq/L
    C. Urine osmolality of 1,000 mOsm/L
    D. Urine specific gravity of 1.005

58. **Your ED was overrun by participants from a riot who had been tear gassed. One of the treatments that should not be used in the treatment of these patients is**
    A. Copious eye irrigation with Lactated Ringers
    B. Wash skin with alkaline soap
    C. Clean the skin with sodium bicarbonate
    D. Copious eye irrigation with normal saline

59. **The specific antidote for methamphetamine is**
    A. Desipramine
    B. Alkalinizing agents
    C. There is no antidote
    D. Naloxone

60. **Patients who are undergoing alcohol withdrawal are frequently hypoglycemic. Their treatment regimen should include**
    A. Bolus of $D_{10}W$, q 2-hour blood glucose monitoring
    B. TPN with high concentrations of sugars, q 2-hour blood glucose monitoring
    C. Maintenance fluids of $D_{25}W$ at 125 ml/hour peripherally
    D. Thiamine, then bolus with $D_{50}W$, then infusion of D_5W

61. **The drug of choice for the treatment of tricyclic antidepressant overdose is**
    A. Atropine
    B. Imipramine
    C. Doxepin
    D. Sodium bicarbonate

62. **A side effect after administration of an antipsychotic drug that causes muscle spasms is known as**
    A. Dystonia
    B. Expression
    C. Latency
    D. Delusion

63. Your patient has been taking an antipsychotic medication. She is now suffering from drooling, muscle tremors, and has difficulty walking. This patient is exhibiting
   A. Boundary effects
   B. Extrapyramidal effects
   C. Dystonic effects
   D. Latent effects

64. Acetaminophen overdose may cause hypoglycemia and should be treated with a
   A. Continuous IV infusion of D_5W at 100 cc/hour
   B. Bolus of $D_{10}W$, continuous infusion of 0.45% normal saline
   C. Bolus of $D_{50}W$, continuous infusion of D_5W
   D. Continuous IV infusion of Lactated Ringer's

65. Your patient is undergoing alcohol withdrawal and exhibits diplopia, peripheral neuropathy, confusion, recent memory loss, and hyperexcitability. You suspect that this patient is suffering from
   A. Jorn's syndrome
   B. Leucine deficiency
   C. Increased carnitine levels
   D. Wernicke-Korsakoff syndrome

66. The effects of the high dosage of bath salts are similar to the symptoms of amphetamines, cocaine, and methamphetamine. Treatment of bath salts overdose would include
   A. Phenylalanines
   B. Phentermines
   C. Benzodiazepines
   D. Ephedrines

67. Alcohol abuse may lead to a deficiency in micronutrients that in turn may cause depression and suicidal behavior. One of these micronutrients is
   A. Potassium
   B. Copper
   C. Sodium
   D. Selenium

68. Which of the following medications is not considered an antimanic drug?
   A. Klonopin
   B. Tegretol
   C. Lithium
   D. Tofranil

69. Which of the following is classified as an antianxiety drug?
   A. Restoril
   B. Elavil
   C. Sinequan
   D. Tofranil

70. Your patient struck a car while riding a bicycle and was thrown over the handlebars. You note the patient is grimacing and will not allow you to assess her abdomen. Except for multiple contusions, the patient was cleared for significant abdominal injuries. The ED attending physician ordered Demerol for pain. Approximately 10 minutes after administration of the Demerol, the patient is combative, has pulled her IV out, has torn off her IV dressing, and is screaming at the staff. Your next action should be to
   A. Apply restraints by yourself as additional staff may scare the patient
   B. Wear personal protective equipment to enter her room to apply restraints
   C. Call security to help subdue the patient
   D. Use a Posey restraint system to subdue the patient

71. **A cyclic antidepressant that may cause cardiovascular effects and will probably cause status epilepticus is**
    A. Amoxapine
    B. Amitriptyline
    C. Desipramine
    D. Doxepin

72. **A patient intoxicated with methamphetamine would exhibit which of the following conditions?**
    A. Elevated liver enzymes
    B. Bradycardia
    C. Hypothermia
    D. Hypotension

73. **An antidote for ethylene glycol toxicity is**
    A. Digoxin
    B. Anisindione
    C. Fomepizole
    D. Narcan

74. **Factors that may affect results of urine morphine levels would not include**
    A. Poppy seed ingestion may produce false-positive results
    B. 10 mg MS IV may be detectable in urine up to 84 hours
    C. Use of stealth adulterant to cause negative results in a positive sample
    D. High levels of lymphocytes will mask morphine in urine

75. **When treating salicylate overdose, which of the following goals is appropriate for this condition?**
    A. A hypocalcemic state
    B. Urine pH of 7–8
    C. Resolution of jaundice
    D. Entry of salicylate into the CNS

76. **Which of the following drugs has a half-life of approximately 24 hours and requires continuous doses of naloxone?**
    A. Demerol
    B. Heroin
    C. Cocaine
    D. Methadone

77. **The triad of symptoms usually associated with opioid overdose is**
    A. Respiratory depression, meiosis, and coma
    B. Obtundation, hypotension, and ventricular arrhythmias
    C. Confusion, slurred speech, and seizures
    D. Stupor, respiratory alkalosis, and hypotension

78. **The specific antidote for a benzodiazepine overdose is**
    A. Calcium chloride
    B. Flumazenil
    C. Atropine
    D. Calcium gluconate

79. **The primary symptoms of cocaine toxicity include hyperthermia, hyperactivity, tachycardia, and hypertension. These symptoms may be managed by administration of**
    A. Morphine
    B. Fentanyl
    C. Codeine
    D. Ativan

80. **Lithium is used as an antipsychotic medication to treat bipolar disorder. Lithium toxicity is deadly. Which of the following statements is true regarding lithium toxicity?**
    A. Toxicity may occur if blood levels reach 1 mEq/L
    B. Signs of lithium toxicity include constipation, hypertonicity, and giddiness
    C. Untreated lithium toxicity may lead to seizures, coma, and cardiac dysrhythmias
    D. Lithium toxicity may be treated safely on a medical–surgical floor

81. **Methamphetamine is officially classified as a(n)**
    A. Stimulant
    B. Euphoric
    C. Hallucinogen
    D. Antidepressant

82. **Ketamine is contraindicated in a patient with**
    A. Bronchospasm
    B. Altered intracranial pressure
    C. Barbiturate overdose
    D. Opioid overdose

83. **Which of the following statements is true regarding the administration of propofol?**
    A. Propofol is used for long-term procedures
    B. Propofol is not indicated for use in a patient with bronchospasm
    C. Propofol is made from eggs and soybeans
    D. Propofol increases cerebral blood flow

84. **Which of the following solutions is usually avoided in patients with kidney failure?**
    A. Hetastarch
    B. Lactated Ringer's solution
    C. 0.45 NaCl
    D. Albumin 5%

85. **Allergic nephritis may be caused by**
    A. Inadequate protein consumption
    B. Weight loss
    C. Cimetidine
    D. Water intoxication

86. **Nephrotoxicity may be caused by which of the following medications?**
    A. Furosemide
    B. Aspirin
    C. Thioguanine
    D. Acyclovir

87. **All of the following are treatments for hyperkalemia except**
    A. Glucose and insulin
    B. Kaon
    C. Calcium gluconate
    D. Bicarbonate administration

88. Your patient has congestive heart failure and was prescribed Lasix for water retention by her nurse practitioner. The patient's feet and legs continued to swell, so she took an extra Lasix this morning. She became dizzy and nauseous and then was admitted to the ED. Now she has profound muscle weakness and flat T waves. You would expect this patient's potassium level at this time to be approximately

   A. 1.8 mEq/L
   B. 3.8 mEq/L
   C. 4.2 mEq/L
   D. 6.1 mEq/L

89. Magnesium is required for all the following physiologic functions except

   A. To act as an antagonist to calcium
   B. Enzyme activation
   C. Synthesis of nucleic acid and proteins
   D. Sodium-potassium pump operation

90. You are caring for a patient in kidney failure. As a trauma nurse, you know one expected side effect of kidney failure is the development of

   A. Anemia
   B. Pulmonary secretions
   C. Hyponatremia
   D. Hypoxia

91. The normal adult glomerular filtration rate (GFR) is

   A. 180 L/day
   B. 600 ml/min
   C. 250 ml/hour
   D. 75 L/day

92. A common cause of hyponatremia is

   A. Saltwater drowning
   B. Overhydration
   C. Administration of hypertonic solutions
   D. Hyperoxia

93. You are receiving report on a patient who was injured when he suffered a seizure while working on his roof. His sodium level on admission was 130 mEq/l. What symptoms of hyponatremia would you expect this patient to exhibit?

   A. Twitching
   B. Tachypnea
   C. Lethargy
   D. Flattened T waves

94. A drug reaction often caused by a Beta-lactam antibiotic that causes an acute inflammation of the kidneys where the primary lesions are in the interstitial space between the nephron is known as

   A. Afferent vasodilation
   B. Progressive nephron loss
   C. Intrarenal failure (AKI)
   D. Amyloidosis

95. The normal range for serum osmolality in a healthy adult is

   A. 163–240 mOsm/kg
   B. 275–295 mOsm/kg
   C. 55–110 mOsm/kg
   D. 120–195 mOsm/kg

96. **Potassium is reabsorbed in which of the areas listed below?**
    A. Proximal tubules
    B. Distal tubules
    C. Ascending colon
    D. Descending colon

97. **Generalized muscle weakness progressing to coma is a late sign of a patient suffering from**
    A. Hyponatremia
    B. Repetitive seizure activity
    C. A lack of ADH
    D. Poor fluid intake

98. **Normal magnesium levels for an adult are in the range of**
    A. 0.5–1.5 mg/dl
    B. 1.5–2 mg/dl
    C. 2–3 mg/dl
    D. 4–5 mg/dl

99. **A nursing consideration when administering magnesium to a patient would include**
    A. Administering an IV dose quickly, over three minutes
    B. Be prepared to give calcium gluconate if needed
    C. Knowing high magnesium levels enhance the action of digitalis
    D. Calcium levels will rise as magnesium is given intravenously

100. **Your patient is becoming confused, is lethargic, and has muscle weakness. A review of her lab reports shows a calcium level of 11.7. A common way to treat this condition is to use**
    A. D_5W and a Kayexalate enema
    B. Normal saline and a loop diuretic
    C. Glucose followed by insulin
    D. Nothing. This is a normal value.

101. **Your patient has a calcium level of 7.8. You would expect which of the following changes to be observed on the EKG tracing?**
    A. Tall, peaked T waves
    B. A prominent U wave
    C. A first-degree AV block
    D. A prolonged QT interval

102. **Apheresis is best defined as**
    A. The removal of plasma and/or proteins from the blood
    B. The selective removal of cells, plasma, and substances from the blood
    C. The selective removal of cellular components from the blood
    D. The removal of an antigen in the blood

103. **Mannitol and loop diuretics may be used in the treatment of AKI. Mannitol is nontoxic but must be used with caution because**
    A. Mannitol may damage the eighth cranial nerve
    B. Mannitol may cause vestibular impairment
    C. Mannitol may produce a hyperosmolar state
    D. Mannitol may bind with proteins in the renal tubule

104. **The use of NSAIDs may cause**
    A. Prerenal AKI
    B. Intrinsic AKI
    C. Postrenal AKI
    D. Increased urine osmolality

105. **This morning a fire broke out in your patient's home. The patient's bed was covered in wool blankets and wool clothing was in the closet. She did not suffer any burns but did inhale large quantities of smoke. What would be the most potent toxin she might have inhaled?**
    A. Carbon monoxide
    B. Smoke
    C. Inhaled nitrates
    D. Cyanide

106. **High levels of carbon monoxide inhalation is expected to cause**
    A. Visual and auditory changes
    B. Headache
    C. Dizziness
    D. Flu-like illness

107. **Side effects of acetylcysteine include**
    A. Red urine
    B. Headache
    C. Hypertension
    D. Bronchospasms

SECTION 9: ANSWERS

1. **Correct answer: B**
    After a patient ingests toxic levels of iron, there is a latent asymptomatic phase that occurs
    2–12 hours after ingestion. After about 12 hours, the patient may enter the next phase, which is an
    abrupt cardiovascular collapse.

2. **Correct answer: D**
    The toxic ingredient in automobile antifreeze is ethylene glycol

3. **Correct answer: B**
    Hydrofluoric acid is absorbed even through intact skin, causing local and systemic effects. Hydrofluoric
    acid is used as a rust remover, metal cleaner, and to etch glass.

4. **Correct answer: B**
    Vascular thrombosis may result from alkaline substances, and liquefaction necrosis will occur. Serious
    injury results from products with a pH higher than 12.

5. **Correct answer: C**
    Oven cleaners contain large amounts of alkali. Additional alkaline substances include dishwasher
    detergent, laundry detergent, drain openers, and ammonia capsules.

6. **Correct answer: D**
    Symptoms of salicylate poisoning include tachycardia and hyperthermia. Additional symptoms
    include tinnitus, tachypnea, LOC changes, respiratory alkalosis, metabolic acidosis, or mixed acid–base
    abnormalities. Occult GI tract bleeding may occur.

7. **Correct answer: C**
    Deferoxamine is used to treat iron poisoning via chelation. It is also possible the patient may have to
    be treated with GI tract decontamination, which may include gastric lavage or whole bowel irrigation.
    Chelation is the bonding of elements, not a treatment.

8. **Correct answer: D**
    Arsenic poisoning may cause convulsions. Arsenic is found in all human tissues as a trace element.
    The levels may become elevated with exposure. About 60% of ingested arsenic is excreted in the urine.
    Arsenic may be found in well water, pesticides, paints, cosmetics, treated wood, and coal. Chronic
    exposure can lead to various types of cancers.

9. **Correct answer: B**
    Renal infarction can occur with cocaine intoxication. The proteinuria and RBCs in the urine are
    indicative of the renal infarction. Cocaine abuse can lead to any infarction, including MI.

10. **Correct answer: C**
    Metabolic acidosis is likely to be seen with an iron overdose. After iron is metabolized, free hydrogen is
    released and leads to metabolic acidosis.

11. **Correct answer: A**
    A possible side effect of cocaine is malignant hyperthermia.

12. **Correct answer: C**
    A pacer should be kept at the bedside for a patient with metoprolol overdose because bradycardia,
    AV block, and hypotension will probably occur.

13. **Correct answer: B**
    Oxygen deprivation is not considered a direct source of energy that would lead to a patient's injury. It
    would be considered a cause of injury or death because of sequelae from the resultant lack of oxygen.

14. **Correct answer: C**
Rocky Mountain spotted fever is spread by ticks that carry a rotavirus. Symptoms include a sudden onset fever for 2–3 weeks and a rash that may cover the entire body. Treatment must include both chloramphenicol and tetracycline.

15. **Correct answer: B**
The antidote for digoxin overdose is digoxin immune fab. Digoxin immune fab reverses hyperkalemia and most dysrhythmias. Patients in renal failure may require dialysis to remove the digoxin immune fab.

16. **Correct answer: C**
Vancomycin-resistant enterococci isolation requires contact isolation. The VRE can survive on surfaces such as your stethoscope for 1 hour and up to 6 days on countertops.

17. **Correct answer: C**
Signs of vitamin D toxicity include azotemia, hypercalcemia, vomiting, and nephrocalcinosis. Vitamin D deficiency will result in hypocalcemia, increased susceptibility to respiratory diseases, lethargy, and seizures.

18. **Correct answer: D**
Rifampin should not be administered to patients receiving diltiazem hydrochloride as the rifampin decreases serum diltiazem levels to undetectable amounts by increasing metabolism of the drug. Nitroglycerin and digoxin therapy may be used concurrently. Insulin use may be required to manage adverse reaction of hyperglycemia, especially in diabetic patients.

19. **Correct answer: D**
Acetaminophen overdose may take as long as 2 weeks to resolve. From 72 to 96 hours after ingestion, the patient's symptoms will include jaundice, confusion, increased ALT and AST, and coagulation disorders. Renal function is possibly decreased.

20. **Correct answer: D**
Cocaine is classified as a Schedule II central nervous system stimulant. It is also used as a local anesthetic, a bronchodilator, and a vasoconstrictor. Cocaine compromises the heart's antioxidant defense system, and an overdose can cause an MI. Cocaine can also cause aortic dissection, stroke, intestinal ischemia, hallucinations, and adverse effects on fetuses.

21. **Correct answer: B**
This patient may have slipped because, even though her lithium level is only 1.7 mmol/L, she may be experiencing ataxia. Lithium is an alkali, a metal salt used mostly in the treatment of bipolar disorder and cluster migraine headaches. In bipolar disorder and alcohol withdrawal, lithium works by altering sodium transport in nerves and muscles, which helps to stabilize mood. Untreated lithium toxicity may lead to seizures, coma, and cardiac dysrhythmias when levels reach greater than 2.5 mEq/L. Toxicity usually occurs with levels of 2 mEq/L, but symptoms may be noted at even lower blood levels with certain body chemistries. Initial toxicity is noted when the patient experiences diarrhea, vomiting, drowsiness, muscular weakness, and disorientation. As toxicity and symptoms worsen, nystagmus, ataxia, giddiness, tinnitus, confusion, and blurred vision may be present. Patients must be managed by close monitoring and immediate intervention of dysrhythmias and electrolyte imbalances.

22. **Correct answer: D**
The causative organism for Lyme disease is *Borrelia burgdorferi*, a spirochete carried by the deer tick.

23. **Correct answer: C**
Increased peripheral vascular resistance is not an action of diltiazem (Cardizem). By blocking calcium transport into cells, coronary and vascular smooth muscles relax, leading to decreased peripheral vascular resistance and vasodilation. Prolonging AV conduction causes a decrease in heart rate and interrupts reentrant tachycardias.

24. **Correct answer: A**
Octreotide acetate (Sandostatin) decreases gastrointestinal motility, it does not increase motility. The suppression of serotonin, as well as GI and pituitary hormones results in increased gastrointestinal water reabsorption, decreasing dehydration.

25. **Correct answer: C**
Adverse reactions to Duramorph (morphine sulfate) administration include respiratory depression, palpitations, and anemia, as well as hypotension, bradycardia, delayed capillary refill, decreased libido, and increased intracranial pressure.

26. **Correct answer: A**
Vasodilation and positive inotropy are the primary actions of milrinone. Milrinone is a cAMP inhibitor used primarily for congestive heart failure.

27. **Correct answer: C**
If a patient with hyperthyroidism on metoprolol suddenly stops taking the drug, the patient may experience a thyroid storm. If metoprolol is to be discontinued, the patient should slowly be weaned off while monitoring T_3 and T_4 levels. Leukopenia and bradycardia are adverse reactions of metoprolol administration.

28. **Correct answer: A**
If metoprolol dosing exceeds 400 mg daily, the patient should be monitored closely for bronchospasms. If the patient has a history of reactive airway disease, metoprolol dosing may need to be reduced. Patients may also experience fatigue, hallucinations, drowsiness, decreased HDP, and dry eyes and mouth.

29. **Correct answer: A**
As a trauma nurse, you would question an order for aspirin for any patient with recent history of varicella outbreak, either as chicken pox or shingles. Administration of aspirin places the patient at risk for Reye's syndrome. Other patients at risk include any patient recovering from viral infection or a patient who exhibits presence of flu-like symptoms. The specific mechanism for the reaction and precipitation of Reye's syndrome and aspirin administration is unknown, but failure to receive early treatment may lead to death. Initial symptoms of Reye's syndrome include persistent vomiting, listlessness, drowsiness, personality changes (irritability), and aggressive behavior.

30. **Correct answer: D**
This patient is having a severe reaction to the black widow bite. He is apneic and bradycardic. Priorities are to maintain the airway to provide ventilation and oxygen therapy. The next step is to administer antivenin as soon as available. Morphine may help with pain but will worsen the bradycardia and hypotension. It is a myth that tying a tourniquet around the affected limb will stop the venom from reaching the bloodstream or lymphatic system. At this point, the venom is already systemic. In minor cases involving healthy patients, symptoms may be managed with pain control, muscle relaxants, and comfort measures. Symptoms should dissipate during the first 3 days after exposure.

31. **Correct answer: A**
Patients suffering from a brown recluse spider bite will not present with dyspnea. Patients may not initially know they were bitten and will seek medical help 12–36 hours after the initial bite. Because treatment is delayed, symptoms may be difficult to treat. Most patients may present with flu-like symptoms such as nausea and vomiting. DIC, hemolysis, and thrombocytopenia are severe symptoms. Treatment includes ice to control inflammation, keeping the area clean and protected, and treating symptoms. No specific treatment has been proven to be 100% effective. Dapsone has limited support for preventing necrosis. Nitroglycerin patches counter the vasoconstrictive properties of the venom and lead to hemodilution in the bloodstream and increased bleeding at the site to wash the venom out.

32. **Correct answer: A**
Cadmium accumulates in the lungs, liver, and kidneys following exposure to cigarette smoke. Cadmium is actually a heavy metal with a half-life of 15–20 years. It is a respiratory irritant and can produce pulmonary edema, interstitial pneumonia, and cardiovascular collapse if inhaled. It is used in the

manufacture of storage batteries, alloys, and in electroplating. If cadmium is ingested, the individual will have severe gastrointestinal symptoms within 30 minutes. Most cadmium collects in erythrocytes and kidney tissues. It is not metabolized in the body.

33. Correct answer: A

Prior to the administration of vancomycin, the trauma nurse should know that vancomycin is nephrotoxic, especially if used in combination with aminoglycosides. Vancomycin is used in the treatment of methicillin-resistant strains (*Staphylococcus epidermidis*) and must be administered by slow intravenous drip.

34. Correct answer: A

Demeclocycline is known to cause nephrogenic diabetes insipidus.

35. Correct answer: B

Calcium channel blockers act primarily on arteriolar tissue. Large lumen vessels in the arterial system are affected. The advantage of this action is that both systolic and diastolic pressures are reduced and the patient will not have a drop in blood pressure. The blood pressure may be lowered slightly and cause a reflex baroreceptor response to speed up the heart rate to maintain cardiac output.

36. Correct answer: A

The sudden collapse of a young woman at a party without explanation is suspicious for gamma-hydroxybutyrate (GHB) or ketamine ingestion. These are known date or party rape drugs. Due to the anesthetic and amnesic effects of the drug, an affected female may be unable to describe events leading up to the collapse. To determine exposure the drug screen should be repeated, looking specifically for gamma-hydroxybutyrate (GHB) and/or ketamine.

37. Correct answer: B

Activated charcoal does not adsorb metals. Activated charcoal adsorbs most poisons. Activated charcoal cannot be mixed with ice cream or syrups because the charcoal adsorbs many of these agents, rendering it less effective. Single doses of activated charcoal are indicated for serious poison exposures.

38. Correct answer: C

This patient suffered a black widow spider bite. Her discharge instructions should include contacting her physician immediately if she has joint or abdominal pain or difficulty breathing. Joint and abdominal pain (pain related to splenomegaly), as well as dyspnea, may be signs of anaphylaxis or serum sickness up to 2–4 weeks after antivenin administration. Patients should be taught to contact their physicians immediately so early treatment can be initiated to prevent complications. Administration of corticosteroids and antihistamines will aid in combating the inflammatory response to the animal proteins in the antivenin. The neurotoxin may cause residual muscle spasms, tingling, weakness, and nervousness for weeks to months after the exposure to the venom. Patients may need to slowly increase activity during their recovery.

39. Correct answer: D

For every 0.5 mg/kg of theophylline given, there should be a 1 mcg/ml increase in blood levels. Study question note: When given a question with numbers, pay close attention to the type of measurement used. If you know that theophylline level is measured in mcg/ml, then you would be able to automatically rule out 0.5 and 0.75 mg/ml as answers.

40. Correct answer: D

Ketamine is both an analgesic and an amnestic.

41. Correct answer: A

Multiple doses of activated charcoal should be used for ingestions of theophylline. Additional drugs for which multiple doses are indicated include digoxin, phenobarbital, and amitriptyline.

42. Correct answer: C

Plague is not transmitted by rats. *Yersinia pestis* is the causative agent for plague. It is often transmitted to humans by rodent fleas, by handling rodents affected with the disease, or by exposure to a person with plague pneumonia. Plague is very rare but occurs mostly in the western United States in rural or semi-rural areas. The *Yersinia pestis* bacterium, and aerosol droplets may spread the disease from person to person. Some countries consider plague as a biologic weapon.

There are three types of plague include bubonic plague, which results from flea bites. It leads to suddenness of fever, chills, weakness, and swollen lymph nodes. Blood cultures are done to identify *Y. pestis*. The patient is treated with gentamicin, streptomycin, tetracycline, third generation cephalosporin, or fluoroquinolones.

Septicemic plague has some of the same symptoms as bubonic plague but with more GI symptoms. Also, the skin can turn black. It can occur as the first symptom of plague and progress to bubonic plague. It is also caused by flea bites and exposure to infected animals.

Pneumonic plague is the most serious form and is the only plague capable of person-to-person infection. The hallmark is a rapidly developing pneumonia with bloody or watery secretions. It can develop after untreated septicemic or bubonic plague.

43. **Correct answer: D**
The probable diagnosis for this patient is mercury poisoning. Fish can contain large amounts of mercury. The concentration in fish can be more than 1,000 times greater than in the surrounding water. People who eat fish as a main component of their diet may be at risk. Organic mercury compounds are very toxic. They are taken into the body by ingestion, inhalation, skin, and eye contact. These mercury compounds can attack all body systems. They can cause nausea, lack of appetite, abdominal pain, kidney failure, swollen gums and mouth sores, tremors, seizures, and numbness and tingling in the lips, mouth, tongue, hands, and feet. The patient can become very uncoordinated and feel disconnected from his surroundings. He may lose part or all of his vision and hearing. Additional neurologic issues may include memory loss, personality changes, and headache. Organic mercury can pass to a baby via breast milk. Methyl mercury may cause serious birth defects.

44. **Correct answer: C**
Western equine encephalitis is a type of encephalitis caused by an arbovirus (togzvirus). An arbovirus means it is carried by arthropods. A horse or small mammal was probably infected and the virus was vectored by a mosquito. This type of encephalopathy is not directly transmitted human to human. This patient is at high risk for aspiration pneumonia and ARDS.

45. **Correct answer: A**
Nonspecific is not a form of anthrax. Cutaneous, pulmonary, and gastrointestinal are all forms of anthrax.

46. **Correct answer: A**
Watery, rice-like diarrhea, nausea, vomiting, irritability, confusion, and paresthesias around the mouth are symptoms of arsenic poisoning. Additional symptoms include headache, a metallic taste, palpitations, and EKG changes.

47. **Correct answer: C**
Aspirin inhibits platelet aggregation by inhibiting thromboxane A2 production. Thromboxane A2 stimulates platelet aggregation.

48. **Correct answer: B**
Duragesic patches contain 2 g of sugar and diabetic patients will likely need a slight increase adjustment to insulin therapy to account for the additional sugar intake.

49. **Correct answer: B**
Gentamycin is an aminoglycoside, as are tobramycin and amikacin. These drugs are used to combat gram-negative bacterial infections such as *E. coli*, but they must be used with caution because they can cause nephrotoxicity.

50. **Correct answer: C**
Phosphodiesterase inhibitors are inotropes that can also cause vasodilation and are referred to as inodilators. Milrinone (Primacor) is an example of an inotrope, as is Amrinone (Inocor). These

medications inhibit phosphodiesterase, and this action results in increased levels of intracellular calcium and adenosine monophosphate. Cardiac output is increased due to an increase in contractility, while the vasodilation reduces afterload. Both of these medications will cause a degree of thrombocytopenia. Milrinone may also cause atrial and ventricular rhythm disturbances.

51. **Correct answer: B**

    The normal range for a serum amiodarone level is 1–2.5 mcg/ml.

52. **Correct answer: B**

    Calcium channel blockers act primarily on arteriolar tissue. Large lumen vessels in the arterial system are affected. The advantage of this action is that both systolic and diastolic pressures are reduced and the patient will not have a drop in blood pressure. The blood pressure may be lowered slightly and cause a reflex baroreceptor response to speed up the heart rate to maintain cardiac output.

53. **Correct answer: B**

    The trauma nurse should monitor closely the urine output and liver function tests of a patient receiving a loading dose of amiodarone. The high concentration of amiodarone may cause renal necrosis and impaired output leading to vascular congestion and respiratory distress. Amiodarone has been linked to hepatocellular damage and impaired liver function. Other side effects include anemia, neutropenia, pancytopenia, and thrombocytopenia. Thyroid levels should also be monitored because amiodarone may cause hypo- or hyperthyroidism. Amiodarone has been linked to bluish-gray pigmentation in long-term patients exposed to sunlight.

54. **Correct answer: A**

    Your patient with an implanted cardiac defibrillator should have thresholds checked frequently during administration of amiodarone. Amiodarone may affect the pacing threshold of implanted cardiac defibrillators, so the pacing settings should be verified prior to and during amiodarone administration. Anisindione is an anticoagulant and administration is contraindicated for a patient with an invasive device such as an implanted cardiac defibrillator.

55. **Correct answer: B**

    Nesiritide is an appropriate drug for heart patients with acute decompensated congestive heart failure. The action of nesiritide is to cause arterial and venous smooth muscle relaxation to decrease cardiac afterload. This relieves pulmonary congestion and cardiac workload. Constrictive pericarditis, obstructive cardiomyopathy, and pericardial tamponade are all examples of preload dependent heart diseases and nesiritide should never be administered. The dilative effects of nesiritide would diminish venous blood to the heart, worsening cardiac function.

56. **Correct answer: C**

    For a patient with atrial fibrillation, a therapeutic range for INR would be 2–3. For prosthetic valves, the therapeutic range would be 2.5–3.5.

57. **Correct answer: A**

    The trauma nurse should immediately report any BUN/creatinine ratio greater than 20 in the presence of decreased urine output to the physician for a patient on nesiritide. The increased creatinine level and decreased urine output are indicators of compromised/diminished blood flow to the kidneys with impending development of prerenal azotemia. Azotemia is an adverse reaction to nesiritide administration. With prerenal azotemia, other lab results to monitor and report include a urine osmolality of less than 500 mOsm/L and a urine specific gravity greater than 1.015.

58. **Correct answer: A**

    Your ED was overrun by participants from a riot who had been tear gassed. One of the treatments that should not be used in the treatment of these patients is copious eye irrigation with Lactated Ringer's. After exposure to tear gas or pepper spray, symptoms will include burning and redness to the nose and eyes, shortness of breath, bronchospasm, respiratory distress, as well as possible skin irritation.

59. **Correct answer: C**

There is no specific antidote for methamphetamine. It is only possible to treat symptoms as they appear. Desipramine may cause sustained activity of amphetamines in the brain. Alkalinizing agents may potentiate the actions of amphetamines.

60. **Correct answer: D**

Patients who are undergoing alcohol withdrawal are frequently hypoglycemic. Treatment should include thiamine, then bolus with $D_{50}W$, and then start an infusion of D_5W.

61. **Correct answer: D**

Sodium bicarbonate is used to treat tricyclic overdose. Imipramine and doxepin are both tricyclics.

62. **Correct answer: A**

A side effect after administration of an antipsychotic drug that causes muscle spasms is known as dystonia.

63. **Correct answer: B**

The patient's drooling, muscle tremors, and difficulty walking are similar to those of patients who suffer from Parkinson's disease and are known as extrapyramidal effects.

64. **Correct answer: C**

Acetaminophen overdose may cause hypoglycemia and should be treated with a bolus of $D_{50}W$, and a continuous infusion of D_5W. Hypoglycemia occurs because of the hepatotoxic effects of acetaminophen. Infusions must also be based on blood glucose results.

65. **Correct answer: D**

The patient undergoing alcohol withdrawal and who exhibits diplopia, peripheral neuropathy, confusion, recent memory loss, and hyperexcitability has Wernicke-Korsakoff syndrome. Wernicke-Korsakoff syndrome is a thiamine deficiency and a metabolic encephalopathy.

66. **Correct answer: C**

The effects of the high dosage of bath salts are similar to the trip of amphetamines, cocaine, and methamphetamine. Treatment of bath salts overdose would include benzodiazepines.

67. **Correct answer: D**

Alcohol abuse may lead to a deficiency in micronutrients that in turn may cause depression and suicidal behavior. One of these micronutrients is selenium.

68. **Correct answer: D**

Tofranil is an antidepressant. Tegretol, klonopin, and lithium are all antimanic drugs.

69. **Correct answer: A**

Restoril is classified as an antianxiety drug. Elavil, sinequan, and tofranil are all classified as tricyclic medications.

70. **Correct answer: B**

When entering this patient's room or any patient's room to apply restraints, wear appropriate personal protective equipment to protect yourself against exposure to bodily fluids. The patient most likely has had a psychotic reaction to the Demerol and has exposed her IV site and removed her IV, resulting in a potential for exposure to bodily fluids. When attempting to place restraints on a combative patient, regardless of the age, at least four staff members should be present—one for each limb. The family should not be asked to participate in placement of the restraints as they are untrained and it may be seen as a betrayal by the patient. Instead, family members should remain at a safe distance to avoid injury or interference with healthcare providers. A Posey is not the best choice because it leaves the patient's hands free to continue pulling on IV lines. Whenever restraints are in use, be vigilant to document continued need of restraints, type used, time placed, vital signs including airway, breathing, and circulation before and after restraints are placed, time of removal, and reassessments. Be sure to follow your facility's restraint protocols and policies. Patient and staff safety is paramount.

71. **Correct answer: A**

Amoxapine is a cyclic antidepressant that may cause cardiovascular effects and will probably cause status epilepticus. The patient often requires intubation and muscular paralysis because of seizures.

72. **Correct answer: A**

A patient intoxicated with methamphetamine exhibits elevated liver enzymes, tachycardia, hyperthermia, and hypertension.

73. **Correct answer: C**

An antidote for ethylene glycol toxicity is fomepizole. Ethylene glycol is a compound found in antifreeze. After ingestion, it is converted to oxalic acid, which is excreted by the kidneys. This causes crystals in the urine, acidosis, tetany, and renal failure. Hemodialysis and peritoneal dialysis will remove ethylene glycol.

74. **Correct answer: D**

Factors that may affect results of urine morphine levels would not include high levels of lymphocytes. The stealth adulterant masks morphine in the urine. Poppy seed ingestion may produce false-positive results. When heroin is taken, it breaks down into morphine. The ten milligrams of morphine is detectable in urine for 84 hours and can be measured in corpses for about a week.

75. **Correct answer: B**

A urine pH of 7–8 is an appropriate goal for a patient treated for salicylate overdose.

76. **Correct answer: D**

Methadone has a half-life of approximately 24 hours and requires continuous doses of naloxone. The continuous doses prevent respiratory depression until the methadone is eliminated from the patient's system.

77. **Correct answer: A**

Respiratory depression, meiosis, and coma are the triad of symptoms associated with opioid overdose.

78. **Correct answer: B**

Flumazenil is a specific antidote for benzodiazepine overdose. This drug should not be used on patients who overdose on tricyclic antidepressants because of an increased risk of seizures.

79. **Correct answer: D**

Ativan may be used to control the symptoms of cocaine toxicity.

80. **Correct answer: C**

Untreated lithium toxicity may lead to seizures, coma, and cardiac dysrhythmias when levels reach greater than 2.5 mEq/L. Toxicity usually occurs with levels of 2 mEq/L, but symptoms may be noted at even lower blood levels with certain body chemistries. Initial toxicity is noted when the patient experiences diarrhea, vomiting, drowsiness, muscular weakness, and disorientation. As toxicity and symptoms worsen, nystagmus, ataxia, giddiness, tinnitus, confusion, and blurred vision may be present. Patients must be managed by close monitoring and immediate intervention of dysrhythmias and electrolyte imbalances.

81. **Correct answer: C**

Methamphetamine is officially classified as a hallucinogen by *The Diagnostic and Statistical Manual of Mental Disorders*. The World Health Organization (WHO) published a list that shows methamphetamine as the second-most-abused chemical substance. The drug may be ingested, smoked, injected, inserted into the anus or urethra, or snorted. Street names include crystal meth, big blue, base, and ice. The base of the drug is pseudoephedrine or ephedrine mixed with common ingredients. The mixture is often highly explosive, and the first warning a meth lab is nearby is when it blows up.

82. **Correct answer: B**

Ketamine is contraindicated in a patient with altered intracranial pressure because it increases ICP and cerebral blood flow.

83. **Correct answer: C**

Propofol is made from egg phosphates and soybeans. It is incumbent on the nurse to determine if the patient has allergies or sensitivities to these ingredients.

84. **Correct answer: B**

Use of Lactated Ringer's solution is often avoided in a patient with kidney failure because LR contains potassium.

85. **Correct answer: C**

Allergic nephritis may be caused by cimetidine. Cimetidine interferes with creatinine excretion in the renal tubule. Renal function does not decrease, but the creatinine does rise. If diminished renal function exists, an allergic nephritis may develop.

86. **Correct answer: D**

Acyclovir is nephrotoxic and can crystallize in the kidney and cause AKI. It is important for the nurse to carefully monitor the infusion time and the amount of fluid used to dilute intravenous drugs. Additional drugs that can crystallize in the kidney are sulfonamides, indinavir, and triamterene.

87. **Correct answer: B**

Kaon is not a treatment for hyperkalemia. Kaon is another name for potassium gluconate, a common potassium replacement medication. Glucose and insulin, calcium gluconate, and bicarbonate all bind or push the potassium back into the cell from the intravascular space and reduce extracellular potassium levels.

88. **Correct answer: A**

This patient is exhibiting signs and symptoms of hypokalemia. Hypokalemia is defined as any potassium level under 3.5 mEq/L. It is important to reinforce teaching patients how diuretics impact electrolyte levels and the underlying condition.

89. **Correct answer: A**

Magnesium does not act as an antagonist to calcium. Magnesium is required for enzyme activation, synthesis of nucleic acid and proteins, and sodium-potassium pump operation. Magnesium is usually synergistic with calcium to control neuromuscular function within all muscle groups.

90. **Correct answer: A**

You are caring for a patient in kidney failure. As a trauma nurse, you know one expected side effect of kidney failure is the development of anemia. If the kidney no longer produces erythropoietin, the bone marrow will not be stimulated to produce red blood cells (erythrocytes). Erythrocytes normally survive 80–120 days. it is important to note that if your patient is on dialysis, the life of these cells is reduced to about 65–80 days. The shortened life span increases the possibility of the development of anemia.

91. **Correct answer: A**

The normal adult glomerular filtration rate (GFR) is 180 L/day or 125 ml/min. Normal adult urine volume is about 1–2 L/day.

92. **Correct answer: B**

Overhydration is a common cause of hyponatremia. The level is below normal due to dilution and not a disease process or injury. Intake of fluids orally or intravenously has caused an artificial drop in sodium. Correction is done through fluid restriction or decreasing IV rates. Other causes of hyponatremia include loss of sodium through sweating or vomiting, shock, bleeding, SIADH, renal failure (inability to save sodium), hypoxia, freshwater drowning, or an over-administration of hypotonic fluids.

93. **Correct answer: A**

With hyponatremia, sodium levels drop below 135 mEq/L. Twitching and seizures are common, as well as apnea (not tachypnea), irritability (lethargy is seen with hypernatremia), and generalized muscle weakness (late sign). Flattened T waves are seen with hypokalemia.

94. **Correct answer: C**

A drug reaction often caused by a beta-lactam antibiotic that causes an acute inflammation of the kidneys where the primary lesions are in the interstitial space between the nephron is known as intra-renal failure (AKI). Other drugs that may cause this reaction are cephalosporins, sulfonamides, rifampin, non-steroidal anti-inflammatories, and diuretics. Additional beta-lactam antibiotics include penicillin, ampicillin, and methicillin.

95. **Correct answer: B**

   The normal range for serum osmolality in a healthy adult is from 275 to 295 mOsm/kg.

96. **Correct answer: B**

   Regulated excretion (absorption) of potassium is in the distal tubules.

97. **Correct answer: A**

   Generalized muscle weakness progressing to coma is a late sign of a patient suffering from hyponatremia. Seizure activity, low ADH levels, and poor fluid intake are signs of hypernatremia.

98. **Correct answer: C**

   The current recommended serum magnesium level is 2–3 mg/dl. This level may be higher for patients with cardiac disease or in their third trimester of pregnancy to treat pregnancy-induced hypertension and to control premature contractions.

99. **Correct answer: B**

   A nursing consideration when administering magnesium to a patient would include being prepared to administer calcium gluconate. Calcium levels fall when magnesium is given IV.

100. **Correct answer: B**

   The patient has hypercalcemia, as evidenced by the calcium level of 11.7. A loop diuretic prevents reabsorption of calcium, and normal saline is used to increase the patient's glomerular filtration rate. If you were to administer a thiazide diuretic, it would actually decrease calcium excretion. Use of glucose, insulin, and Kayexalate are not indicated because they are treatments for hyperkalemia.

101. **Correct answer: D**

   This patient is hypocalcemic. Lack of calcium slows cardiac contractility (the prolonged QT) and the patient might develop Torsades de pointes (polymorphic ventricular tachycardia). Torsades is also caused by hypomagnesemia.

102. **Correct answer: B**

   Apheresis is the general term used for all pheresis techniques and encompasses any selective removal of cells, plasma, and substances from blood with the return of remaining components and volume to the patient. Plasmapheresis is the removal of plasma and/or proteins from the blood or as a plasma exchange. Cytapheresis is the selective removal of cellular components from the blood (i.e., WBC). Leukocytopheresis is the specific removal of WBCs. Erythrocytapheresis is the removal of RBCs. Plateletpheresis is the removal of platelets. Plasma adsorption/perfusion is the filtering and treatment of plasma via adsorptive fiber filters. Immunoadsorption is the removal of an antigen via an antibody filter. Photopheresis is the removal and return of blood after exposure to ultraviolet light to destroy specific cells (in solid organ transplant rejection).

103. **Correct answer: C**

   Mannitol is nontoxic but must be used with caution because it may produce a hyperosmolar state. Damage to the eighth cranial nerve, vestibular impairment, and renal tubule binding of proteins are characteristics of loop diuretics. Loop diuretics include furosemide, bumetanide, and torsemide.

104. **Correct answer: A**

   NSAIDs block prostaglandin production, which alters glomerular arteriolar perfusion and may cause prerenal AKI.

105. **Correct answer: D**

   Wool and silk give off cyanide gas. Nitriles, like the gloves we wear, will burn and give off cyanide. Household plastics like melamine dishes, plastic cups, polyurethane foam in furniture cushions, and many other synthetic compounds may produce lethal concentrations of cyanide when burned under appropriate circumstances. Cyanide inhibits cellular respiration, even with enough oxygen stores. Cellular metabolism changes from aerobic to anaerobic and produces lactic acid. The organs with the highest oxygen requirements are the most affected by cyanide inhalation.

Hydrogen cyanide is an odorless, pale blue gas that affects the oxygenation of nearly every organ. It is used in many commercial industries. it smells like bitter almonds or it can have a musty scent. It is found in cigarettes, used in pest control, the making of paper and plastics, and by photographic developers. It also occurs in nature in apple seeds and peach pits.

A person can be exposed through many routes including inhalation, ingestion, skin contact, or eye contact. Most are never aware they have been exposed to hydrogen cyanide until it is too late. If cyanide gas is accidentally released the safest place is to get close to the ground and leave the area as soon as possible.

This type of exposure should be treated as a hazardous materials exposure. Full protective gear must be worn at all times to prevent cross contamination.

Inhalation causes the most problems, with ingestion a close second. The patient experiences shortness of breath, weakness, nausea, vomiting, tachycardia. As the conditions worsen the patient develops lung injury, loss of consciousness, and low blood pressure. Eventually there is bradycardia and respiratory failure leading to death.

106. **Correct answer: A**
High levels of carbon monoxide inhalation are expected to cause visual and auditory changes. Additional findings include:

- Cherry red skin
- Retinal hemorrhages
- Tachycardia
- Tachypnea
- Vomiting
- Confusion
- Syncope
- Slurred speech
- Cyanosis
- Myocardial ischemia
- Coma
- Death

Low level exposure is likely to cause

- Headache
- Flu-like illness
- Dyspnea with exertion
- Dizziness

Management:

- One hundred percent oxygen
- Hyperbaric oxygen
- Hospitalization is indicated if
  CO-Hgb levels > 25%
  CO-Hgb levels > 10% during pregnancy
  History or presence of neurologic symptoms
  Presence of metabolic acidosis
  ECG changes are present

Additional information:
Delayed permanent neuropsychiatric syndrome, consisting of memory loss, personality changes, deafness, and seizures, may occur in some victims up to 4 weeks after CO exposure.

107. **Correct answer: D**
Side effects of acetylcysteine include bronchospasms. Thinning the mucus may promote excessive coughing with resultant bronchospasms. Additional side effects include rhinorrhea, stomatitis, nausea, and vomiting.

Special Populations I

- **Bariatrics**
- **Geriatrics**
- **Pediatrics**

INTRODUCTION

	Infant	Child	Adult	Score
Eye Opening	Spontaneous To voice or sound To pain None	Spontaneous To voice To pain None	Spontaneous To voice To pain None	4 3 2 1
Verbal Response	Coos, babbles, fixes and follows Cries, but consolable Persistently irritable Restless and agitated None	Oriented appropriate for age Confused Inappropriate words Incomprehensible None	Oriented Confused Inappropriate words Incomprehensible None	5 4 3 2 1
Motor Response	Spontaneous movement Localizes pain Withdraws to pain Abnormal flexion Abnormal extension None	Obeys commands Localizes pain Withdraws to pain Abnormal flexion Abnormal extension None	Obeys commands Localizes pain Withdraws to pain Abnormal flexion Abnormal extension None	6 5 4 3 2 1

ENA (2013). *Certified Pediatric Emergency Nurse CPEN Review Manual.* Sudbury, MA: Jones & Bartlett Learning.

SECTION 10: QUESTIONS

1. **EMS just radioed the ED and reports they are en route with a 5 year old female who was struck by a car. As a trauma nurse, you know to expect which of the following injuries?**
   A. Head neck, spinal column
   B. Head, chest, abdomen, lower extremities
   C. Head, chest, upper extremities
   D. Chest, pelvis, and upper extremities

2. **In geriatric blunt trauma victims, the normal presenting vital signs and symptoms are not necessarily reliable. Which statement is true about this phenomenon in older adults?**
   A. Geriatric patients are at greater risk for fractures at C1
   B. Geriatric patients are more likely to sustain linear fractures and epidural hemorrhages
   C. MRI imaging is the preferred scanning method for adults over age 65
   D. Two thirds of all rib fractures are sustained from simple falls from a standing position

3. **A 4 year old was involved in a high-speed collision. The child sustained a right pneumothorax, facial, mandibular, and chest injuries, unilateral limb weakness, and a carotid bruit. While performing a secondary survey, a cervicothoracic seat belt abrasion was noted. There was a decline in neurological status, but the results of a CT scan were unremarkable. As a trauma nurse, you believe this child is probably suffering from**
   A. A hemothorax
   B. A C4 vertebral fracture
   C. A blunt carotid artery injury
   D. A partially crushed larynx

4. **A fire department rescue vehicle has transported a child from an accident scene who is still in his car seat. The most appropriate way to safely remove the child from the car seat would be for the team leader to give orders and**
   A. Carry the car seat
   B. Support the head
   C. Support the torso
   D. Support the legs

5. **Calculate the body mass index for a person weighing 220 pounds (100 kg) and is 5 feet 6 inches (1.7 m) tall.**
   A. 47.2
   B. 26.4
   C. 31.1
   D. 34.6

6. **An elderly trauma patient as defined by the American College of Surgeons is over**
   A. 60 years old
   B. 55 years old
   C. 70 years old
   D. 75 years old

7. **A 14 year old patient has been consuming large quantities of power drinks and has been having intermittent episodes of SVT. Today while riding a bike the patient felt light-headed and fell onto the street. The only injuries the patient sustained were minor bruising and lacerations. Which of the following medications is specific to the treatment of sustained supraventricular tachycardia?**
   A. Atropine
   B. Theophylline
   C. Amiodarone
   D. Adenosine

8. Infants with CHF are at high risk during interventional procedures because of
   A. Transcatheter defect occlusion
   B. Prolonged testing times
   C. Balloon atrial septostomy
   D. Contrast dye

9. It is incumbent on the trauma nurse to be familiar with frequently used pediatric medications. For example, intravenous hydralazine is incompatible with
   A. Furosemide
   B. Hydrocortisone
   C. Potassium chloride
   D. Heparin

10. If infiltration of a dopamine infusion occurs, the suggested treatment is to inject which of the following medications into the affected area?
    A. Epinephrine
    B. Phentolamine
    C. Lidocaine
    D. Atropine

11. A toddler was climbing on a step stool in the kitchen then slipped and fell hitting his chest on the kitchen cabinet. The child did not lose consciousness and was brought to the emergency department by his mother. The anterior chest is bruised and the patient is found to have diffuse chest pain and tachycardia. Upon auscultation, you hear muffled heart sounds and note an increased JVD. You suspect the patient has developed a cardiac tamponade. If your patient does have a cardiac tamponade, which of the following findings would you expect on a chest X-ray?
    A. A dilated superior vena cava
    B. Pneumothorax
    C. Narrowed mediastinum
    D. Delineation of the pericardium and epicardium

12. A mother and 4 month old infant were in a car accident. The infant was restrained in a car seat and is now being evaluated in your trauma bay. The mother reports that the infant has a history of Ebstein anomaly and is on cardiac glycosides. A major effect of this class of medications is
    A. Increased conductivity
    B. Positive chronotropism
    C. Its usefulness as a ventricular antiarrhythmic
    D. Inotropism

13. A junior high school student has been experimenting with multiple drugs. She was admitted to your ED after a cocaine overdose. The patient has been diagnosed with an anterolateral myocardial infarction. As a trauma nurse, where do you expect to see changes on the 12-lead EKG that indicate the patient is having an anterolateral MI?
    A. $V_1, V_2,$ I, and AVL
    B. $V_2, V_3, V_4,$ I, and AVL
    C. $V_2, V_3, V_4,$ II, III, and AVF
    D. $V_1, V_2,$ II, III, and AVF

14. A 10 year old was struck by a car and subsequently received morphine IV for pain. He is now unresponsive and his respiratory rate and depth are diminished. As a trauma nurse, you know that the antagonist for morphine is
    A. Naloxone
    B. Atropine
    C. Regitine
    D. Bicarbonate

15. A teenager just gave birth in your ED. The teen has lupus, so the newborn is at risk for cardiomyopathy and
    A. Myocarditis
    B. Blisters on the skin
    C. Congenital heart block
    D. Weight gain

16. You are mentoring a new nurse in the ED. The patient you will be caring for is receiving lidocaine via a continuous infusion. The new trauma nurse must know that lidocaine may cause adverse effects such as
    A. Hyperexcitability
    B. CNS toxicity
    C. Ventricular tachycardia
    D. Premature atrial complexes

17. The most common mechanisms of unintentional injury in the elderly are
    A. Hypertension and motor vehicle crashes
    B. Cardiac issues and ETOH abuse
    C. Falls and motor vehicle crashes
    D. Polypharmacy and hypertension

18. You have been selected to present a cardiac assessment class at your facility. You are asked the location of the PMI in an infant. As a trauma nurse, you know newborns and infants usually demonstrate right ventricular dominance. The location of the PMI in this case would be
    A. At the lower left sternal border
    B. At the right midclavicular line
    C. At the second right intercostal space
    D. At the right lower sternal border

19. The patient had a syncopal episode during a pep rally at school and fell against one of the bleachers and struck her head. There was no LOC and she was transported to the ED by ambulance. She has been diagnosed with refractive SVT that did not respond to either adenosine or cardioversion. She is awaiting transfer to your PICU for monitoring prior to ablation therapy. Tachy arrhythmias that are refractive to conventional therapies may have to be treated with radio-frequency ablation. This treatment is usually successful on reentry tachy arrhythmias. The radio-frequency destroys myocardial tissue via
    A. Radiation
    B. Heat
    C. Cold
    D. An overriding signal to ablate the pacemaker

20. A 14 year old took his brother's motorcycle out for a ride. The patient lost control of the motorcycle in the rain. He was wearing a helmet and protective gear. The patient suffered a fractured left femur, left flail chest, a cervical sprain, and road rash on his face and neck. He is admitted with a blood pressure of 82/42, HR 102, RR 26 and shallow, and T 98.2°F. His 12-lead EKG shows ST elevation in the anterior leads. His CXR shows a normal cardiac silhouette and no infiltrates. His Hgb is 9.0, Hct is 31. MB is 18%. The patient is restless and complains of pain in his chest and left leg. As a trauma nurse, you know this patient is probably suffering from
    A. Pulmonary edema
    B. Hypovolemic shock
    C. Systolic dysfunction
    D. Pulmonary hypertension

21. **Your pediatric trauma patient had an arterial line and is being mechanically ventilated. You note very pronounced phasic variations in the arterial line and suspect that**
    A. The patient's ETT is becoming dislodged
    B. The patient has tricuspid regurgitation
    C. The patient is suffering from heart failure
    D. The patient's arterial line is kinked

22. **You are preparing to give adenosine to a 3 year old exhibiting recurrent SVT. It is important that adenosine be given rapidly. Why?**
    A. If given slowly, the adenosine will probably fail to convert the SVT
    B. Adenosine is incompatible with adrenalin
    C. If given slowly, adenosine may cause systemic vasodilation and reflex tachycardia
    D. If given slowly, adenosine may cause blurred vision

23. **Dobutamine is used to improve cardiac output primarily by**
    A. Causing profound peripheral vasodilation
    B. Acting on alpha-adrenergic receptors in the heart
    C. Acting on beta-1 adrenergic receptors in the heart
    D. Acting on both alpha- and beta-adrenergic receptors in the cardiovascular tissue

24. **Your pediatric trauma patient has been started on dobutamine for blood pressure support. Which of the following lab results should you monitor closely for life-threatening effects from the dobutamine?**
    A. Calcium levels
    B. Potassium levels
    C. Magnesium levels
    D. Chloride levels

25. **High-dose epinephrine was started for your 7 year old patient post–cardiac arrest due to beta blocker overdose. Which of the following lab results should you monitor closely?**
    A. Glucose levels
    B. Calcium levels
    C. Chloride levels
    D. Sodium levels

26. **Atropine was given to an 8 year old during an episode of bradycardia that resulted in a heart rate in the 20s. The patient had just been deeply suctioned. The low heart rate was unresponsive to oxygen support, so assisted ventilation via a bag-valve mask was provided. The patient's heart rate improved to pre-bradycardic levels. Which of the following potential complications of atropine administration may now occur?**
    A. Diuresis
    B. Hypertension
    C. Rebound bradycardia
    D. Headache

27. **During a code, it is discovered that your pediatric patient was given IV heparin instead of epinephrine. Protamine sulfate was ordered to counter the effects of the heparin. Which of the following places the patient at an increased risk for an allergic reaction to protamine sulfate?**
    A. Influenza vaccine
    B. Type 2 diabetes
    C. A history of PKU
    D. Allergy to fish

28. **Your bariatric patient was involved in a frontal collision between two cars. Which of the following statements is false regarding injury and comorbidity with bariatric patients involved in motor vehicle collisions?**
    A. Length of stay, especially in the ICU, is decreased by one third
    B. In frontal collisions, there is increased mortality for bariatric patients
    C. In frontal collisions, bariatric patients suffer more head, thoracic, abdominal, and lower extremity fractures
    D. Bariatric patients suffer fewer injuries, but they are usually more severe injuries

29. **Burns are the third leading cause of death in the elderly. Which of the following statements is least likely to be a cause of these fatalities?**
    A. Elderly victims are less able to evacuate the area of fire
    B. The elderly possess less fire extinguishers
    C. Many elderly live in older housing
    D. Elderly are less likely to have smoke detectors

30. **You are training a new trauma nurse regarding administration of IV drugs to the pediatric trauma patient. You explain that Lasix must be given slowly because**
    A. Lasix may cause nausea
    B. A rash may develop
    C. Hyperkalemia may occur
    D. A rapid infusion can lead to hearing loss

31. **Which of the following medications is contraindicated for use in children younger than 1 year of age?**
    A. Verapamil
    B. Adenosine
    C. Procainamide
    D. Esmolol

32. **A 15 year old gamer was participating in a 24-hour tournament. He tried to walk to the restroom and collapsed. He is being brought to your ED via ambulance for chest pain and severe hypertension. Upon arrival to the ED, a nitroglycerin drip is ordered. Which of the following statements is true regarding nitroglycerin administration?**
    A. Use polyvinyl chloride tubing
    B. Nitroglycerine may be piggybacked to Isolyte P
    C. Nitroglycerine should be filtered prior to delivery
    D. Have normal saline or other volume expander available at the bedside

33. **A 6 year old comes to the ED after falling from the monkey bars while at school. He sustained a fractured left tibia and fibula and a fractured left clavicle. The patient has to remain in the ED holding overnight due to a lack of available beds in the PICU. Your initial assessment results are as follows:**
    EKG: ST at 115 with isolated PVCs
    Art line BP 70/50
    Cuff BP 76/50
    Skin pale, cool, clammy
    RR 26, breath sounds clear, slightly diminished RLL
    O_2 2 L/min via NC
    Mentation: responds to questions slowly, oriented to self and time
    Pulmonary artery catheter readings:
    PAP 24/8
    PAOP 5
    RAP 4

Cardiac output 3.3
Cardiac index 1.7

Which of the following conditions do you believe the patient is developing?

A. Cardiogenic shock

B. Hypovolemic shock

C. Septic shock

D. Left ventricular failure

34. Your patient is a 15 year old freshman football player. When he returned home from school this afternoon, he was short of breath and overly fatigued. Several bruises were noted on his arms and lower legs. His mother mentioned that his ankles were quite swollen at that time. The patient uncharacteristically went to bed; when his mother could not arouse him, she called paramedics. They arrived in your ED approximately 30 minutes ago. The patient is being mechanically ventilated at TV 650, FiO_2 0.80, and AMV 14. He remains unresponsive. A pulmonary artery catheter was placed. His assessment findings are as follows:

EKG: ST at 124
Art line BP 68/42
Cuff BP 64/46
Doppler only to dorsalis pedis, no pressure obtained
Skin pale, cool, clammy
RR 15, breath sounds = crackles LLL, RLL
Marked pretibial and pedal edema
Mentation: unresponsive to painful stimuli
Pulmonary artery catheter readings:
PAP 46/28
PAOP 26
RAP 18
Cardiac output 3.2
Cardiac index 1.2

The patient is probably developing

A. Pulmonary hypertension

B. Cardiac tamponade

C. Cardiogenic shock

D. Right heart failure

35. **Malignant hyperthermia is most likely to occur after the administration of**

A. Morphine

B. Tetracycline

C. Halothane

D. Lidocaine

36. **A late sign of malignant hyperthermia is**

A. Jaw rigidity

B. Rhabdomyolysis

C. Tachycardia

D. Metabolic acidosis

37. **An early sign of malignant hyperthermia is**

A. Rhabdomyolysis

B. Bleeding from venipuncture sites

C. Increased temperature

D. Elevated serum creatinine phosphokinase

38. **Which of the following is the first functional organ during embryonic development?**
    A. Heart
    B. Lungs
    C. Kidneys
    D. Liver

39. **According to American Heart Association 2015 guidelines, when providing chest compressions to infants and children, recommendations are to compress one-third the anterior–posterior depth of the chest. What approximate chest depth is this?**
    A. ½ inch for infants, 1 inch for older children
    B. 1 inch for infants, 1.5 inches for older children
    C. 1.5 inches for infants, 2 inches for older children
    D. 2 inches for infants, 2.5 inches for older children

40. **Signs of potential elder maltreatment would not include**
    A. The caregiver allows the elderly patient to be seen and treated alone
    B. The caregiver belittles, controls, or threatens the patient
    C. The patient mimics dementia by mumbling to themselves, sucking, or rocking
    D. A history of repeated injuries and visits to multiple EDs

41. **Which of the following is true regarding management of a child who has died after a sudden and unexpected cardiac arrest?**
    A. Provide grief counseling for staff members
    B. Do not allow anyone to touch the body until after a clergy member has spoken with the family
    C. Remove all tubes, treatment devices, and monitors prior to allowing the family to see the patient
    D. Notify the family that a complete, unrestricted autopsy should be done

42. **According to the American Heart Association 2015 guidelines, healthcare providers should begin chest compressions immediately on infants and children if they cannot palpate a pulse within how many seconds?**
    A. 3
    B. 6
    C. 10
    D. 15

43. **Per the American Heart Association 2015 guidelines, which of the following statements is true regarding calculation of pediatric emergency drugs?**
    A. If the patient is obese, calculate the drug dosage based on the ideal weight using the patient's body length as measured on a resuscitation tape
    B. If the patient is obese, calculate the drug dosage based on the actual weight minus half the ideal weight based on body length
    C. If the patient is obese, calculate the drug dosage based on the actual body weight and administer the calculated dose, even if it exceeds the adult dose recommendation
    D. If the patient is obese, administer the recommended adult dosage

44. **You are attempting to draw an arterial blood gas sample from an arterial line. The syringe requires a lot of force to move the cylinder. What effect will this high friction on the syringe have on the blood gas results?**
    A. It will put the artery into spasm
    B. It will increase the $PaCO_2$
    C. It will decrease the PaO_2
    D. No effect

45. **Chronic hypoxia usually results in which of the following electrolyte imbalances?**
    A. Decreased chloride
    B. Decreased potassium
    C. Decreased calcium
    D. Decreased bicarbonate

46. **An example of a comorbidity that would directly impact the potential for a traumatic injury would include**
    A. Diabetes
    B. GERD
    C. Sleep apnea
    D. Kidney disease

47. **Your patient is a 16 year old being treated in the ED for a left Colles' fracture and status asthmaticus. She has been taking Accolate, Allegra and using a Proventil HFA rescue inhaler at home. Today she was skateboarding with her friends and tripped over a curb. After falling she could not catch her breath. Her bronchospasms worsened, and she was transported to the ED. In the ED, the patient received albuterol, oxygen, and epinephrine without significant improvement. You note that she is using accessory muscles for respiration and is tachycardic and tachypneic. On auscultation, inspiratory and expiratory wheezing with a prolonged expiratory phase is heard throughout the lung fields. Your patient is placed on 2 L/min via NC, and ABGs are drawn. Blood gas results are as follows: pH 7.53, PaO_2 104 mmHg, $PaCO_2$ 27 mmHg, and HCO_3 23 mEq/L. These blood gas results indicate**
    A. Compensated metabolic alkalosis
    B. Uncompensated respiratory acidosis
    C. Compensated metabolic acidosis
    D. Uncompensated respiratory alkalosis

48. **Which of the following conditions would be the most probable cause of the acid–base imbalance of uncompensated respiratory alkalosis?**
    A. Kidney failure
    B. A side effect of theophylline
    C. Hyperventilation
    D. Hypoventilation

49. **A new ED resident orders Inderal (propranolol) for your patient who is an asthmatic. As a trauma nurse, you know that propranolol is contraindicated for asthmatics because**
    A. It will lead to severe respiratory acidosis
    B. It will exacerbate the tachycardia
    C. Pneumonia may result
    D. Bronchospasm may worsen

50. **Your 13 year old trauma patient needs to be placed on mechanical ventilation. The trauma physician uses pancuronium bromide (Pavulon) to paralyze the respiratory muscles. Which of the following drugs will counteract the effects of Pavulon?**
    A. Atropine
    B. Neostigmine
    C. Narcan
    D. Regitine

51. **Patients can develop pulmonary air leaks while on mechanical ventilation. A risk factor for the development of an air leak would be**
    A. PEEP set too low
    B. Asynchrony
    C. Use of SIMV
    D. A malfunctioning ETT

52. **Pulmonary consideration in the elderly does not include**
    A. Bony abnormalities
    B. Increased surfactant
    C. Decreased PaO_2
    D. Sleep apnea

53. **If you hear faint breath sounds on the left side of the chest and normal sounds on the right side of the chest immediately after your pediatric trauma patient has been intubated, most likely**
    A. The ETT has an air leak
    B. The physician has intubated the esophagus
    C. The ETT is at the carina
    D. The right mainstem bronchus has been intubated

54. **On a ventilator, a high-pressure limit alarm may sound if**
    A. The ventilator tubing contains excess water
    B. A leak occurs in a chest tube
    C. A pneumothorax occurs
    D. The tubing is disconnected

55. **An adverse effect of excessive CPAP is**
    A. A continuous need to increase oxygen over time
    B. A rise in intrathoracic pressure
    C. Intraventricular hemorrhage
    D. A sudden change in cerebral blood flow

56. **Your patient is 6 years old and requires mechanical ventilation. If positive inspiratory pressure (PIP) is increased on a mechanical ventilator, what effect should this change have on the patient's blood gases?**
    A. It will increase the $PaCO_2$ and decrease the PaO_2
    B. It will decrease the $PaCO_2$ and decrease the PaO_2
    C. It will decrease the $PaCO_2$ and increase the PaO_2
    D. It will decrease the pH and decrease the $PaCO_2$

57. **Analyze the following arterial blood gas results from a toddler on 2 L O_2 via a nasal cannula:**

pH	7.48
CO_2	31
HCO_3	22

    A. Normal
    B. Compensated respiratory acidosis
    C. Uncompensated respiratory alkalosis
    D. Uncompensated metabolic alkalosis

58. **Analyze the following arterial blood gas results from a term infant on room air**

pH	7.15
CO_2	57
HCO_3	21

    A. Uncompensated metabolic alkalosis
    B. Uncompensated (mixed) respiratory/metabolic acidosis
    C. Compensated metabolic acidosis
    D. Uncompensated respiratory acidosis

59. **When caring for an infant with an expiratory grunt, the infant**
    A. Needs to be intubated immediately
    B. Requires monitoring of vital signs every hour
    C. Is exhaling against a closed glottis
    D. Is exhibiting a neurological sign due to hypoxia

60. A patient recently admitted to the ED requires immediate intubation. The physician orders succinylcholine. Which of the following conditions is not a side effect of succinylcholine?
    A. Hypotension
    B. Malignant hypothermia
    C. Hypokalemia
    D. Smooth-muscle contraction

61. Vecuronium (Norcuron) is eliminated primarily via the
    A. Hepatic/biliary system
    B. Spleen
    C. Renal glomerulus
    D. Large bowel

62. One cause of decreased SVO_2 in a pediatric patient would be
    A. An increased metabolic rate
    B. Sedation
    C. A decreased metabolic rate
    D. Increased cardiac output

63. As patients age from birth through young adulthood, chest wall compliance decreases. One reason for this change is
    A. Increased arterial oxygen tension
    B. Decreased total lung capacity
    C. Costal cartilage degeneration
    D. Decreased residual volume

64. Elderly patients will always have a diminished PaO_2, even if they possess healthy lungs. They also have a diminished reserve. Try to solve this equation: Patient is 70 years old. Assuming healthy lungs, their calculated new normal PaO_2 would be
    A. 60 mmHg
    B. 55 mmHg
    C. 65 mmHg
    D. 70 mmHg

65. The oxyhemoglobin dissociation curve may be shifted to the right by
    A. Alkalosis, hyperthermia, and hypercapnia
    B. Acidosis, hypocarbia, and hypothermia
    C. Acidosis, hypercarbia, and hyperthermia
    D. Alkalosis, hypothermia, and hypercapnia

66. The nursing student assigned to you for the day asks you to explain the oxyhemoglobin dissociation curve. You reply that the oxyhemoglobin dissociation curve is
    A. A relation between dissolved oxygen and the affinity for oxygen by the hemoglobin molecule
    B. A graphic representation of carbon dioxide content versus oxygen content in arterial blood
    C. A measure of methemoglobin
    D. A way to calculate gas transport across the alveoli

67. Mask continuous positive airway pressure (CPAP) should be used with caution if a pediatric patient has
    A. A low functional residual capacity (FRC)
    B. A basilar skull fracture
    C. Sinusitis
    D. Pneumonia

68. **What is the purpose of grunting?**
    A. Grunting increases lung compliance
    B. Grunting pushes more air through an ETT
    C. Grunting decreases the need for abdominal muscle use
    D. Grunting helps maintain functional residual capacity

69. **Which of the following medications is both an analgesic and an amnestic?**
    A. Barbiturates
    B. Propofol
    C. Atropine
    D. Ketamine

70. **Which of the following statements about infant and child airways is false?**
    A. The chest wall is composed of more cartilage than bone
    B. Because of rib pliability, the ribs may fail to support the lungs
    C. A pneumothorax is easy to auscultate because breath sounds are easily transmitted
    D. Internal injury may be present without extreme signs

71. **The volume of gas remaining in the lungs at the end of one normal expiration is called**
    A. Residual volume
    B. Capacitance
    C. Total lung capacity
    D. Functional residual capacity

72. **Your patient's father was driving his car through an intersection when the vehicle was T-boned by another car. The patient suffered a fractured pelvis and left femur and was stabilized in the ED. The patient is now awaiting surgical fixation of the fractures. When auscultating lung sounds, you hear what you believe to be bowel sounds in his chest. The patient also states he has moderate shoulder pain on the left side and he is mildly tachypneic. The patient will probably be diagnosed with**
    A. A fractured scapula
    B. A hemothorax
    C. Diaphragmatic rupture
    D. Bowel rupture

73. **Endotracheal cuff pressures should not exceed**
    A. PAOP
    B. Tracheal capillary filling pressure
    C. RAP
    D. Pulmonary artery diastolic pressure

74. **You suspect your patient is developing a pulmonary embolism. Signs and symptoms of a pulmonary embolus can include**
    A. Sinus bradycardia or a normal EKG
    B. Pleuritic chest pain, decreased cardiac output
    C. ABGs showing respiratory acidosis, increased respiratory rate
    D. Decreased PAS pressure

75. **Which of the following statements is true when a patient has a pulmonary embolism?**
    A. Respiratory acidosis will occur
    B. Heparin is used to dissolve clots
    C. Normal d-dimer results can rule out a pulmonary embolism
    D. Metabolic alkalosis will develop

76. **Elderly patients have a decrease in functioning nephrons and a reduced capacity to filter and clear drugs. Examples of hospital-acquired renal failure would not include**
    A. Nephrotoxicity from IV contrast
    B. Surgery
    C. Hypertension
    D. Hypotension

77. **Your patient was admitted to the ED following a fall from a tree. She complains of stabbing substernal pain each time she changes her position. She has been diagnosed with a pneumomediastinum. A common significant finding is**
    A. Cullen's sign
    B. Grey-Turner's sign
    C. Hamman's sign
    D. Handes' sign

78. **Pulse oximetry should never be used**
    A. To determine oxygen saturation values
    B. During a cardiac arrest
    C. As a determinant for predicting hemoglobin affinity for oxygen
    D. To determine a patient's activity tolerance

79. **To determine if your patient has a genetic predisposition toward malignant hyperthermia, which of the following drugs might be used for sensitivity testing?**
    A. Halothane
    B. Caffeine
    C. Accolate
    D. Singulair

80. **Pertussis in infants younger than one month old who received erythromycin may mean the infants are at increased risk for**
    A. Infantile hypertrophic pyloric stenosis
    B. Toxoplasmosis
    C. Rubella
    D. Pulmonary hypertension

81. **Which of the following statements about respiratory diphtheria is true?**
    A. Protection against respiratory diphtheria is predominantly provided by immunoglobulin G antibodies
    B. Respiratory diphtheria occurs only during the third trimester of pregnancy
    C. The mortality rate of respiratory diphtheria is approximately 90% if left untreated
    D. Maternal antitoxin is not transferred to the fetus

82. **Death in the hypothermic infant is caused by**
    A. The underlying disease process
    B. Aerobic metabolism
    C. Bradycardia
    D. Hypoglycemia and hypoxemia

83. **Temperature regulation in the infant is controlled by the hypothalamus through the release of which of the following hormones?**
    A. Dopamine
    B. Norepinephrine
    C. Cortisol
    D. Epinephrine

84. A bariatric patient has arrived in your ED after a fall at home. As a trauma nurse, you know the patient is likely to suffer from respiratory compromise, just because of anatomic changes. The patient may develop obesity hypoventilation syndrome (OHS). This syndrome is not characterized by
   A. Increased systemic pulmonary artery pressures
   B. Increased right and left ventricular pressures
   C. Decreased cardiac output
   D. Right-sided heart failure

85. What are the two most common causes of a comatose state in a child younger than 5 years of age?
   A. Falls and drowning
   B. Inappropriate use of car seats and trauma
   C. Nonaccidental trauma and near-drowning
   D. Accidental overdose and head injury

86. What does the Pediatric Glasgow Coma Scale measure?
   A. Eye opening, deep tendon reflexes, verbal response
   B. Eye opening, motor response, verbal response
   C. Eye opening, motor response, cranial nerve response
   D. Eye opening, cranial nerve response, verbal response

87. Normal intracranial pressure in a 3 year old child is
   A. 0–5 mmHg
   B. 3–7 mmHg
   C. 16–20 mmHg
   D. 20–40 mmHg

88. When should a lumbar puncture be done on a patient with increased intracranial pressure?
   A. Once the patient has completed a CT or MRI scan
   B. A lumbar puncture should always be done to check intracranial pressure
   C. The decision to do a lumbar puncture should be made on a case-by-case basis
   D. Never

89. What is the ideal range for cerebral perfusion pressure for a 4 year old child?
   A. 50–60 mmHg
   B. 20–40 mmHg
   C. 10–20 mmHg
   D. 70–90 mmHg

90. In a child older than 6 years of age, a positive Babinski or plantar reflex indicates
   A. A reflex elicited with a reflex hammer to the Achilles tendon
   B. Normal neurologic functioning
   C. An upper motor neuron lesion of the pyramidal tract
   D. A lower motor neuron lesion of the pyramidal tract

91. A relative contraindication for administration of methylprednisolone following a spinal injury would be
   A. A spinal cord injury less than 4 hours old
   B. Pregnancy
   C. A patient younger than the age of 8 years
   D. An intubated patient

92. **Your patient is a 6 year old who had a subarachnoid hemorrhage after being struck by a car while riding his bicycle. Which of the following conditions is most likely to occur with this injury?**
    A. Communicating hydrocephalus
    B. Diabetes mellitus
    C. Seizure disorder
    D. Nystagmus

93. **What is an early sign of uncal herniation?**
    A. Contralateral pupil dilation
    B. Ipsilateral pupil dilation
    C. Contralateral pupil constriction
    D. Ipsilateral pupil constriction

94. **What is the "purple glove syndrome"?**
    A. A complication of intravenous phenytoin administration
    B. A complication of intravenous lopressor administration
    C. A complication of intravenous adenosine administration
    D. A complication of intravenous phenobarbital administration

95. **In children, in which age range are febrile seizures most likely to occur?**
    A. Newborn infants to 6 months
    B. 6 months to 6 years of age
    C. 10 months to 10 years of age
    D. Infants up to 1 year of age

96. **Your elderly patient was trying to sit at his desk chair, but misjudged the distance and sat down hard. He is now complaining of increased pain while walking. The patient's posture is noted to be slightly kyphotic. As a trauma nurse, you suspect this patient has suffered a**
    A. Fractured coccyx
    B. High cervical injury
    C. Compression fracture
    D. Pelvic fracture

97. **You are to administer mannitol to your patient with cerebral edema. Which precautions should you take when giving this drug?**
    A. No precautions are necessary
    B. Mannitol must be administered quickly over 1–2 minutes
    C. Mannitol must be administered slowly through an in-line 5-micron filter
    D. Mannitol is contraindicated in children

98. **How quickly should phenobarbital sodium be administered intravenously to a 15 year old patient?**
    A. Phenobarbital should be given at less than 30 mg/min
    B. Phenobarbital should be given via rapid intravenous push
    C. Phenobarbital should be given in a drip chamber over 1 hour
    D. Phenobarbital should not be given to children

99. **Your pediatric trauma patient has sustained a head injury and is demonstrating blood collection behind the tympanic membrane. This symptom usually indicates a**
    A. Skull base fracture
    B. Temporal bone fracture
    C. Middle fossa basilar fracture
    D. Parietal skull fracture

100. Your patient is 8 years old and has an epidural hematoma. His symptoms include hemiplegia, hemiparesis, and an inequality of his pupils greater than a 1 mm difference. This inequality in the pupils is known as
    A. Miosis
    B. Ford's sign
    C. Anisocoria
    D. Hill's sign

101. Depressed skull fractures in infants may result in indentation or pliable skull bone(s) without loss of bone integrity. This condition is known as
    A. "Ping-Pong" depression
    B. Diastasis
    C. Medullary bulge
    D. Walker fracture

102. Which of the following statements about taking the temperature of a geriatric patient is true?
    A. Axillary temperatures are the most accurate
    B. Oral temperature is decreased with age
    C. Core measurements are the preferred route to obtain temperature measurements
    D. Increased stroke volume increases core temperature

103. Normal ICP in children ranges from
    A. 1.5–6 mmHg
    B. 3–7.5 mmHg
    C. 8–10 mmHg
    D. 11–15 mmHg

104. In an older child, approximately what percentage of cardiac output is delivered to the brain?
    A. 5%
    B. 10%
    C. 15%
    D. 20%

105. Jugular venous oxygen saturation (SjO_2) is used to
    A. Identify patients at risk for cerebral ischemia
    B. Monitor brain temperature
    C. Measure the balance between cerebral oxygen delivery and cerebral oxygen consumption
    D. Identify complications of catheter insertion

106. The normal range for SjO_2 is between
    A. 60% and 75%
    B. 70% and 85%
    C. 80% and 90%
    D. 85% and 95%

107. Which of the following statements about SjO_2 monitoring is true?
    A. SjO_2 monitoring should be used for patients older than age 8 and/or who weigh 30 kg
    B. SjO_2 monitoring is not used in conjunction with ICP or CPP monitoring
    C. SjO_2 values may be abnormally low in patients with nonviable brain tissue
    D. The SjO_2 catheter does not need to be calibrated

108. Which of the following signs or symptoms will differentiate a generalized seizure from syncope?
    A. Incontinence
    B. Sense of an impending loss of consciousness
    C. A headache
    D. An actual loss of consciousness

109. **Normal cerebrospinal fluid (CSF) flow in a toddler should be approximately _____ per hour**
    A. 3–5 ml
    B. 10–15 ml
    C. 5–10 ml
    D. 15–20 ml

110. **Absence seizures are characterized by**
    A. No postictal state
    B. Discharge of neurons in one hemisphere
    C. Loss of posture
    D. Increased thoracic muscle tone

111. **At what stage of fetal development does the GI tract begin to develop?**
    A. 2–4 weeks gestational age
    B. 4–8 weeks gestational age
    C. 6–10 weeks gestational age
    D. 12–16 weeks gestational age

112. **You have been tasked with starting a peripheral IV on an obese patient. Which of the following techniques is the most likely to be successful?**
    A. Use a smaller gauge catheter
    B. Start the IV in the patient's foot
    C. Use a tight tourniquet
    D. Have the patient clench the fist and use a loose tourniquet

113. **Your patient is a 17 year old student who weighs 85 pounds. She was found unconscious in the bathroom and was admitted for severe dehydration and starvation. Which of the following symptoms would you expect to observe with this patient?**
    A. Decreased serum lactate
    B. Normal urinary nitrogen excretion
    C. Conservation of body fluids with third spacing
    D. Decreased serum catecholamines, glucagon, and cortisol

114. **Your patient, a 16 year old student with cirrhosis, was admitted to the ED after a weekend party where he indulged in alcohol, drugs, and smoking. His lab results were as follows:**

    ALT 245 U/L   AST 147 U/L
    PT 24 seconds   PLT 75 × 10³/mm³
    Hgb 8.4 g/dl   Hct 31%.
    Bilirubin 10 mg/dl
    These results indicate that patient is at high risk for
    A. Variceal bleeding
    B. Peptic ulcer disease
    C. Gastritis
    D. Boerhaave syndrome

115. **Which of the following lab results would contraindicate administration of peritoneal lavage?**
    A. RBC 5.2 million/mm³
    B. PLT 79,000 mm³/ml
    C. PT 12.5 seconds and PTT 75 seconds
    D. Hgb 14.7 g/dl and Hct 46%

116. Your 15 year old patient was involved in a motor vehicle accident and suffered blunt abdominal trauma related to the seat belt placement. He begins complaining of severe abdominal pain around the epigastric area that is knife-like and twisting. You also note that he has a low-grade fever with diaphoresis, abdominal distention, decreased bowel tones, and rebound tenderness. You suspect this patient is suffering from
    A. Pancreatitis
    B. Acute liver failure
    C. Gastrointestinal bleeding
    D. Abdominal bruising

117. Despite being only 12 years old, your patient is frequently in the ED for alcohol-induced comas. Just prior to his transfer to a step-down unit, he begins projectile vomiting bright red blood. Your first action should be to
    A. Position the patient flat
    B. Obtain and insert a Linton-Nachlas tube
    C. Make the patient NPO and verify IV access
    D. Start dopamine at 5 mcg/kg/min

118. Your 13 year old patient is 7 months pregnant and presents in the ED with severe HELLP syndrome. She is also at risk for which of the following conditions?
    A. Intra-abdominal hypertension (IAH) and abdominal compartment syndrome (ACS)
    B. Decreased intracranial pressure (ICP)
    C. Hypocarbia
    D. Increased platelets

119. Drug dosages for the geriatric patient are often less than normal dosages. Which of the follow explains this reasoning?
    A. The geriatric patient has a faster rate of absorption
    B. The geriatric patient GI motility rate is accelerated
    C. The geriatric patient has a decreased first pass effect
    D. The geriatric patient has a decreased gastric pH

120. The BUN may be elevated in geriatric patients because they
    A. Are undergoing steroid treatments
    B. Are taking streptomycin
    C. Are taking chloramphenicol
    D. Have a low protein intake

121. Which of the following is the most common cause of intestinal obstruction in the newborn?
    A. Intussusception
    B. Meconium ileus
    C. Intestinal atresia
    D. Volvulus

122. Your patient is an 8 year old boy who was hit in the lower back while playing football with friends. His X-ray shows T11 and T12 transverse process fractures. Which of your patient's symptoms probably indicates renal injury?
    A. Flank pain
    B. 2 ml/kg/hr of urinary output
    C. Urinary incontinence
    D. Urine osmolarity of 300 mOsm/L

123. **Which of the following statements is true regarding kidney function in the pediatric population?**
    A. Nephrons continue to develop until age 8
    B. Kidney location is fixed at L1–L3
    C. Infant kidneys are less susceptible to fluid changes
    D. Approximately 20% to 25% of cardiac output is directed to the kidneys

124. **Which of the following statements is true regarding kidney structure in the pediatric population?**
    A. Cortical nephrons account for 99% of all nephrons
    B. Cortical nephrons have long Loops of Henle for water conservation
    C. The tubular components of the nephron include the proximal tubule, Loop of Henle, and distal tubule
    D. Afferent arterioles take blood from the glomerulus to the second capillary bed

125. **Which of the following statements about creatinine is true?**
    A. A normal range is 0.8–1.4 mg/dl
    B. Creatinine levels are higher in females
    C. Lower than normal levels may indicate pyelonephritis
    D. Low levels are a precursor to eclampsia

126. **The most common cause of hypermagnesemia is**
    A. Gastrointestinal bypass
    B. Gastrointestinal fistulas
    C. Renal failure
    D. Overdose

127. **The normal glomerular filtration rate for a 1 year old child is**
    A. 35–40 ml/min
    B. 60 ml/min
    C. 80–120 ml/min
    D. 140–180 ml/min

128. **Your patient is 14 years old and is an alcoholic. Chronic use of alcohol will have which of the following effects on the patient's potassium levels?**
    A. Potassium moves out of the vascular circulation and into the cells
    B. Potassium moves out of the cells and into the vascular circulation
    C. Potassium moves out of the cells and into the interstitium
    D. Potassium moves out of the vascular circulation and into the interstitium

129. **Your patient is receiving a magnesium drip to control premature contractions. As a trauma nurse, you know magnesium alters intracellular calcium by influencing**
    A. Parathyroid function
    B. Aldosterone secretion
    C. Cortisol secretion
    D. Glycosol production

130. **Your patient is becoming confused, is lethargic, and has muscle weakness. A review of her lab report shows a calcium level of 11.9. A common method of treatment for this condition is to use**
    A. Normal saline and a loop diuretic
    B. D_5W and a Kayexalate enema
    C. Glucose followed by insulin
    D. Nothing; this is a normal value

131. **The normal specific gravity of urine at 1.002–1.012 reflects the normal value of urine**
    A. 50–100 mOsm/L
    B. 100–300 mOsm/L
    C. 200–500 mOsm/L
    D. 200–400 mOsm/L

132. **Serum calcium is increased by which of the following conditions?**
    A. Increases in vitamin D
    B. Renal tubular excretion
    C. Gastrointestinal excretion
    D. Bone demineralization

133. **An elderly patient has a fever, chills, dysuria, frequency, and pain at the costovertebral angle. It is likely this patient is suffering from**
    A. Pyelonephritis
    B. Urinary calculi
    C. A lower urinary tract infection
    D. AKI

134. **The primary causative organism for urinary tract infections is**
    A. *Escherichia coli*
    B. *Staphylococcus aureus*
    C. *Proteus* species
    D. *Klebsiella*

135. **An elderly male patient requires urinary catheterization. As you attempt to advance the catheter, you meet resistance and cannot advance the catheter more than about 3 inches into the urethra. The probable cause of this blockage is**
    A. A urinary calculus
    B. Benign prostatic hyperplasia
    C. A large catheter
    D. A small catheter that has curled on itself

136. **Your patient is an elderly diabetic with congestive heart failure. After 4 days of no contact, her daughter found her in bed, unresponsive. She has a red, dry, swollen tongue, temperature of 102ºF, and flushed dry skin. She is tachycardic, hypotensive, and has decreased reflexes. Her urine specific gravity is 1.050. You suspect this patient is suffering from**
    A. Hypernatremia
    B. Hypocalcemia
    C. Hypermagnesemia
    D. Hypokalemia

137. **Which of the following statements is false regarding water and sodium regulation in the elderly?**
    A. The sensation of thirst, renal function, concentration, and hormonal modulators of salt and water balance are often impaired in the elderly patient
    B. Elderly patients have fewer problems with sodium and water balance secondary to nutritional deficits
    C. Elderly patients are highly susceptible to iatrogenic events involving salt and water
    D. Age-related changes, chronic diseases, and lapses in care are often associated with impairment of sodium and water metabolism in elderly patients

138. **Your patient had gastric bypass surgery 2 weeks ago. Which of the following electrolytes is she at most risk for an imbalance?**
    A. Potassium
    B. Magnesium
    C. Calcium
    D. Sodium

139. Your patient eats a diet high in calcium because her family has a history of osteoporosis. She was admitted to the ED for a fractured pelvis and pulmonary embolism suffered when she fell down her stairs. She has been experiencing increasing weakness and muscle tremors. She has noted an increase of "skipping" beats. She stated she was very dizzy and disoriented just before she fell. Based on the symptoms, which of the following lab values should you assess immediately?

    A. Calcium level
    B. Sodium level
    C. Hemoglobin and hematocrit
    D. Magnesium level

140. The older adult trauma patient may have altered cardiac physiology, which may contribute to the reasons for sustaining an injury and increasing the difficulty of an accurate assessment. Which statement is false regarding alterations in cardiac physiology in the older adult:

    A. Myocytes increase and replace fibrous tissue
    B. Maximum heart rate, ejection fraction, stroke volume, and cardiac output decrease
    C. Blood loss will decrease cardiac filling pressures, reducing peripheral oxygen delivery
    D. Elasticity of vessels decreases, afterload increases

141. The most common injuries that result from falls by geriatric patients include:

    A. Head injuries, liver lacerations, and humerus fractures
    B. Hip fractures, liver lacerations, and sepsis
    C. Rib fractures, hypovolemic shock, and liver lacerations
    D. Rib fracture, wrist injury, and broken toes

142. The most commonly injured areas sustained in a motor vehicle crash involving an older adult would be

    A. Rib fractures and hip fractures
    B. Cervical spine, head, and chest
    C. Sternal fractures and thoracic injuries
    D. Head, knees, calcaneus

143. Because an injury in an older adult, regardless of the severity, may result in a poor outcome, the trauma nurse must take several factors into account when assessing and treating the elderly trauma patient. Which of the following factors is not considered a priority in this process:

    A. Medications
    B. A lower physiologic reserve
    C. Comorbidities
    D. Consumption of resources

144. Because of the normal age-related physiological changes that occur, the trauma nurse has an opportunity to reinforce knowledge about self-protection for an elderly patient. This teaching is unlikely to include

    A. Avoidance of driving at night
    B. Carrying fewer passenger
    C. Avoidance of driving on freeways
    D. Driving a smaller vehicle

145. You are attempting to obtain a blood pressure on your new admission, an elderly patient. After obliterating the radial pulse, an attempt is made to palpate the radial pulse. The area feels like a firm tube. This finding

    A. Is not significant
    B. Indicates hypotension
    C. Indicates pseudohypertension
    D. Means the radial pulse was not obliterated

SECTION 10: ANSWERS

1. **Correct answer: B**
   EMS just radioed the ED and reports they are en route with a 5 year old female who was struck by a car. As a trauma nurse, you know to expect injuries to the head, chest/abdomen, and lower extremities. This combination is often referred to as Waddell's triad. If the front bumper impacts the child, injuries are likely to include abdominal, pelvic, and/or femur fractures. Chest and head injuries may be sustained if the child is propelled onto the hood of the car. If the child strikes the windshield, head and facial injuries may occur. If the car stops or decelerates, the child may roll off or slide onto the street, and head injuries may be due to striking the roadway.

   The type and severity of injuries are the result of the mechanism of injury (MOI), such as type of vehicle, acceleration/deceleration forces, speed, and age of the child.

2. **Correct answer: A**
   Geriatric patients are at greater risk for fractures at C1 and odontoid fractures at C2. Geriatric patients are actually less likely to sustain linear fractures and epidural hemorrhages, but more likely to have subdural hematomas and subarachnoid hemorrhages. As the brain shrinks, bleeding may occur in the spaces around vessels, so symptoms may be delayed. CT is the preferred scanning method for adults over the age of 65. Half of all rib fractures are sustained from simple falls from a standing position.

3. **Correct answer: C**
   This child is exhibiting classic signs of a blunt carotid artery injury. The child sustained a right pneumothorax, facial, mandibular, and chest injuries, unilateral limb weakness, and a carotid bruit. While performing a secondary survey, a cervicothoracic seat belt abrasion was noted. There was a decline in neurological status, but the results of a CT scan were unremarkable.

4. **Correct answer: B**
   The most appropriate way to safely remove the child from the car seat would be for the team leader to give orders and support the head. Other team members should position themselves around the child. The child should be slid from the car seat and placed on a backboard. The person closest to the cervical spine and airway should control the movement of the head.

5. **Correct answer: D**
   The body mass index (BMI) is used to not only define the degree to which a person is overweight but also to estimate the potential risk of diseases. The World Health Organization uses the following ranges to classify the degree of obesity:

   - Underweight: BMI less than 18.5 kg/m^2
   - Normal weight: BMI between 18.5 and 24.9 kg/m^2
   - Overweight: BMI between 25 and 29.9 kg/m^2
   - Obese: BMI is 30 kg/m^2 or greater
   - Morbidly obese: BMI is greater than 40 kg/m^2

   For purposes of the TCRN exam, a bariatric patient has a BMI of 30 kg/m^2 or greater.
   To calculate a BMI, use (weight in kg)/(height in meters)^2.

6. **Correct answer: B**
   An elderly trauma patient as defined by the American College of Surgeons is over 55 years old.

7. **Correct answer: D**
   Adenosine is used for the suppression or elimination of sustained supraventricular tachycardia (SVT). It can also be used in diagnostic studies to establish the cause of SVT. Adverse effects may include transient arrhythmias, flushing, dyspnea, and (rarely) apnea. It is important to note that in approximately 30% of patients, SVT recurs. Caffeine and theophylline act by competitive antagonism to diminish the effects of adenosine.

8. **Correct answer: D**
Infants with CHF are at high risk during interventional procedures because of the use of contrast dye. Contrast dye has a high sodium content. Sodium contributes to myocardial depression and creates an osmotic effect that temporarily increases intravascular volume. Transcatheter defect occlusion and balloon atrial septostomy are procedures, not risks.

9. **Correct answer: A**
Hydralazine is incompatible with furosemide, phenobarbital, aminophylline, and ampicillin. Hydralazine is compatible with heparin, dobutamine, hydrocortisone, potassium chloride, prostaglandin E_1, and dextrose/amino acids (TPN).

10. **Correct answer: B**
Phentolamine (Regitine) 1 mg/ml solution should be injected into the affected area if infiltration of dopamine occurs. It may take as much as 5 ml to treat the affected area.

11. **Correct answer: A**
A dilated superior vena cava would appear on X-ray if the patient had a cardiac tamponade. The vena cava is dilated because blood cannot empty into the right atrium. The mediastinum would be widened. A CXR will not show delineation of the pericardium or epicardium. A pneumothorax may exist, but would not be an expected finding on X-ray.

12. **Correct answer: D**
Cardiac glycosides possess positive inotropic activity, which is mediated by inhibition of sodium-potassium adenosine triphosphatase. Also, cardiac glycosides reduce conductivity in the heart, particularly through the atrioventricular node, and therefore have a negative chronotropic effect. The cardiac glycosides have very similar pharmacological effects but differ considerably in terms of their speed of onset and duration of action. They are used to slow the heart rate in supraventricular arrhythmias, especially atrial fibrillation, and also are used in patients with chronic heart failure.

13. **Correct answer: B**
Changes in leads V_2, V_3, V_4, I, and AVL are indicative of an anterolateral MI. The MI could also include changes in V_5 and V_6, which are also lateral leads.

14. **Correct answer: A**
The antagonist for morphine and other opioids is Narcan (naloxone). Generally, for a patient over 5 years old, the naloxone dose is 2 mg IV. This dose can be repeated about every 3–4 minutes, for a total of three times. When you give naloxone, you must always be alert for the patient's potential relapse once the dose wears off. Administering multiple follow-up doses is not uncommon.

15. **Correct answer: C**
The newborn is at risk for cardiomyopathy and congenital heart block because the mother has lupus. Neonatal congenital heart block is thought to occur when maternal antibodies pass through the placenta into the fetal circulation. Some infants with congenital heart block are treated with corticosteroids and have limited mediation of symptoms; these symptoms may include thrombocytopenia, skin rash, and hepatitis. Even if the symptoms resolve, some research has shown that affected infants often develop a variety of autoimmune disorders later in life. If the congenital complete heart block does not resolve, it will become permanent. In approximately two-thirds of all infants with complete heart block, a pacemaker is required.

16. **Correct answer: B**
Signs of CNS toxicity from lidocaine may include agitation, vomiting, drowsiness, and muscle twitching. Later signs may include loss of consciousness, seizures, respiratory depression, and apnea. Cardiac toxicity may develop and cause hypotension, bradycardia, and heart block, ultimately leading to cardiovascular collapse.

17. **Correct answer: C**
The most common mechanisms of unintentional injury in the elderly are falls, motor vehicle crashes, burns, and pedestrian injuries.

18. **Correct answer: A**

The PMI in a newborn is usually located at the lower left sternal border. The apical impulse of a newborn is usually felt at the fourth intercostal space, just to the left of the midclavicular line.

19. **Correct answer: B**

Radio-frequency waves destroy myocardial tissue with heat. These waves actually heat the tissue around the active sites and prevent the occurrence of a reentry loop. Once the temperature reaches 50°C, cell damage and death occur. The continuing heat creates a lesion approximately 2–5 mm in diameter. This "burned" area is characterized by necrosis and will not conduct electricity.

20. **Correct answer: C**

The patient is in the first stage of cardiogenic shock secondary to systolic dysfunction. The injuries to his chest may have caused a pulmonary artery laceration or a cardiac contusion (the latter is more likely). His blood pressure is low, and the EKG shows ST-segment elevation in the anterior leads. If the myocardium is contused, it will react the same way as if an MI had occurred. The ST elevation may be the result of a physiologic insult to a coronary artery, with an area of the myocardium becoming ischemic as a result. The pumping function of the myocardium is compromised and may need additional support with inotropes and possibly an intra-aortic balloon pump (IABP). The patient may undergo angiography and/or surgery. Volume replacement may be necessary.

21. **Correct answer: C**

Phasic variations in an arterial pressure waveform during mechanical ventilation usually indicate hypovolemia or heart failure.

22. **Correct answer: C**

If adenosine is given slowly, it may cause systemic vasodilation and reflex tachycardia, further compromising cardiac output. Blurred vision is an expected adverse reaction. The patient should be monitored for development of atrial fibrillation, bradycardia, and heart blocks. Withhold adenosine if the patient experiences atrial fibrillation, atrial flutter, second-degree type II heart block, or complete heart block. Adenosine slows conduction via the AV node, and these rhythms may degrade to ventricular fibrillation.

23. **Correct answer: C**

Dobutamine improves cardiac output by acting on beta-$_1$ adrenergic receptors in the heart. It may cause minimal peripheral vasodilation, but primarily acts to increase contractility, coronary blood flow, and heart rate, thereby improving cardiac output. Dopamine acts on alpha-adrenergic receptors in the heart. Norepinephrine is a catecholamine that acts on both alpha- and beta-adrenergic receptors in the cardiovascular tissue.

24. **Correct answer: B**

Dobutamine has been linked with profound hypokalemia in some patients due to beta-$_2$ adrenergic stimulation. Monitor the patient's urine output to determine renal function prior to implementing any potassium replacement. Consider alternative vasoactive drugs if blood pressure support continues to be required. Long-term dobutamine use may result in tolerance and decreased effectiveness after the medication is administered for several days.

25. **Correct answer: A**

In patients receiving high-dose epinephrine, glucose levels should be monitored closely for potential hyperglycemia. The risk for hyperglycemia is even greater if the patient is diabetic. Potassium levels—not calcium, chloride, or sodium—should also be monitored for potential hyperkalemia or hypokalemia.

26. **Correct answer: D**

Atropine administration may result in headaches, dizziness, and coma. You should also assess the patient for urinary retention, hypotension, and tachycardia due to blocking of parasympathetic receptor sites.

27. **Correct answer: D**

An allergy to fish places patients at an increased risk for an allergic reaction to protamine sulfate. Patients who have undergone other cardiac procedures or patients with diabetes who have used protamine insulin are also at risk for experiencing an allergic reaction to protamine sulfate. Protamine may also cause rebound bleeding as long as 18 hours postoperatively. Although not on the TCRN exam, it is interesting note that males who have undergone a vasectomy or who are infertile may have developed antibodies to protamine.

28. **Correct answer: A**
Bariatric patients who are involved in frontal vehicular collisions result in a decreased length of stay (LOS) in the ICU is a false statement. The LOS has actually been shown to increase due to type of injury and existing comorbidities. In frontal collisions, the bariatric patient suffers fewer injuries, but they are usually more severe; suffer more head, thoracic, abdominal, and lower extremity (especially the distal femur) fractures and proximal arm injuries. Bariatric patients also suffer increased mortality.

29. **Correct answer: B**
Burns are the third leading cause of death in the elderly. That elderly patients possessing fewer fire extinguishers is not a true statement. However, the elderly are less able to evacuate, tend to live in older housing, possess fewer smoke detectors, and suffer more serious inhalation injuries and burns.

30. **Correct answer: D**
Rapid infusion of Lasix can cause tinnitus and hearing loss.

31. **Correct answer: A**
Verapamil is contraindicated in children younger than 1 year of age because it has been linked to cardiovascular collapse and death. Adenosine, procainamide, and esmolol may all be used in children younger than 1 year.

32. **Correct answer: D**
When administering nitroglycerin, it is important to have normal saline or another volume expander available at the bedside in case of vascular collapse. The potential for collapse results from the possibility of peripheral venous and arterial dilation (relative hypovolemia). Only non-polyvinyl chloride tubing may be used for infusion: Nitroglycerin may absorb PVC if that type of tubing is used. Filtration is not required prior to infusion. Nitroglycerin is compatible only with D_5W, normal saline, Lactated Ringer's solution, D_5NS, and half normal saline for infusion.

33. **Correct answer: B**
The patient's blood pressure, PAS/PAD pressures, and RAP are low. The cardiac output and cardiac index are low, the heart and respiratory rates are elevated. The patient's mentation is diminished. Collectively, these symptoms indicate hypovolemic shock.

34. **Correct answer: C**
The patient is developing cardiogenic shock. When the left ventricle fails, fluid backs up into the pulmonary vasculature. In this case, the high wedge pressure indicates that the fluid is already backed up in the patient's left heart. The PAP and RAP are high, indicating pulmonary congestion. Cardiac output and cardiac index are low, and the BP is not being maintained.

35. **Correct answer: C**
Use of induction agents such as halothane, succinylcholine, and desflurane may initiate an episode of malignant hyperthermia (MH). Stress and depolarizing muscle relaxants may also trigger MH. In malignant hyperthermia, excess calcium builds up in the mycoplasm. The patient then suffers from sustained skeletal muscular contractions, which ultimately leads to a hypermetabolic state.

36. **Correct answer: B**
Late signs of malignant hyperthermia include rhabdomyolysis, increased temperature, and bleeding from venipuncture sites.

37. **Correct answer: D**
Early signs of malignant hyperthermia include elevated serum creatinine phosphokinase (CPK), jaw rigidity, tachycardia, and respiratory and metabolic acidosis. Malignant hyperthermia can develop up to 24 hours after exposure to the causative agent.

38. **Correct answer: A**

The heart is the first organ to become functional during embryonic development. It begins to beat from the sinus venosus once the endothelial tubes fuse to form the heart tube, around day 21 of development. The lungs become functional as soon as 23–24 weeks gestation, with vascularization and alveolar development occurring at delivery. The kidneys begin to form urine and perform glomerular filtration at 9–10 weeks gestation. The liver is a multifunctional organ whose actions support gastrointestinal, endocrinologic, and hematological functions that emerge at different intervals in fetal development. For example, the liver synthesizes and secretes bile as soon as 16 weeks gestation. From weeks 6–20 of gestation, the liver functions as the primary source of hematopoiesis until the fetal bone marrow matures and dominates production.

39. **Correct answer: C**

According to the American Heart Association 2015 guidelines, one-third of the anterior-posterior chest depth equates to approximately 1.5 inches in most infants and 2 inches in most older children. Compressions of less than the minimum one-third anterior–posterior chest depth will not provide sufficient compression of the heart to produce the needed blood flow to maintain circulation to the heart, lungs, and brain.

40. **Correct answer: A**

Signs of potential elder maltreatment would not include the caregiver allowing the elderly patient to be seen and treated alone. Signs of potential abuse would include the caregiver belittling, controlling or threatening the patient. If the patient mimics dementia by mumbling to themselves, sucking or rocking, and a history of repeated injuries and visits to multiple EDs, are indications of potential abuse.

41. **Correct answer: D**

It is important that the family be notified that a complete, unrestricted autopsy be done on the child as soon as possible, preferably by a pathologist with training and experience in cardiovascular pathology. According to the American Heart Association 2015 guidelines, a child who has died suddenly and unexpectedly from a cardiac arrest may have had an underlying condition called "channelopathy." This genetic calcium-channel ion irregularity may predispose other family members to cardiac arrhythmias leading to sudden death. Therefore when sudden unexplained cardiac arrest occurs in children and young adults, obtain a complete past medical and family history (including a history of syncopal episodes, seizures, unexplained accidents or drownings, or sudden unexpected death at < 50 years old) and review previous ECGs.

42. **Correct answer: C**

According to the American Heart Association 2015 guidelines, healthcare providers should begin chest compressions immediately on infants and children if they cannot palpate a pulse within 10 seconds. Research has shown that both laypeople and healthcare personnel are unable to accurately palpate pulses in arrested and compromised patients in less than 30 seconds. Therefore, compressions should be started in any patient who is unresponsive, fails to demonstrate effective breathing (i.e., agonal respirations), and has no palpable pulse.

43. **Correct answer: A**

Per the American Heart Association 2015 guidelines, if the patient is obese, the healthcare provider should calculate the drug dosage based on the ideal weight and using the body length measured on a resuscitation tape if the weight is unknown or the actual weight if known, as long as the dose does not exceed the standard adult dosage. Subsequent administrations of medications can be titrated for effect and observation of toxicity. Drug dosages should never exceed the adult dosage. If the patient is within the ideal body weight range for his or her length, medications should be administered based on body length using the resuscitation tape.

44. **Correct answer: C**

Using a vacutainer or a high-friction syringe will create a vacuum. When that occurs, dissolved gases come out of solution, which decreases PaO_2 and $PaCO_2$. The increased effort to move the cylinder may cause the artery to spasm and impede obtaining the sample, but will not directly affect the test results.

45. **Correct answer: A**

Chronic hypoxia usually results in decreased chloride levels. The kidneys try to correct the imbalance by retaining bicarbonate. Chronic hypoxia results in increased CO_2, leading to chronic respiratory acidosis. The bicarbonate is exchanged for the chloride to maintain a balance.

46. **Correct answer: C**

An example of a comorbidity that would directly impact the potential for a traumatic injury would include sleep apnea. Patients who suffer from sleep apnea have about a seven times greater risk for vehicular collisions due to drowsiness. The comorbidities of diabetes, GERD, and kidney disease are more likely to delay or complicate healing.

47. **Correct answer: D**

Your patient is a 16 year old being treated in the ED for a left Colles' fracture and status asthmaticus. She has been taking Accolate, Allegra and using a Proventil HFA rescue inhaler at home. Today she was skateboarding with her friends and tripped over a curb. After falling she could not catch her breath. Her bronchospasms worsened, and she was transported to the ED. In the ED, the patient received albuterol, oxygen, and epinephrine without significant improvement. You note that she is using accessory muscles for respiration and is tachycardic and tachypneic. On auscultation, inspiratory and expiratory wheezing with a prolonged expiratory phase is heard throughout the lung fields. Your patient is placed on 2 L/min via NC and ABGs are drawn. Blood gas results are as follows: pH 7.53, PaO_2 104 mmHg, $PaCO_2$ 27 mmHg, and HCO_3 23 mEq/L. These blood gas results indicate an uncompensated respiratory alkalosis.

The pH is elevated, indicating alkalosis. The HCO_3 is normal and the $PaCO_2$ is decreased.

48. **Correct answer: C**

Hyperventilating will cause respiratory alkalosis because the patient is unable to get enough oxygen due to bronchial constriction. Hypoventilation would cause a buildup of CO_2, leading to respiratory acidosis.

49. **Correct answer: D**

Propranolol is contraindicated for asthmatics because it may cause bronchospasm. Propranolol works by blocking the beta-adrenergic effects of the sympathetic nervous system (like bronchodilation). Some antihypertensive drugs are cardioselective, such as atenolol. Newer agents, such as nebivolol, provide for cardioselective beta blockade with vasodilation.

50. **Correct answer: B**

Neostigmine will counteract the effects of Pavulon. Neostigmine is an enzyme that prevents the breakdown of acetylcholine into its enzyme, thereby improving impulse transmission. Sometimes neostigmine causes bradycardia and increases bronchial secretions; atropine may be used with neostigmine to mitigate these effects. Narcan is an opioid antagonist.

51. **Correct answer: B**

Asynchrony is a risk factor for the development of an air leak. Use of conventional mechanical ventilators that deliver intermittent positive-pressure inflations and positive end-expiratory pressure at a preset rate may be out of synch with the patient's respiratory efforts. The resulting barotrauma may increase pulmonary injury.

52. **Correct answer: B**

Pulmonary consideration in the elderly does not include increased surfactant. Surfactant decreases with age. Bony abnormalities, decreased PaO_2, sleep apnea, COPD, decreased expansion, asthma, bronchitis, and decreased cilia should always be considered in pulmonary management of an elderly patient.

53. **Correct answer: D**

If you hear faint breath sounds on the left side of the chest and normal sounds on the right side immediately after the patient has been intubated, most likely the tube has been placed in the right mainstem bronchus. The right mainstem bronchus is somewhat wider and has less of an angle off the mainstem bronchus, so it is much more readily intubated.

54. **Correct answer: C**
On a ventilator, a high-pressure-limit alarm may sound if a pneumothorax has occurred. The increases and changes in thoracic pressure in the presence of a pneumothorax will set off a high-pressure alarm to alert staff. In addition, alarms for saturation and possibly heart rate may sound on the cardiorespiratory monitor. A low-limit alarm may sound if tubing is disconnected and a leak in the chest tube occurs.

55. **Correct answer: B**
Excessive CPAP may increase intrathoracic pressure to the point of compressing the right atrium and vena cava. The preload will be decreased and cardiac output will be reduced.

56. **Correct answer: C**
If positive inspiratory pressure (PIP) is increased on a mechanical ventilator, the result will be a decrease in $PaCO_2$ and an increase in PaO_2.

57. **Correct answer: C**
This result is uncompensated respiratory alkalosis. The pH is greater than 7.45, so the value is an uncompensated alkalosis. To determine whether the alkalosis is respiratory or metabolic, find the value that represents alkalosis—in this case, $CO_2 < 35$ mmHg.

58. **Correct answer: B**
This result is an uncompensated (mixed) respiratory/metabolic acidosis. The pH is less than 7.35, so the value is uncompensated acidosis. To determine whether the acidosis is respiratory or metabolic, find the value that represents acidosis—in this case, $HCO_3 < 22$ mEq/L and $CO_2 > 45$ mmHg. Thus, the cause of the acidosis is both respiratory and metabolic in nature.

59. **Correct answer: C**
An infant with an expiratory grunt is performing a Valsalva maneuver in which the infant exhales against a closed glottis, producing a sound similar to a moan. With this behavior, transpulmonary pressure is increased, which decreases or prevents atelectasis. Oxygenation and alveolar ventilation are improved. Intubation should not be tried unless the infant's condition is rapidly deteriorating, because the ETT prevents the Valsalva maneuver and the alveoli will collapse.

60. **Correct answer: D**
Succinylcholine combines with acetylcholine to cause smooth-muscle relaxation, not contraction. Prolonged use may change the blocking action and result in potassium-regulated alterations in electrical activity. Other side effects of succinylcholine include malignant hyperthermia, either hypertension or hypotension, hyperkalemia, anaphylaxis, and increased intraocular pressure.

61. **Correct answer: A**
Norcuron is eliminated via the hepatic/biliary system. Use this agent with caution in patients with known or suspected hepatic or biliary compromise, such as cirrhosis or hepatitis. Norcuron may take twice as long to clear a patient's system.

62. **Correct answer: A**
One cause of decreased SVO_2 would be an increased metabolic rate. An increased metabolic rate would increase the O_2 uptake by tissues, resulting in a lower value measured by venous blood gases. The other answers result in a lower tissue oxygen requirement, so that a larger concentration of oxygen remains in the bloodstream.

63. **Correct answer: C**
From birth, chest wall compliance decreases. Much of this decrease is due to calcification of the costal cartilage, but the elasticity decreases as well. Vertebrae develop osteoporosis and a degree of kyphosis can occur. Weight gain is common and posture is affected. In today's society, children are more commonly suffering from obesity and frequently develop back problems. The chest wall compliance decreases, as does vital capacity. Residual volume increases, PaO_2 decreases, and $PaCO_2$ increases.

64. Correct answer: D
If the patient is 70 years old, assuming healthy lungs, their calculated new "normal" PaO_2 would be 70 since an elderly patient will always have a diminished PaO_2, even if they possess healthy lungs. They also have a diminished reserve. Use the following formula to calculate the PaO_2 for a 70 year old patient.
> *The formula works well for patients between 60 and 90 years of age.*

Subtract 1 mmHg from the minimal 80 mmHg level for every year over 60 years of age. That will give you a value of 70 mmHg, which would be that person's "normal." So, even with relatively healthy lungs, they are compromised with stiffer lungs and less oxygen available for extraction.

Until the PaO_2 gets to about 60%, the oxygen saturation stays above 90% and 90% is not good.

65. Correct answer: C
Acidosis, hypercarbia, and hyperthermia will all lead to a rightward shift in the oxyhemoglobin dissociation curve. Hemoglobin in this instance has a decreased affinity for oxygen and enhances tissue uptake of oxygen.

66. Correct answer: A
The oxyhemoglobin dissociation curve reflects the patient's physiological circumstances and their effect on hemoglobin's affinity for oxygen.

67. Correct answer: B
CPAP should be used with caution in patients with basilar skull fractures. Research has shown that pneumocephalus may occur if a basilar skull fracture exists. CPAP increases the functional residual capacity by helping to re-expand the alveoli. Patients who have acute cardiogenic pulmonary edema may also benefit from the use of CPAP.

68. Correct answer: D
Grunting helps the patient maintain functional residual capacity.

69. Correct answer: D
Ketamine is an analgesic and an amnestic.

70. Correct answer: C
A pneumothorax is difficult to auscultate because breath sounds are easily transmitted.

71. Correct answer: D
Functional residual capacity is the volume of gas remaining in the lungs at the end of one normal expiration.

72. Correct answer: C
The patient's abdominal contents have probably entered the thoracic cavity secondary to a diaphragmatic tear. If air also enters the thoracic cavity, it will increase the intrathoracic pressure and help to transmit sound. It is usually the left side of the diaphragm that ruptures—and the patient was injured on the left. It is postulated that perhaps the liver, because it is large, protects the right side of the diaphragm. A fractured pelvis increases the probability of a ruptured diaphragm by 50%.

73. Correct answer: B
The endotracheal cuff pressure should not exceed the tracheal capillary filling pressure. Blood flow to the trachea requires a tracheal filling pressure of approximately 15–25 mmHg. If the cuff pressure exceeds this amount, complications such as a tracheoesophageal fistula may occur. The overinflated cuff may also cause ischemia and possibly necrosis.

74. Correct answer: B
An acute pulmonary embolism can be associated with right heart failure. The PAS and PVR will be elevated. The patient may develop chest pain, dyspnea, tachycardia, hypotension, shock, and possibly coma.

75. **Correct answer: C**

If the d-dimer is elevated, it may be caused by multiple other conditions. A normal d-dimer rules out a pulmonary embolism. Hyperventilation will occur subsequent to hypoxemia, so respiratory alkalosis will occur. Heparin does not dissolve existing clots.

76. **Correct answer: C**

An example of hospital-acquired renal failure would not include hypertension. Potential causes would include surgery, hypotension, nephrotoxic drugs, and hypovolemia

77. **Correct answer: C**

A very common and significant finding in a patient with a pneumomediastinum is Hamman's sign. Hamman's sign is a "crunching" sound or a slight clicking sound with each heart sound auscultated over the apex of the heart.

78. **Correct answer: B**

During resuscitation, blood pressure and blood flow may vary. The pharmacologic effects of medications such as vasoactive drugs used during resuscitation will compromise SpO$_2$ values.

79. **Correct answer: B**

In malignant hyperthermia, the use of anesthetic agents such as halothane causes muscles to contract and the patient to become hypothermic. Caffeine is used diagnostically because it can contract muscles at higher doses without the danger of depolarizing cell membranes. The antidote for malignant hyperthermia is dantrolene.

80. **Correct answer: A**

Infants younger than 1 month who receive erythromycin are at increased risk of infantile hypertrophic pyloric stenosis. For this reason, and because azithromycin is associated with fewer adverse effects than erythromycin, azithromycin is the preferred antimicrobial for prophylaxis of newborns exposed to pertussis. A macrolide antibiotic (erythromycin, azithromycin, or clarithromycin) is preferred for postexposure prophylaxis and treatment of pertussis. Antimicrobials generally do not affect the severity or course of this illness after paroxysmal cough has begun, but they can eliminate the pathogen, *Bordetella pertussis,* and stop transmission to newborns. A macrolide should be given to women with pertussis that is acquired late in pregnancy, to their household contacts, and to their infants. Early recognition of pertussis is necessary to ensure the effectiveness of this approach.

81. **Correct answer: A**

Protection against respiratory diphtheria is provided predominantly by the immunoglobulin G antibody. During pregnancy, the maternal antitoxin is transferred to the fetus. Transplacental maternal antitoxin provides newborns with protection against diphtheria if the mother is immune. Respiratory diphtheria can occur during any trimester of pregnancy, at term, or in the postpartum period. The mortality rate of obstetric respiratory diphtheria is estimated at 50% when no antitoxin is administered.

82. **Correct answer: D**

Infants experiencing severe hypothermia cannot provide a sufficient oxygen supply to meet the demand by the tissues; they also have hypoglycemia related to an increase in glycogen metabolism, which cannot be satisfied by their body's diminishing supply. In the absence of both oxygen and glucose, anaerobic metabolism is used to create energy. This metabolism is achieved at great cost to tissues, as lactic acid builds up in the body. As pH decreases and lactic acid increases, tissues throughout the body are destroyed. Bradycardia, apnea, renal failure, and altered neurologic function worsen as tissues are destroyed, and hypoxia and hypoglycemia continue.

83. **Correct answer: B**

Norepinephrine is released by the hypothalamus in response to chemical and temperature receptors in the skin, face, and along the spinal column. Norepinephrine triggers a cascade of actions within the body to retain or create heat in the core. The efficiency of this cascade is impaired by factors relating to the patient's weight, disease process, and respiratory function. Peripheral vasoconstriction shunts blood flow to internal organs in an effort to control heat loss through the massive surface area of the infant. Unfortunately, in attempting to raise temperature, the metabolic rate is also increased, resulting in a significant increase in consumption of oxygen and glycogen. The child's body responds by burning brown fat or moving and flexing the extremities in an attempt to generate heat. Norepinephrine also causes pulmonary vasoconstriction that inhibits normal blood flow through the lungs, inhibiting blood oxygenation. The best treatment for hypothermia or cold stress is appropriate and timely prevention.

84. **Correct answer: C.**

   In obesity hypoventilation syndrome, cardiac output is actually increased, not decreased. The weight of the chest wall causes an increased work of breathing. The diaphragm becomes displaced because of the abdominal size and pressure. Sometimes this syndrome is called Pickwickian syndrome. Causes may include

   - Obstructive sleep apnea, aka OHS
   - Increased adipose chest tissue = diminished respiratory excursion
   - Decreased vital capacity (20–30%) and reduction in functional and residual lung capacity
   - Increased systemic pulmonary artery pressures
   - Increased right and left ventricular pressures
   - Right-sided heart failure
   - Increased work of breathing
   - Hypoxemia, hypercarbia, and polycythemia (monitor for PE)
   - Pulmonary hypertension
   - Larger tongue and increased fat distribution in oropharynx
   - Additional weight of the chest wall
   - Increased cardiac output (compensation for low O_2)

85. **Correct answer: C**

   Among children younger than 5 years of age, nonaccidental trauma and near-drowning are the two most common reasons for a comatose state. Nearly 6 million cases of child abuse are reported each year in the United States, according to Child Help. In children older than 5 years of age, the most common causes of coma are drug overdose and accidental head injury.

86. **Correct answer: B**

   The Pediatric Glasgow Coma Scale (GCS) is commonly used to assess a patient's neurologic status. It also gives clues about survivability. The scale assesses the patient's ability to open their eyes spontaneously, to react to voice commands, to react to painful stimuli, or not to react at all. The motor response tests the patient's ability to follow commands, localize to pain, flexion withdraw from pain, demonstrate decorticate or decerebrate posturing, or show no response to pain. The verbal response assesses orientation or appropriateness or responses, disorientation, inappropriate speech, incomprehensible words, or no response. The lower the GCS score, the worse the outlook for the patient. A consistent score of 6–7 indicates coma.

87. **Correct answer: B**

   Normal intracranial pressure for a young child is 3–7 mmHg. Sustained intracranial pressures greater than 10 mmHg may lead to severe neurologic damage or herniation.

88. **Correct answer: D**

   Lumbar puncture in a patient with increased intracranial pressure can lead to herniation of the tentorium or brain stem and, subsequently, death.

89. **Correct answer: A**

   The ideal range of CPP for a 4 year old child is 50–60 mmHg. This value actually applies to all children in the 2 to 4 year old age range. In children, the CPP goal is 40–70 mmHg, and the goal ranges are higher in older children and teens. The CPP may also be calculated using the CVP instead of the ICP, because it is a measure of vascular resistance.

90. **Correct answer: C**
A positive Babinski or plantar reflex is a sign of an upper motor neuron lesion in children who are older than 6 years of age. Prior to the child reaching 6 years of age, the nervous system has not fully matured and the Babinski reflex elicited may be positive without being a pathologic sign. In contrast, a positive Babinski or plantar reflex in an older child may be seen with spinal cord compression, head injury, and stroke. It is a pathologic sign.

91. **Correct answer: B**
A relative contraindication for administration of methylprednisolone following a spinal injury would be pregnancy. Additional relative contraindications would be an injury more than 8 hours old, mediation allergy, and uncontrolled diabetes mellitus.

92. **Correct answer: A**
Communicating hydrocephalus is the most common sequela after a subarachnoid hemorrhage (SAH). This type of hemorrhage moves through the subarachnoid space, where it may clog the arachnoid villi, preventing absorption of cerebrospinal fluid. This condition may be permanent, requiring placement of a ventriculo peritoneal shunt.

93. **Correct answer: B**
Ipsilateral (same-side) pupil dilation is evidence of increasing ICP in the lateral middle fossa of the brain, creating a shift in the temporal lobe. This area contains the uncus, which is forced through the dura mater that supports the temporal lobe. The herniation catches cranial nerve III (oculomotor) and the posterior cerebral artery on the same side as the lesion. In the pediatric population, if cranial sutures have not fused, then herniation is unlikely. Presentation would include an increase in head circumference representing hydrocephaly.

94. **Correct answer: A**
Purple glove syndrome is a potential complication of phenytoin administration that can lead to fasciotomy or amputation of a limb.

95. **Correct answer: B**
Febrile seizures are the type of seizure most likely to occur in children between 6 months and 6 years of age. They are usually seen in children with no prior history of febrile seizures, central nervous system infection, or inflammation. The seizures may last 15 minutes or longer.

96. **Correct answer: C**
Your elderly patient was trying to sit at his desk chair, but misjudged the distance and sat down hard. He is now complaining of increased pain in the thoracic while walking. The patient's posture is noted to be slightly kyphotic. As a trauma nurse, you suspect this patient has suffered a compression fracture. Normally, if acute, this type of fracture occurs from a fall or axial loading when landing on the feet. If chronic, the patient often is quite kyphotic and suffers from osteoporosis. The information given is not sufficient to differentiate between acute and chronic with certainty as we do not have a complete history. In the elderly, it is imperative to provide early mobility, PT, and rehabilitation.

97. **Correct answer: C**
Mannitol is a powerful osmotic diuretic. It can induce cardiovascular collapse if given too quickly. Mannitol is always given via the in-line 5 micron filter over 20–30 minutes or a time appropriate for the patient's age.

98. **Correct answer: A**
Phenobarbital should be given as a slow intravenous push at a rate less than 30 mg/min. Rapid infusion may lead to extravasation and tissue destruction.

99. **Correct answer: B**
Blood collection behind the tympanic membrane in a patient post–head injury indicates a temporal bone fracture. If the dura matter is also torn, CSF may leak out of the patient's ear.

100. **Correct answer: C**

Inequality of pupils greater than a 1 mm difference is known as anisocoria. Some people normally have unequal pupils, however, they usually demonstrate less than a 1 mm difference.

101. **Correct answer: A**

Depressed skull fractures in infants may result in indentation or pliable skull bone(s) without loss of bone integrity, a phenomenon known as a "Ping-Pong" depression.

102. **Correct answer: B**

Oral temperature in the elderly is lower because blood flow to the buccal area is decreased. If an elderly person exhibits what would usually be considered a normal temperature, that reading could indicate an elevation in temperature. It is a good idea to not take axillary temperatures in anyone except a neonate because of interference from ambient temperatures.

103. **Correct answer: B**

Normal ICP in children is 3–7.5 mmHg. Normal ICP in newborns is 0.7–1.5 mmHg. In infants, the normal ICP is 1.5–6 mmHg. In an adult, the ICP should be less than 10 mmHg.

104. **Correct answer: D**

Approximately 20% of cardiac output is delivered to the brain of an older child.

105. **Correct answer: C**

Jugular venous oxygen saturation (SjO_2) is used to measure the balance between cerebral oxygen delivery and cerebral oxygen consumption.

106. **Correct answer: A**

The normal range for SjO_2 is between 60% and 75%.

107. **Correct answer: A**

SjO_2 monitoring should be used for patients who are older than age 8 or who weigh at least 30 kg. SjO_2 monitoring is used in conjunction with ICP or CPP monitoring. SjO_2 values may be abnormally high in patients with nonviable brain tissue, because nonviable brain tissue does not abstract oxygen. The SjO_2 catheter should be calibrated at regular intervals with venous blood gas analysis.

108. **Correct answer: A**

Incontinence occurs only very rarely with syncope. A sense of an impending loss of consciousness, an actual loss of consciousness, and a headache can be associated with both conditions. Additional signs and symptoms of a prodromal period, including nausea, diaphoresis, and pallor, are common to both conditions. Recovery is usually rapid with syncope, and the child often feels fatigued.

109. **Correct answer: A**

Normal cerebral spinal fluid (CSF) flow should be approximately 3–5 ml/hr in a toddler and 10–15 ml/hr in an adolescent.

110. **Correct answer: A**

Absence seizures are characterized by the lack of a postictal state. The seizures last less than 15 seconds and there is no loss of posture. A discharge of neurons in one hemisphere cause focal (partial) seizures.

111. **Correct answer: B**

The organs of the GI system begin developing at 4 weeks gestation and are generally well defined by 8 weeks. At 10 weeks, the midgut moves to the abdomen. It is during this time that a problem may occur with herniation of some or all of the GI contents. At 12 weeks gestation, the GI tract begins peristalsis.

112. **Correct answer: A**

You have been tasked with starting a peripheral IV on an obese patient. Use of a smaller gauge catheter is often successful because smaller diameter vessels are generally found in adipose tissue. Sometimes, if you use a longer catheter, it may reach through the adipose tissue to underlying vessels. You might also consider using a BP cuff in lieu of a rubber tourniquet to help visualize peripheral veins.

113. **Correct answer: C**

Prolonged starvation and protein loss result in fluid shifting and third spacing. Muscle wasting results in an increase in serum lactate levels, not a decrease. Initially, there is an increased urinary nitrogen excretion, which is then followed by a decrease in the excretion rate. Increases in serum catecholamine, glucagons, and cortical levels occur as the body releases elements to maintain energy and make glucose available to the cells.

114. **Correct answer: A**

Fifty percent of deaths of patients with cirrhosis are from variceal bleeding. These lab tests are used to differentiate causes of bleeding. The history and lab values both lean toward a diagnosis of varices. Although the Hgb and Hct levels would be decreased in peptic ulcer disease and gastritis, the other changes in the lab results would not be occurring. Boerhaave syndrome is a full-thickness rupture or perforation of the esophageal wall due to prolonged and frequent vomiting related to eating disorders.

115. **Correct answer: B**

A patient with a platelet count of 79 mm^3/ml is thrombocytopenic and at risk for coagulation complications. Heparin is normally added to the solution to prevent clotting and can lead to further complications of bleeding. The other lab values are within the normal range for either males or females.

116. **Correct answer: A**

Acute pancreatitis may occur as a result of seat belt trauma to the pancreatic duct or abdominal ischemia. Acute liver failure is characterized by flu-like symptoms, jaundice, confusion, and enlarged liver. Gastrointestinal bleeding is often associated with a history of ulcers and/or esophageal varices with hemodynamic changes, narrowing pulse pressures, hematemesis, and hyperactive bowel tones. Abdominal trauma does not produce the knife-like and twisting pain, and tenderness and a marbled appearance would be noted.

117. **Correct answer: C**

This patient has likely ruptured a varix (the singular form of "varices"). Priorities are to maintain the airway, stop bleeding, and verify venous access for blood replacement, fluid management, and homeostasis. Placing the patient NPO and obtaining IV access is the first correct answer listed. You would want to position the patient upright (not flat) to prevent aspiration. You would anticipate the placement of a Minnesota tube, not a Linton-Nachlas tube. Dopamine at 5 mcg/kg/min would better support renal function—not blood pressure, as is needed in this patient.

118. **Correct answer: A**

Due to the pregnancy and resulting HELLP syndrome, there is an increased risk for fluid to collect in the abdominal cavity and for development of tissue edema. Signs and symptoms of IAH and ACS include an increased ICP, hypercarbia, decreased platelet values, decreased cardiac output, poor or absent urinary output, and abdominal wall rigidity.

119. **Correct answer: C**

Drug dosages for the geriatric patient are often less than normal dosages due to the decreased first pass effect. The first pass effect is the amount of drug that is processed by the liver into a nonviable metabolite. As the first pass effect decreases, the amount of drug available in the bloodstream to cause an effect is higher. To counter this effect, the amount of drug administered is decreased. Other factors that impact drug absorption in the geriatric patient include a slower rate of GI motility rate, a slower rate of absorption, and an increased gastric pH.

120. **Correct answer: A**

The BUN may be elevated in patients undergoing steroid treatments. The BUN may also be elevated in cases of GI or mucosal bleeding or excessive protein intake. For the geriatric patient, a decrease in cardiac output, reduced GFR, and reduced tubular secretion further impairs the patient's ability to eliminate drugs and metabolites from the bloodstream.

121. **Correct answer: C**

Intestinal atresia is the most common cause of intestinal obstruction in the newborn. Bile-colored vomitus is the hallmark of intestinal atresia. The site of the obstruction may occur anywhere in the small or large bowel. Symptoms depend on the obstruction's location. Duodenal atresia is often seen with Down syndrome. Malrotation with volvulus usually occurs at the duodenal–jejunal junction and is a surgical emergency. Jejunal atresia, often seen with meconium ileus, presents with bile vomitus at birth. Meconium plug syndrome is often seen with Hirschsprung's disease and cystic fibrosis and causes diffuse distention of the bowel.

122. **Correct answer: A**

A report of flank pain indicates renal injury in pediatric patients who experience blunt trauma and transverse and vertebral body fractures to the T11–12 and L1–L4 levels. The kidneys in pediatric patients are proportionally larger than the kidneys in adults and move freely with respiration. As a result, the kidneys are more prone to injury in children. A urinary output of less than 0.5-1 ml/kg/hr and the presence of hematuria also would indicate renal impairment. Urinary incontinence may indicate spinal cord injury (not renal injury), so it should definitely be reported. A urine osmolarity of 300 mOsm/L is normal.

123. **Correct answer: D**

In pediatric patients, 20% to 25% of cardiac output is directed to the kidneys. Nephrons are completely formed at 28 weeks gestation. Kidney location is not fixed, but moves easily with the diaphragm within the abdominal cavity between T11 and L4. Infant kidneys are more vulnerable to fluid changes, including dehydration and over-hydration, due to their inability to concentrate urine effectively.

124. **Correct answer: C**

The tubular components of the nephron include the proximal tubule, Loop of Henle, and distal tubule. Cortical nephrons account for approximately 85% of all nephrons. The juxtaglomerular nephrons account for the other 15%. Cortical nephrons have long Loops of Henle—a factor that is important for water conservation. Afferent arterioles bring blood to the glomerulus, and efferent arterioles take blood from the glomerulus to the second capillary bed.

125. **Correct answer: A**

A normal range for creatinine is 0.8-1.4 mg/dl. Females have less muscle mass than males, so they have lower levels of creatinine. Higher levels than normal may indicate pyelonephritis or eclampsia.

126. **Correct answer: C**

Renal failure is one of the most common causes of hypermagnesemia. The patient is unable to excrete excess magnesium via the urine. Gastrointestinal bypass and fistulas lead to hypomagnesemia.

127. **Correct answer: C**

The normal glomerular filtration rate (GFR) for a 1 year old is 80–120 ml/min. The normal GFR for a newborn at the second week of life is 35–40 ml/min. A GFR of 60 ml/min is normal for a 6 month old. GFR peaks in the 20s at 120–130 ml/min, then declines with age. A GFR of < 60 ml/min indicates likely renal impairment and should be reported in any patient who is more than 1 year old.

128. **Correct answer: A**

Chronic alcohol use leads to an alkalotic state. Potassium has a positive charge and hydrogen moves in the opposite direction to potassium. Thus, when potassium moves into the cell, hydrogen moves out to correct the alkalosis.

129. **Correct answer: A**

The parathyroid controls the calcium level within the body. Magnesium has been found to influence the secretion rate of the parathyroid and, therefore, influence calcium levels.

130. **Correct answer: A**

This patient has hypercalcemia, as evidenced by the calcium level of 11.9. A loop diuretic prevents reabsorption of calcium, and normal saline is administered to increase the patient's glomerular filtration rate. If a thiazide diuretic were used, it would actually decrease calcium excretion. Use of glucose, insulin, and Kayexalate is not indicated, because they are treatments for hyperkalemia.

131. **Correct answer: B**

The normal specific gravity of urine for a 12 year old should reflect a normal value of urine osmolality in the range of 100–300 mOsm/L. This value is accurate if the patient does not have blood, glucose, or protein in the urine.

132. **Correct answer: A**
Vitamin D increases serum calcium levels.

133. **Correct answer: A**
A patient presenting with fever, chills, dysuria, frequency, and pain at the costovertebral angle is likely suffering from pyelonephritis. The patient will also likely present with orthostatic vital signs and pain on palpation or urination that may radiate toward the umbilicus or lower abdomen.

134. **Correct answer: A**
The primary causative organism for urinary tract infections is *Escherichia coli*. Newer studies have shown that adenovirus-related hemorrhagic cystitis is becoming a more frequently diagnosed cause of UTIs.

135. **Correct answer: B**
Benign prostatic hyperplasia is common in elderly men. The prostate gland enlarges and impinges on the urethra.

136. **Correct answer: A**
Because of her diabetes, this patient was unable to drink sufficient fluids, leading to dehydration, hemoconcentration, and resultant hypernatremia. Due to her diabetes she may have additional renal injury. Because of the decreased blood flow through the kidneys from the CHF, the kidneys were unable to filter the excess sodium from her body.

137. **Correct answer: B**
"Elderly patients have fewer problems with sodium and water balance secondary to nutritional deficits" is a false statement.
    True statements include:
"The sensation of thirst, renal function, concentration, and hormonal modulators of salt and water balance are often impaired in the elderly patient."
"Elderly patients are highly susceptible to iatrogenic events involving salt and water."
"Age-related changes, chronic diseases, and lapses in care are often associated with impairment of sodium and water metabolism in elderly patients."

138. **Correct answer: B**
Because magnesium is absorbed in the small intestines, surgeries, such as gastric bypass, that remove or alter the small intestines place the patient at risk for hypomagnesemia. Gastric surgeries also impact water reabsorption, time processing in the intestines, calcium level, and amount of lactose in the diet.

139. **Correct answer: D**
This patient is exhibiting signs and symptoms of hypomagnesemia. This is related to the high calcium intake. Calcium and magnesium are absorbed in the small intestines. Calcium consumed in extremely high doses competes with magnesium absorption. The patient needs nutritional teaching to balance her diet.

140. **Correct answer: A**
Myocytes actually decrease, not increase, and are replaced with fibrous tissue and fat. Maximum heart rate, ejection fraction, stroke volume, and cardiac output decrease while the end systolic and diastolic volumes increase. Blood loss will decrease cardiac-filling pressures, reducing peripheral oxygen delivery. Elasticity of vessels decreases while afterload increases.

141. **Correct answer: D**
The most common injuries that result from falls by geriatric patients include fractures (especially hip), traumatic brain injuries, and lacerations. Keep in mind that most of these patients will not be able to get up without assistance. If they lay motionless for hours, their body weight will lie on muscle tissue. The patient will then be at grave risk for rhabdomyolysis with its multiple sequelae.

142. **Correct answer: B**
The most commonly injured areas sustained in a motor vehicle crash involving an older adult are the head, cervical spine, and chest.

143. **Correct answer: D**

Because an injury in an older adult, regardless of the severity, may result in a poor outcome, the trauma nurse must take several factors into account when assessing and treating the elderly trauma patient. Potential consumption of resources is not considered a priority in this process.

Priorities would include medications, comorbidities, a lower physiologic reserve, and normal pathophysiologic changes.

144. **Correct answer: D**

Because of the normal age-related physiological changes that occur, the trauma nurse has an opportunity to reinforce knowledge about self-protection for an elderly patient. This teaching is unlikely to include information about driving a smaller vehicle. A larger vehicle would be most beneficial for safety because of size, occupant protection, and visibility to other traffic. Statistics show most crashes involving the elderly involve good weather, daylight, left turns into traffic, and close proximity to home. Patient teaching should include decreasing daily and nighttime driving, avoiding freeways and peak hours, using lower speeds, carrying fewer passengers, and driving a larger car.

145. **Correct answer: C**

You are attempting to obtain a blood pressure on your new admission, an elderly patient. After obliterating the radial pulse, an attempt is made to palpate the radial pulse. The area feels like a firm tube. This finding indicates pseudohypertension. The elderly often have stiff arterial walls due to atherosclerosis. Sometime calcification prevents the artery from being compressed by the blood pressure cuff. The readings may be falsely high if auscultated, but if an arterial line is used, a more accurate measurement can be obtained.

Special Populations II

- Delivery/Neonatal Management
- Gynecological Issues
- Obstetrical Issues

Quick note from the author...Even on the best of days, the presence of an obstetric patient, regardless of the reason for the ER visit, can strike terror in the hearts of even seasoned nurses. The fear, stress, and anxiety are even more heightened when that pregnant patient is a trauma victim. For those with maternal and neonatal services in-house, you have resources to call on and know that this patient may not be staying in the ER for very long. For those without support services you may find yourself on your own when managing obstetric patients and the potential, consequential neonatal delivery. This chapter will cover the key concepts of assessment, management, and treatments of the unique obstetric patient as well as potential neonatal resuscitation. It is this author's intention that you not only learn what is needed to pass the TCRN exam, but learn core concepts and tools that will make you a better practitioner to save both mother and fetus.

SECTION 11: QUESTIONS

1. **When managing the care of a pregnant trauma victim, which of the following is a key concept?**
    A. The pregnant patient may be treated the same as any other trauma victim until 22 weeks gestation
    B. As the pregnancy progresses, hemodynamic parameters are easier to manage
    C. The fetus is not considered a patient until viability
    D. Efficient and prompt resuscitative care of the mother increases fetal survival

2. **Your patient is 7 months pregnant and admitted to your ED for severe HELLP syndrome. She is also at risk for which of the following conditions?**
    A. Intra-abdominal hypertension (IAH) and abdominal compartment syndrome (ACS)
    B. Decreased intracranial pressure (ICP)
    C. Hypocarbia
    D. Increased platelets

3. **Your patient was prescribed steroids by the obstetrician while awaiting transfer to a facility with obstetrical services. Antenatal corticosteroids affect fetal lung maturation and help prevent respiratory distress syndrome. Steroids work by**
    A. Decreasing the size of the alveoli
    B. Accelerating the rate of glycogen depletion
    C. Reducing the number of lamellar bodies inside the cells
    D. Thickening the intra-alveolar septa

4. **The leading cause of non-obstetric maternal death is**
    A. Intimate partner violence
    B. Suicide
    C. Motor vehicle crashes
    D. Fall

5. **Your patient has been diagnosed with maternal hyperglycemia. Maternal hyperglycemia ultimately causes**
    A. Increased hepatic glucose uptake
    B. Microsomia
    C. Pierre Robin sequence
    D. Decelerated lipogenesis

6. **The Kleihauer-Betke test identifies**
    A. Sickle-cell trait in utero
    B. Common blood group antigens
    C. Bone marrow lymphocyte precursors
    D. Fetal hemoglobin in maternal blood

7. **Your patient plans to breastfeed her newborn, just delivered in your emergency department. A mother's breast milk contains the immunoglobulin known as**
    A. IgG
    B. IgA
    C. IgM
    D. IgE

8. **Which of the following statements about human breast milk is true?**
    A. Human breast milk contains insoluble proteins
    B. Human breast milk is always the best choice for an infant
    C. Human breast milk is high in cytokines
    D. Human breast milk provides absolute protection against bronchopulmonary dysplasia

9. You just received a call that paramedics are bringing in a driver in a motor vehicle crash. She is pregnant at 32 weeks gestation. On scene it was noted that the patient was unrestrained and the airbag was deployed. The patient is complaining about abdominal pain. Which of the following statements is true about unrestrained pregnant drivers and passengers?

   A. Fetal death is more likely when the patient is unrestrained

   B. The airbag alone is protective and sufficient when traveling at speeds over 32 mph

   C. Risk of delivery is likely within 72 hours

   D. Maternal and fetal survival is higher when the mother is unrestrained after 20 weeks gestation

10. Rhesus (Rh) hemolytic disease of the newborn is a severe, often fatal disease caused by

    A. An Rh-negative mother alloimmunized during the first Rh-incompatible pregnancy

    B. An Rh-positive mother with an Rh-negative fetus

    C. An allergy to rhesus serum

    D. IgG Rh antibodies are unable to cross the placenta

11. Your patient has a diagnosis of placenta previa. As a trauma nurse, you know this means

    A. Your patient was previously pregnant and has retained placental material

    B. Your patient is pregnant and the placenta has partially separated from the uterine wall

    C. Your patient is pregnant and the placenta is partially implanted into the endometrium

    D. Your patient is pregnant and the placenta is partially implanted over the inferior uterus and/or the cervix

12. Calculation of fetal gestational age is based on

    A. 210 days from conception

    B. 40 premenstrual weeks

    C. 10 lunar months counted from the first day of the last menstrual period

    D. A 29-day cycle

13. You are teaching trauma prevention to a group of pregnant teens as part of a hospital outreach program. Which of the following is a key point when teaching about motor vehicle safety?

    A. When driving, make sure to sit at least 13 inches from the steering wheel or dashboard

    B. The shoulder strap may be safely positioned under the arm

    C. The seat belt is optional when pregnancy is past 20 weeks due to potential injury from that lap belt

    D. It is okay to tuck the lap belt under the dome of the belly

14. Your patient is being seen in the emergency department for hyperemesis. She reports she is in her 2nd trimester of pregnancy. You know the 2nd trimester includes which of the following ranges for weeks of gestation?

    A. 6–24 weeks

    B. 13–27 weeks

    C. 15–30 weeks

    D. 20–29 weeks

15. Your patient asks what causes her morning sickness. You explain that morning sickness is affected by

    A. Increased human chorionic gonadotropin (hCG) levels

    B. Decreased progesterone levels

    C. Decreased estrogen levels

    D. Increased glucose levels

16. Your patient is 5 months pregnant and presents to the emergency department with constant abdominal pain at the right costal margin, nausea, and low-grade fever. You note muscle rigidity and rebound tenderness. You suspect your patient may have

    A. Appendicitis

    B. Preterm labor

    C. Abruption

    D. Braxton-Hicks contractions

17. **Falls sustained due to nonviolent causes are more common in which gestational month?**
    A. 5th month
    B. 6th month
    C. 7th month
    D. 9th month

18. **Your patient has a diagnosis of HELLP syndrome. What do the letters HELLP stand for?**
    A. Headaches, emesis, lethargy, liver enzymes elevated, petechiae
    B. Headaches, elevated liver enzymes, lethargy, petechiae
    C. Hemolysis, emesis, lethargy, liver enzymes elevated, platelet deficiency
    D. Hemolysis, elevated liver enzymes, low platelets

19. **Which of the following complications has not been associated with HELLP syndrome?**
    A. DIC
    B. Abruption
    C. Placenta previa
    D. Acute renal failure

20. **The hormone most responsible for increasing gait instability during pregnancy is**
    A. Relaxin
    B. Relaxa
    C. Relacin
    D. Relacina

21. **Which of the following statements regarding HELLP syndrome is true?**
    A. HELLP syndrome can occur in the postpartum patient
    B. HELLP syndrome has a clearly defined etiology
    C. Classic symptoms of preeclampsia, hypertension, and proteinuria are always associated with HELLP syndrome
    D. Low platelet count in HELLP syndrome is caused by decreased production

22. **Which of the following disease processes can mimic HELLP syndrome?**
    A. Hepatitis and preterm labor
    B. ITP and preeclampsia
    C. Preterm labor and ITP
    D. Preeclampsia and abruption

23. **Your patient is a 28 year old gravida 8, para 1, and has been pregnant 33 weeks. She presents to the emergency department with headache, blurred vision, increased fatigue, +3 pitting edema, nausea, vomiting, and right abdominal pain. Which of the following lab results indicates a need for immediate intervention?**
    A. Bilirubin 1 mg/dl
    B. Serum aspartate aminotransferase 120 units/L
    C. Lactate dehydrogenase 480 units/L
    D. Platelet count 200 mm^3

24. **Your patient is suspected of having HELLP syndrome. What initial action should be taken by the emergency department nurse before transfer to the Labor and Delivery department?**
    A. Insert an IV
    B. Ensure a BMP is drawn
    C. Place a Foley catheter
    D. Verify history and physical—gravida, para, and gestation

25. Corticosteroids were ordered for a 30 week gestation, gravida 5, para 2, 32 year old in labor. Why was this patient prescribed corticosteroids as part of her therapy?
    A. To decrease inflammation in the feet and ankles
    B. To decrease destruction of platelets
    C. To increase fetal lung maturity
    D. To prevent seizures

26. Your patient is being transferred to a higher level medical center for treatment for HELLP syndrome. Her blood pressure is 150/88, heart rate 120, respiratory rate 28, and temperature 99.2°F. The physician orders a magnesium sulfate infusion. The magnesium is given to
    A. Treat hypertension
    B. Prevent seizures
    C. Decrease respiratory distress
    D. Decrease contractions

27. Your facility does not have maternal child services. Should a laboring mother come to the emergency department, which of the following pieces of equipment is not usually needed in the first 15 minutes of a neonatal resuscitation?
    A. Epinephrine, naloxone, normal saline
    B. Self-inflating or flow-inflating bag
    C. Warming device and blankets
    D. Bulb syringe

28. Your patient is a 25 year old presenting to the emergency department with mild respiratory distress, cough, night sweats, and fatigue. She reports she is 23 weeks pregnant. You receive orders to discharge her home for flu management (rest, fluids, and antivirals). Before the patient's discharge, what additional action should be performed?
    A. Discharge as ordered, nothing else is needed
    B. Ask the physician for a cough suppressant
    C. Ask the physician for an antibiotic for secondary infection
    D. Request that labor and delivery provide a nurse to assess fetal health

29. Your patient is a 19 year old presenting to the emergency department with unilateral pelvic pain, palpable pelvic mass, and abnormal vaginal bleeding. You should anticipate orders to
    A. Request an hCG test
    B. Administer glycerin suppository
    C. Suggest the patient walk the hall
    D. Request a CT scan

30. When managing the hemodynamics of a pregnant patient in a trauma, it is important to keep in mind which of the following cardiovascular changes?
    A. Blood volume for a pregnancy with one fetus (is singleton) increases by 15%
    B. Cardiac output increased by 60%
    C. Anemia is common with a hematocrit of around 35%
    D. Systemic vascular resistance is normally increased

31. Your patient is a 20 year old presenting to the emergency department in active labor. You are told that she is a gravida 2, para 3. This means
    A. The patient has been pregnant twice and delivered three viable children
    B. The patient has been pregnant three times and delivered two viable children
    C. The patient has been pregnant three times and has had three miscarriages
    D. The patient has been pregnant twice and has had three miscarriages

32. **Your patient is 30 years old. She presents with abdominal pain and vaginal bleeding. The physician writes that she is a nullipara, gravida 5, para 0. This means**
    A. The physician wrote her history wrong and will need to correct it
    B. The patient has never been pregnant
    C. The patient has been pregnant five times but has never delivered a viable fetus
    D. The patient has been pregnant five times but has had five abortions

33. **Your patient is a 32 year old presenting to the emergency department with vaginal bleeding, cramping, and abdominal pain. She is 20 weeks pregnant. During the vaginal exam, the physician reports that your patient's cervical os is dilated to 5 cm. Your patient is experiencing a(n)**
    A. Threatened abortion
    B. Inevitable abortion
    C. Incomplete abortion
    D. Missed abortion

34. **Your patient was brought into the emergency room by family members for heavy vaginal bleeding and severe cramping. Her hCG test is positive, the vaginal exam shows an open cervical os, and an enlarged uterus is noted. She is AB negative, serology negative, Hepatitis B negative, and GBS positive. Your patient reports passing larger blood clots than normal in the last few days. Which of the following orders is contraindicated at this time?**
    A. Place an IV for fluid resuscitation with Lactated Ringer's
    B. Administer Rho(D) immune globulin
    C. Consult the obstetrical surgeon
    D. Infuse oxytocin 200 units per 1000 ml of Lactated Ringer's

35. **What is the most common cause of spontaneous abortion in the 1st trimester?**
    A. Trauma
    B. Maternal anatomic abnormalities
    C. Infection
    D. Embryonic chromosomal defects

36. **Complete abortions left untreated may result in a(n)**
    A. Incomplete abortion
    B. Missed abortion
    C. Septic abortion
    D. Threatened abortion

37. **With the increase in circulating vascular volume, the maternal heart rate**
    A. Remains the same as pre-pregnancy baseline
    B. Decreases to allow for increased fetal perfusion
    C. Remains the same as stroke volume increases with increased cardiac contractility
    D. Increases as cardiac output increases

38. **Which of the following organisms is not considered normal vaginal flora?**
    A. *Escherichia coli*
    B. Alpha-hemolytic *streptococci*
    C. Beta-hemolytic *streptococci*
    D. *Candida albicans*

39. **Your patient presents with severe abdominal distention, constant pelvic pain, fever, chills, and uterine tenderness. She reports that she had a dilation and curettage 3 days ago. She also reports passing green and black tissue clots. You should immediately**
    A. Contact a surgical consult and prepare the patient for surgery
    B. Observe the patient for anaphylactic shock
    C. Administer spectinomycin hydrochloride
    D. Administer ganciclovir

40. **Which of the following discharge instructions for a post-abortion patient is true?**
    A. Vaginal bleeding should stop within 4–5 days
    B. Slight cramping that lasts for 1–2 weeks is normal
    C. Avoid intercourse, douching, and tampons for at least 2 weeks
    D. Monitor blood pressure for 5 days

41. **PIH stands for**
    A. Pregnancy-induced hypoglycemia
    B. Pregnancy-induced headaches
    C. Pregnancy-induced hyperemesis
    D. Pregnancy-induced hypertension

42. **What is the primary difference between preeclampsia and eclampsia?**
    A. The systolic blood pressure of the preeclamptic patient is less than 180 mmHg and greater than 180 mmHg for the eclamptic patient
    B. Albuminuria is only noted with preeclampsia
    C. Seizures are noted only with eclampsia
    D. HELLP syndrome is only noted with preeclampsia

43. **Paramedics transported your patient to the emergency department for seizures. She had a seizure immediately upon arrival in the patient treatment area. The seizure has lasted for minutes. Your patient is 30 weeks pregnant. Her BP is 210/130, RR is 40, and she has +4 pitting edema. After you administer magnesium sulfate, your patient stops seizing. What position should you place her in while waiting for transfer to the high-risk obstetrical unit?**
    A. Supine
    B. Prone
    C. Right
    D. Left

44. **Why is placenta previa a concern during late pregnancy?**
    A. The placenta pulls away from the uterus with fetal growth
    B. As the fetus grows, the os thins and leads to bleeding
    C. High placenta implantation pulls away with contractions
    D. As the fetus grows the placenta thins and leads to preterm labor

45. **Which signs and symptoms are consistent with placenta previa presentation?**
    A. Sudden painless bleeding of bright red blood, hypotension, tachycardia, delayed capillary refill
    B. Sharp abdominal pain without bleeding, tachycardia, and tachypnea
    C. Uterine rigidity, frank red blood, hypotension, tachycardia, back pain
    D. Foul vaginal discharge, constant pelvic pain, fever, chills

46. **Your patient is 47 years old and pregnant at 35 weeks gestation. She was brought in to the ED after a motor vehicle accident. She was driving when the vehicle she was driving was T-boned on the passenger side. Your patient has multiple lacerations to the face, chest, and abdomen. Her pants are saturated with blood and you note an open femur fracture to her right leg. She is at high risk for which of the following life-threatening conditions?**
    A. Compartment syndrome
    B. Preterm labor
    C. Abruption
    D. Infection

47. **Which of the following is an expected finding when interpreting a blood gas of a pregnant patient?**
    A. Respiratory acidosis
    B. Respiratory alkalosis
    C. Metabolic acidosis
    D. Metabolic alkalosis

48. **Which of the following actions is a nursing priority when caring for a mother experiencing abruption?**
    A. Two large-bore IVs with 1/2 normal saline infusions
    B. Consider administration of 0+ blood
    C. Set up for intermittent fetal monitoring
    D. Mark fundal height and assess frequently

49. **Fetal _____ improves fetal survivability until maternal oxygen drops below _____ of normal.**
    A. Shunts; 70%
    B. Circulation; 40%
    C. HbF; 50%
    D. HbF; 20%

50. **Which of the following signs is not an indication of impending delivery?**
    A. Bloody show
    B. Bulging membranes
    C. Desire of the mother to void
    D. Crowning

51. **Your patient just delivered a term male infant with clear amniotic fluid in the emergency department. What is your immediate priority?**
    A. Call nursery or NICU to come get the baby
    B. Remove wet blankets after drying
    C. Tracheal suctioning to clear airway
    D. Use hot water bottles or gloves to warm baby

52. **Your patient just delivered a term infant in the emergency department. The umbilical cord was wrapped twice around the infant's neck. After you dried, stimulated, and suctioned the infant's airway with a bulb syringe, you determine the heart rate as 40 bpm. Your next action should be to**
    A. Suction the airway using wall suction
    B. Begin chest compressions at a 15:2 ratio
    C. Use your fingertips to vigorously stimulate the infant
    D. Provide positive pressure ventilation at 40–60 bmp for 30 seconds and then reassess the heart rate

53. **You are providing positive pressure ventilation (PPV) to an apneic newborn. You note increasing difficulty with obtaining chest rise. After repositioning the mask and head, your next action should be to**
    A. Use wall suction to clear the mouth
    B. Place an orogastric tube
    C. Place a nasogastric tube to low intermittent wall suction
    D. Increase positive inspiratory pressure to greater than 40 mmHg

54. **Your patient is in active labor. Friends report she was "using this morning." She delivers a preterm female infant in the emergency department. The infant is apneic, floppy, cyanotic, and has a heart rate of 70. Which of the following actions is contraindicated in the care of this infant?**
    A. Provide positive pressure ventilation for 30 seconds and then reassess HR, respiratory, and color
    B. Administer Narcan (naloxone) at 0.1 mg/kg
    C. Use pulse oximetry to titrate FiO_2 to keep oxygen saturation between 85% and 95%
    D. Wrap the infant in a polyethylene bag and place under a heat source

55. Childbearing age for any female trauma victim is defined as a woman between the ages of
    A. 10–60
    B. 12–55
    C. 15–50
    D. 10–55

56. Your patient is a 35 year old seen in the emergency department for low back pain, severe muscle spasms, malaise, and dysmenorrhea. Her temperature is 102°F, HR 120, and RR 19. Assessment reveals an enlarged uterus with purulent, foul-smelling vaginal discharge. Which of the following diagnoses is likely given your patient's symptoms?
    A. Atrophic vaginitis
    B. Chancroid
    C. Endometritis
    D. Gonorrhea

57. Paramedics transported a 29 year old admitted to the emergency department after the metro train she was riding in derailed. She appears to be approximately 30 weeks pregnant. Witnesses reported that she was thrown into the back of the seat in front of her and she had initially complained of severe abdominal pain. She is now unresponsive and hypotensive. You are unable to detect fetal heart tones. You suspect uterine rupture. What findings support your suspicions?
    A. Copious vaginal bleeding
    B. Footling breech presentation in the vaginal canal
    C. Fetal legs in the abdominal cavity demonstrated by ultrasound
    D. A clot identified behind the placenta demonstrated by ultrasound

58. Your patient is a 40 year old who was struck in the head by a stray bullet during the July 4th holiday. She was brought into the emergency department with chest compressions in progress. Paramedics reported that CPR was started 2 minutes ago for ventricular fibrillation. Your patient is 35 weeks pregnant. After 2 more minutes of CPR in the ED, she becomes asystolic. The physician decides a postmortem cesarean delivery is indicated. Which of the following statements regarding postmortem cesarean delivery is true?
    A. Fetal outcome is best if postmortem cesarean delivery occurs within 10 minutes of maternal death
    B. Perimortem delivery may only be performed in surgery
    C. A neonatal resuscitation team should be on call should the infant survive delivery
    D. A classical abdominal incision is the best method for delivery

59. How soon after birth should you obtain an infant's blood glucose?
    A. Within 10 minutes
    B. Within 30 minutes
    C. Within 45 minutes
    D. Within 60 minutes

60. Paramedics just brought in a 30 year old, 38 weeks pregnant patient. She was a passenger in a rear-end MVA. She is brought in on a backboard. While waiting for a CT scan, she reports feeling light-headed. On monitor, her heart rate keeps dropping, her pulse oximetry is 88–92% and she is dyspneic. What initial action would improve this patient's condition?
    A. Start oxygen at 10 L nonrebreather
    B. Angle the backboard onto the left side
    C. Administer IV bolus of 2 L NS
    D. Provide orange juice to improve blood glucose

61. **Hypotonia, jitteriness, poor suck, apnea, and seizures indicate a hypoglycemic state in the**
    A. Lungs
    B. Muscles
    C. Heart
    D. Brain

62. **Initial IV fluids should be calculated at _____ for an infant newly born.**
    A. 40 ml/kg/d
    B. 50 ml/kg/d
    C. 60 ml/kg/d
    D. 80 ml/kg/d

63. **Which of the following initial reactions occurs with an infant suffering from cold stress?**
    A. Hypotonia, peripheral vasoconstriction
    B. Increased metabolism of brown fat, decreased O_2 consumptions
    C. Increased glucose consumption, hypertonia
    D. Increased O_2 consumption, hypotonia

64. **Effects of cold stress in infants is caused by a release of**
    A. Norepinephrine
    B. Epinephrine
    C. Dopamine
    D. Glycogen

65. **Which of the following warming methods is contraindicated for the care of a newborn?**
    A. Heat stethoscope in hands before auscultation
    B. Use warmed, humidified oxygen
    C. Servo set radiant warmer
    D. Heat lamp set 6 inches away from the infant

66. **A neonate was just born in the emergency department. He demonstrates cyanosis, tachypnea, and depressed mentation, and his PCO_2 is 30. The likely cause for his symptoms is**
    A. Respiratory distress syndrome
    B. Congenital heart disease
    C. Aspiration
    D. Pneumothorax

67. **Which acronym can be used to remember what information should be prepared prior to transport of a newborn infant days from the emergency department to a higher level of care within or outside the facility?**
    A. S.T.A.B.L.E.
    B. TRANSPORT
    C. INFANT
    D. SEND

68. **You are assisting with an emergency vaginal delivery in your ED. When the head is delivered, you note that the cord is wrapped tightly around the throat. What action should be performed at this time?**
    A. Hold a hand to the head to prevent the infant from delivering until you can move the mother to labor and delivery
    B. Stretch the cord over the head
    C. Continue to deliver the infant and untangle the cord once the body is delivered
    D. Clamp the cord in two places and use sterile scissors to cut between the two clamps

69. **Actions should be taken to maintain an infant's blood glucose level at**
    A. 40–100 mg/dl
    B. 50–120 mg/dl
    C. 60–160 mg/dl
    D. 80–150 mg/dl

70. **Your patient is a 46 year old seen in the emergency room for cyclical abdominal cramping that is increasing in frequency and severity. When you assist her to undress you note a bulging bag with what appears to be a foot moving in it. As she lays down on the gurney, the rest of the bag delivers onto the bed. You should**
    A. Rupture the amniotic sac and peel it away from the face and begin resuscitation
    B. Leave the sac intact and call Labor and Delivery
    C. Leave the sac intact and call the Neonatal Care Unit
    D. Wait for the physician to determine viability before starting resuscitation

71. **Risk for abdominal trauma increases with gestation. Which of the following statements is correct regarding changes in maternal gastrointestinal system during pregnancy?**
    A. Gastric motility is increased with delayed emptying
    B. The gastroesophageal sphincter is tighter
    C. Small bowel injury is less common
    D. Splenic and liver trauma is rare

72. **Why is fetal breech positioning dangerous?**
    A. Fetal breech positioning results in irreparable muscular skeletal damage
    B. Fetal breech positioning causes an increased risk of shoulder dystocia
    C. Fetal breech positioning causes an increased risk of uterine rupture
    D. Fetal breech positioning causes an increased risk of strangulation

73. **Your patient is 36 years old and pregnant at 39 weeks. She is in active labor and reports that her water broke an hour ago. Since then she has not felt the baby move. On inspection, you see the head engaged in the vagina with the umbilical cord pinched between the head and the wall of the vagina. Your first action should be to**
    A. Transport the mother to the obstetrical unit
    B. Administer oxygen
    C. Use a gloved hand to support the head off the cord and leave it in place
    D. Push the cord back into the vagina

74. **A ruptured ovarian cyst often presents with similar symptoms to which of the following conditions?**
    A. Appendicitis, ectopic pregnancy, and PID
    B. PIE, diverticulitis, and appendicitis
    C. Appendicitis, PDI, and ectopic pregnancy
    D. Ectopic pregnancy, appendicitis, and PID

75. **Which of the following actions is not helpful with controlling post-delivery bleeding?**
    A. Administer oxytocin at 20 units per 1000 ml Lactated Ringer's at 250-500 ml/hr
    B. Massage the fundus to keep it firm
    C. Assist the mother in breastfeeding
    D. Encourage the mother to drink ginseng tea to increase comfort after delivery

76. **Fetal bradycardia is classified as a heart rate less than**
    A. 60
    B. 80
    C. 100
    D. 120

77. **Which organism is likely to cause toxic shock syndrome?**
    A. *Staphylococcus aureus*
    B. *Escherichia coli*
    C. *Candida albicans*
    D. *Pseudomonas aeruginosa*

78. **Which of the following is an appropriate treatment of toxic shock syndrome?**
    A. Stabilize vascular pressure using colloids
    B. Provide O_2 support to maintain PaO_2 greater than 80 mmHg
    C. Transfer patient to an isolation room
    D. Remove identifiable sources of infection

79. **Your patient is admitted to the emergency room via ambulance after being found in a side ditch. Her clothing is torn and she has bruising noted to her face, chest, inner thighs, and buttocks. Her left eye is swollen shut and she is missing teeth. She has vaginal and rectal bleeding. Although she denies sexual assault, you should**
    A. Contact police
    B. Provide medical care only
    C. Allow the patient to void if desired
    D. Begin washing and cleaning wounds

80. **All the following professionals are considered a part of SART except**
    A. Police officers
    B. Forensic examiners
    C. Laboratory personnel
    D. Patient advocates

81. **The SART process should follow which of the following orders?**
    A. Notify police, forensic evidence is collected, patient advocate is notified, counselors provided
    B. Notify police, SANE initiates assessment, evidence is transferred to attorney, patient is transferred to psych unit for evaluation and counseling
    C. Police are notified, patient advocate arrives to assist patient through process of hospitalization, disclosure is completed between hospital staff and police agency
    D. Police are notified, patient advocate and SANE are notified, initial disclosure with police and hospital staff, forensic evidence is collected

82. **A woman has just been brought in by friends after she was sexually assaulted at a club. After initiating the SART process, you should**
    A. Place the woman in a private room by herself until she can be examined
    B. Withhold notifying police until a history and physical can be taken
    C. Offer information on sexual assault attorneys
    D. Have a social services representative stay with the victim

83. **Your 37 week pregnant patient sustained a pelvic fracture when she struck a bench after being hit by a truck in the pedestrian walkway. Although she sustained no other remarkable injuries, she displays symptoms of hypovolemic shock. Which of the following statements is true regarding pelvic fractures and hemorrhagic shock in the pregnant patient?**
    A. Is associated with a 35% maternal mortality rate
    B. Fracture type and severity have no impact on maternal or fetal mortality
    C. Always result in fetal death, regardless of gestation at the time of injury
    D. Pelvic fractures are a common occurrence

84. **Which of the following statements is true about the collection of evidence?**
    A. Clothing should be removed via unbuttoning or unzipping if possible; if clothing must be cut, avoid cutting through bullet holes, knife cuts, tears, or button holes
    B. Collected evidence should be labeled with patient name, hospital name, collection site (ED), date and time of collection, description of specimen, and collector's initials
    C. All items released to police should be documented on the police report only
    D. Any biohazard materials related to the victim's care should be disposed of through hospital policy

85. **Which of the following statements is false regarding consent when caring for a sexual assault victim?**
    A. Additional medical care consents must be obtained before treating a sexual assault victim
    B. A consent for or against must be signed prior to an official forensic examination
    C. The consent for forensic examination implies consent to transfer evidence to police
    D. General medical consent implies permission to obtain photographs of injuries for documentation

86. **Which of the following reactions is the best way to determine if ventilations with a bag-mask-valve are effective?**
    A. Visible chest rise
    B. Visible abdominal movement
    C. Spontaneous breathing occurs within 30 seconds
    D. Heart rate improves over 90 seconds

87. **You are monitoring a pregnant patient in the ED until a labor room is available. You note three 4-minute drops fetal heart rate to 68. The infant delivers apneic without tone. After drying the baby and removing blankets, your initial assessment indicates a heart rate of 70, apnea despite stimulation, and the baby remains limp and cyanotic. This baby is**
    A. In primary apnea
    B. In secondary apnea
    C. In tertiary apnea
    D. Is stillbirth

88. **Which of the following neonates should be intubated immediately?**
    A. An apneic, term infant with poor chest rise despite positive pressure ventilation
    B. A 26 week gestation neonate crying with minimal retractions
    C. A 31 week gestation neonate with a marked inguinal hernia
    D. A 36 week gestation neonate with a small umbilical hernia

89. **You are participating in the delivery and resuscitation of a 28 week gestation neonate. The heart rate is 140 with a respiratory rate of 80 with moderate retractions and circumoral cyanosis. Your next step is to**
    A. Provide positive pressure ventilation with 100% FiO_2
    B. Provide CPAP using a self-inflating bag-mask-valve
    C. Provide PPV with a flow-inflating bag-mask
    D. Provide CPAP using a T-piece resuscitator

90. **You are participating in a multidisciplinary community ride-along with local EMS when a call is received for an MVA involving a pregnant patient. What are key factors when deciding to transfer the patient to the nearest community hospital versus traveling an additional 10 miles to the closest trauma center?**
    A. The facility offers neonatal emergency services only
    B. The facility offers maternal emergency services only
    C. The gestation age is relevant
    D. EMTALA requires transfer to the closest medical facility, irrespective of services provided

91. **Transition to extrauterine life begins when**
    A. The baby's head is delivered
    B. The baby takes the first breath
    C. The baby takes the first breath and the cord is clamped
    D. The cord is clamped

92. **You are using a flow-inflating bag-mask-valve to resuscitate a 32 week gestation neonate. The bag fails to inflate and the chest does not rise. What action should you take first to resolve this problem?**
    A. Reposition the head and verify the mask seal
    B. Verify the tubing is connected to the air line
    C. Get a new bag-mask-valve device
    D. Increase the flow meter to 15 Lpm

93. **Which of the following is not an important part of the history assessment of a victim of a sexual assault?**
    A. Sexual history
    B. Childhood vaccinations
    C. Post-assault activities
    D. Last menstrual period

94. **You are preparing to give epinephrine to a premature infant with a heart rate of 40 bpm despite well-coordinated positive pressure ventilation via an endotracheal tube and adequate chest compressions. Which of the following statements regarding epinephrine administration is true?**
    A. The correct epinephrine dose is 0.1-0.3 ml/kg via the umbilical venous line
    B. Epinephrine is just as effective whether administered endotracheally or via an umbilical venous line
    C. The endotracheal tube placement does not need to be confirmed prior to administering epinephrine via the endotracheal tube
    D. Use 1:1000 concentration of epinephrine when administering via ETT

95. **Intubation of a term infant was just completed. The infant has a heart rate of 20 bpm, no spontaneous respiratory effort, and he is flaccid and mottled. The chest rises equally and breath sounds are auscultated in all lung fields. The CO_2 detector does not indicate the presence of exhaled CO_2. What is the next step in this resuscitation?**
    A. Remove the endotracheal tube and insert a combitube
    B. Remove the endotracheal tube and reintubate after 30 seconds of positive pressure ventilation
    C. Remove the endotracheal tube and insert a laryngeal-mask airway
    D. Continue to provide positive pressure ventilation and observe for a rise in heart rate

96. **While shopping at a local department store, a fellow shopper's amniotic sac ruptures. The mother tells you she has had three previous children and this child should be due this week. You realize delivery of a single, term infant appears imminent. EMS have been contacted and the unit en route is 5 minutes away. Before EMS arrives, a female infant is delivered. What is the first action you should take?**
    A. Dry and stimulate the infant using available clothing articles
    B. Leave the cord attached and focus on establishing ventilation
    C. Place the infant on the floor and pile clothing on top
    D. Do not dry the infant, just place on the mother's chest and cover with a blanket

97. A pregnant mother arrives in the ED. She is 38 week gestation and complains of absent fetal movement for 5 minutes. The infant delivers vaginally and is noted to be apneic, flaccid, and cyanotic. After drying, suctioning, and positioning, the infant remains apneic without a heartbeat and is gray. Over the next few minutes, the team intubates the infant, provides effective positive pressure ventilation, and begins well-coordinated chest compressions. An umbilical venous line is placed by the ED physician for epinephrine and volume replacement. Throughout the resuscitation, the team has never been able to establish a heartbeat in the infant. At what point may the team stop resuscitation?
    A. After 5 minutes of resuscitation
    B. After 10 minutes of resuscitation
    C. After 15 minutes of resuscitation
    D. After 20 minutes of resuscitation

98. An ED visitor brings an infant to the desk that was just found outside the ED doors. The infant's first temperature was 35.4°C. During your assessment, you find the blood glucose to be 17 mg/dl. The ED physician orders Dextrose 25% at 2 ml/kg IV STAT. You should
    A. Administer the dextrose as ordered
    B. Refuse the order and hang a $D_{10}W$ continuous drip at 150 mg/kg/d
    C. Politely refuse the order, notify your transport neonatologist and follow standard stabilization protocol of using Dextrose 10% at 2 ml/kg IV
    D. Correct the physician; the correct concentration is Dextrose 15%

99. Death of the hypothermic infant may be caused by
    A. Aerobic metabolism
    B. Hypoglycemia and hypoxemia
    C. Bradycardia
    D. Decreased fill time due to tachycardia

100. Which of the following is a correct method to take the temperature of a neonate?
    A. Rectally, with the tip of a standard thermometer inserted 5 cm into the anus
    B. In the axillary area, by holding the standard thermometer for 3–5 minutes
    C. Use a tympanic thermometer for 1–10 seconds
    D. Use a skin probe

101. Your 19 week pregnant patient sustained a pelvic fracture when her vehicle was t-boned by a moving van. Where would you anticipate blood to pool if she was hemorrhaging?
    A. There would not be pooling, as the fetus provides a tamponade on the bleed
    B. Retroperitoneal space
    C. Anterior to the bladder
    D. Blood would not pool, but present as vaginal bleeding only

102. A 47 year old trauma patient in active labor is a gravida 10, para 5. She received late prenatal care, seeing the obstetrician only once. Estimated gestation is 21 weeks and 450 g on ultrasound. The mother believes she is at 23 weeks. Upon delivery, the infant is dried, positioned, and placed on the warmer. Weight is estimated to be 350 g. The skin is friable and sticky, the eyelids are tightly fused, and the heel–toe length is 45 mm. These findings suggest
    A. The parents should be allowed to choose what resuscitation measures should be taken or continued
    B. The infant is viable and all resuscitation measures should be initiated
    C. The infant is not viable and resuscitation efforts should be withheld
    D. The infant is viable, but the prognosis is poor, so resuscitation should be withheld

103. **The bladder in a pregnant trauma patient is at higher risk for injury due to which of the following factors?**
    A. The bladder is displaced to the posterior and inferior abdomen and is at high risk secondary to pelvic fracture injuries
    B. The bladder capacity increases five fold
    C. Decrease in GFR results from impaired blood flow to the kidneys
    D. Mechanism of injury involving a shearing force may tear the ureters from the bladder

104. **Which of the following findings is normal in the pregnant patient?**
    A. Increased creatinine due to fetal growth
    B. Glycosuria
    C. Increased BUN due to fetal urea production
    D. Proteinuria

105. **Prioritization of care during resuscitation should focus on the ABCs. ABC stands for**
    A. Airway, breastfeeding, crying
    B. Airway, breathing, circulation
    C. Appearance, breathing, color
    D. Activity, bradycardia, crying

106. **A 16 year old female is a passenger in a truck that rolled over an embankment when the vehicle was sideswiped. Which of the following assumptions should be made?**
    A. The patient is pregnant
    B. Drugs were involved in the accident
    C. Alcohol was consumed prior to the accident
    D. The patient will bleed due to energy drink consumption

107. **Your patient is a 20 year old seen in the emergency department 5 days ago for streptococcal pharyngitis. She returned with complaint of profuse, white, curd-like vaginal discharge. A vaginal exam shows vulvular inflammation and redness with red dermatitis and weeping areas on the inner thighs. Your patient also reports painful urination with itching and burning. You suspect she is suffering from**
    A. A trichomoniasis infection
    B. A gonorrheal infection
    C. Genital herpes
    D. A candidiasis infection

108. **You are mentoring a nursing student and discussing the importance of obtaining a maternal history prior to delivery. Maternal health during the pregnancy is extremely important in the development of the fetus and directly affects the post-delivery management of the neonate. Which are the most important maternal factors you should discuss with the nursing student?**
    A. Placental function and inherent maternal resources
    B. Placental location and overall maternal health
    C. Maternal socioeconomic and physiologic status
    D. Family support system and community resources

109. **Infants are at great risk for heat loss at a rate of three to four times that of an adult because**
    A. The infant has a greater surface-to-body ratio
    B. Infants cannot shiver
    C. Infants cannot regulate body temperature
    D. High water content

110. Paramedics are transporting a 21 week pregnant patient that was thrown 20 feet due to a car bombing. She has first-degree burns to her legs and arms, scattered bruising to her arms and torso, and a scalp abrasion. Paramedics are providing oxygen via a nonrebreather mask. On arrival to your ED, the patient reports that it is difficult to breathe. As a trauma nurse, you know the first action you should take is to
    A. Position the patient right lateral to avoid pressure to her burned skin and improve venous return
    B. Prepare for intubation with a slightly smaller ETT
    C. Place an NGT for gastric decompression
    D. Start a levophed drip for blood pressure support

111. Paramedics are en route with a 35 week pregnant gunshot victim. On arrival, CPR has been in progress for the past minute. After primary survey, the trauma attending determines that maternal resuscitation is not likely and the obstetrician agrees. To improve fetal survival, a postmortem cesarean section should occur within _____ of _____ maternal rhythm.
    A. 3 minutes; bradycardic
    B. 4 minutes; life-threatening
    C. 5 minutes; agonal
    D. 6 minutes; absent

112. Complete the statement. The number one cause of fetal death when trauma is involved is due to
    A. Direct fetal injury
    B. Maternal hypoxia
    C. Maternal shock
    D. Fetal hypoxia

113. A pregnant trauma victim has an estimated 1750 ml blood loss. What maternal physiologic compensatory actions should you expect to see?
    A. Mild tachycardia with a MAP of 50–60 mmHg
    B. Cold, pale extremities with a MAP of 72 mmHg
    C. Altered LOC with tachycardia greater than 120 beats per minute
    D. Hemorrhagic shock with oliguria

SECTION 11: ANSWERS

1. **Correct answer: D**
   Efficient and prompt resuscitative care of the mother increases fetal survival is a key concept when managing the care of a pregnant trauma victim. By focusing on maternal ventilation, oxygenation, and perfusion, blood flow and oxygen to the fetus is improved, thus decreasing the risk of premature labor and delivery. Primary assessment and management initially focuses on maternal needs as with other trauma victims, but then management focuses on the actions that could impact both maternal and fetal survival irrespective of gestation. Although viability is not until 22–23 weeks gestation, profound physiologic development occurs during the 1st trimester with both development and growth occurring in the 2nd trimester. Medications, asphyxia, and impaired maternal hemodynamics can negatively impact fetal development and growth. As the pregnancy progresses, hemodynamic parameters are much more difficult to manage and even slight drops in blood pressure can compromise placental blood flow making hemorrhagic hypovolemic shock more challenging to detect.

2. **Correct answer: A**
   Due to the pregnancy and resulting HELLP syndrome, there is an increased risk for fluid to collect in the abdominal cavity and for development of tissue edema resulting in intra-abdominal hypertension (IAH) and abdominal compartment syndrome (ACS). Signs and symptoms of IAH and ACS include an increased ICP, hypercarbia and decreased platelet values, decreased cardiac output, poor or absent urinary output, and abdominal wall rigidity.

3. **Correct answer: B**
   Antenatal corticosteroids affect fetal lung maturation and help prevent respiratory distress syndrome. Steroids work by accelerating the rate of glycogen depletion and glycerophospholipid biosynthesis. This process results in thinning the intra-alveolar septa and increases the size of the alveoli.

4. **Correct answer: C**
   Motor vehicle crashes account for just over 50% of all non-obstetric maternal death regardless of geographic location. As pregnancy progresses, women may not use or position seatbelts correctly. One study found that almost half of the women killed in MVCs were positive for an intoxicant. Intimate Partner Violence (IPV) is now used interchangeably with domestic violence and accounts for approximately 20% of non-obstetric maternal trauma leading to death. Falls, particularly in the 5th–8th months, accounts for approximately 25% of maternal deaths, while suicide accounted for up to 10% of maternal deaths depending upon the study.

5. **Correct answer: A**
   Maternal hyperglycemia ultimately causes increased hepatic glucose uptake secondary to fetal hyperinsulinemia and hyperglycemia. Increased glycogen synthesis, accelerated lipogenesis, and macrosomia will also occur.

6. **Correct answer: D**
   The Kleihauer-Betke test identifies fetal hemoglobin in maternal blood. The results of this test allow for calculations to determine the amount of fetal-maternal hemorrhage and the amount of immune globulin (RhoGAM) necessary to prevent sensitization. If a patient has a positive test, follow-up testing at a postpartum checkup should be done to rule out the possibility of a false-positive result. For example, a false-positive result in the mother could be caused by a sickle-cell trait, which causes persistent elevation of fetal hemoglobin.

7. **Correct answer: B**
   A mother's breast milk contains the immunoglobulin known as immunoglobulin A (IgA). This immunoglobulin is also secreted in human colostrum. IgA does not cross the placental barrier and is the most common immunoglobulin in the gastrointestinal and respiratory tracts.
   During pregnancy and lactation, because of hormonal stimuli, IgA B lymphocytes colonize mammary glands and produce a specific secretory IgA that may bind to a pathogen and prevent

infection. The antimicrobial effects of IgA antibodies are related to immune exclusion, interference, or an inhibited ability to adhere to the epithelial cell wall. This helps provide protection to the neonate. Agglutination, neutralization, and immune elimination by phagocytosis and cytotoxicity may enhance the antimicrobial effects as well. HIV-infected mothers do not evidence protection. IgA antibodies may enhance transmission of HIV infection.

8. **Correct answer: C**
Human breast milk is high in cytokines. Cytokines are soluble proteins that help stimulate the chemotaxis of neutrophils and help in epithelial cell propagation. Of all the factors associated with immunity—immunological, hormonal, and enzymatic—cytokines are believed to play a significant role in the immune modulation and immune protection of breast milk. Most cytokines that are known to be deficient in the neonate, particularly in preterm infants, have been found in significant amounts in breast milk. There are certain circumstances where human breast milk is not safe for infant consumption.

9. **Correct answer: A**
Fetal death is four times more likely when the patient is unrestrained. Seatbelt restraints should be used during the entire pregnancy and are known to prevent severe head injury, ejections, and lowers mortality rate. Maternal and fetal survival is higher when seat belts and airbags are used together. With motor vehicle crashes, delivery is over two times more likely within 48 hours. It is vital that a fetal assessment should be completed as soon as possible.

10. **Correct answer: A**
Rhesus (Rh) hemolytic disease of the newborn (HDN) is a severe, often fatal disease caused by incompatibility between an Rh-negative mother and her Rh-positive fetus. The mother becomes alloimmunized to the D antigen present on fetal red blood cells (RBCs) during the first Rh-incompatible pregnancy. The first pregnancy is rarely affected because the number of Rh antibodies produced by the mother is low and the antibodies are usually IgM. When the mother is exposed to D-positive fetal RBCs during a subsequent Rh-incompatible pregnancy, the mother develops a secondary immune response. A large number of IgG Rh antibodies are produced that cross the placenta and make fetal red cells susceptible to attack by antibodies. The mother may also be alloimmunized from fetal-maternal hemorrhage, bleeding that occurs during normal delivery, ectopic pregnancies, spontaneous or induced abortions, and abdominal trauma.

11. **Correct answer: D**
A diagnosis of placenta previa indicates the patient is pregnant and the placenta is partially implanted over the inferior uterus and/or over the cervix. This is highly dangerous as the patient enters the second and third trimesters when the uterus stretches and thins under the low implanted placenta. If the uterus stretches or the cervix thins, the placenta may separate and lead to bleeding. Partial separation from the uterine wall is abrupt placenta. A placenta that partially implants into the endometrium, and possibly the myometrium, is called a placenta accreta.

12. **Correct answer: C**
Calculation of fetal gestational age is based on 10 lunar months counted from the first day of the last menstrual period. Other calculations include 280 days and 40 postmenstrual weeks. Assumption on months based on a 28-day cycle.

13. **Correct answer: D**
Tucking the lap belt under the dome of the belly, low on the hips and upper thighs, and the shoulder belt strap between the breasts and midclavicular is the best way to wear a seat belt throughout pregnancy. The seat should be positioned at least 10 inches from the steering wheel or dashboard. It is very important to stress the need to wear a seat belt any time a pregnant woman is in a car to increase the maternal and fetal survival rates should a motor vehicle crash occur.

14. **Correct answer: B**
The 2nd trimester includes the range of 13–27 weeks of fetal gestation. It is during this trimester that a fetus reaches viability at 23 weeks. Unless the exact date of conception is known, weeks of fetal

gestation may be off by ±3 weeks. The 1st trimester encompasses 0–12 weeks and the 3rd trimester from 28–40 weeks, or until delivery.

15. **Correct answer: A**

Increased human chorionic gonadotropin (hCG) levels contribute to morning sickness. Increased progesterone and estrogen levels as well as decreased glucose levels contribute to morning sickness.

16. **Correct answer: A**

Although the patient is pregnant, the patient's presenting symptoms indicate appendicitis. Due to fetal positioning the appendix is displaced to the right costal margin, shifting the location of the rebound tenderness and pain. Pain would not be constant if the patient was in labor. An abruption presents with sudden, colicky abdominal pain and frank vaginal bleeding.

17. **Correct answer: C**

During the 7th month of pregnancy, the risk of falls due to nonviolence peaks. Between the trimesters, the last trimester sees the overall greater risk for falls due to increasing levels of relaxin and the inability to see where the woman is walking.

18. **Correct answer: D**

HELLP syndrome stands for hemolysis, elevated liver enzymes, and low platelets. This life-threatening condition occurs in approximately 4–12% of women with severe preeclampsia.

19. **Correct answer: C**

Placenta previa has not been associated with HELLP syndrome. HELLP syndrome has been associated with DIC, uterine abruption, and acute renal failure as well as premature delivery, intrauterine asphyxia, and ruptured liver hematoma. Placenta previa is not co-maternal morbidity.

20. **Correct answer: A**

Relaxin is the hormone most responsible for the increasing gait instability during pregnancy. Relaxin causes cartilage softening resulting in joint hypermobility to allow for passage of the infant through the pelvic inlet. The effect also causes loosening in the hips, knees, and ankles, which combined with the shift in center of gravity, increases the risk of falls.

21. **Correct answer: A**

HELLP syndrome can occur in the postpartum patient. Specific causes of HELLP syndrome are unknown. Although common, hypertension and proteinuria are not always seen in the patient with HELLP syndrome. Decreased platelet count is related to increased platelet consumption and not due to platelet production.

22. **Correct answer: B**

Idiopathic thrombocytopenic purpura (ITP), preeclampsia, hepatitis, and gallbladder diseases can present with symptoms similar to HELLP syndrome.

23. **Correct answer: B**

A serum aspartate aminotransferase level of 120 units/L indicates immediate intervention is required. This patient is developing HELLP syndrome. Findings that indicate possible HELLP syndrome include a serum aspartate aminotransferase > 70 units/L, bilirubin > 1.2 mg/dl, lactate dehydrogenase > 600 units/L, and platelets < 150 mm^3. Women who are multiparous (more than one pregnancy), older than 25 years, and who suffered previous miscarriages are at higher risk of HELLP syndrome. If the patient has a history of HELLP syndrome, then the patient is at even higher risk of developing HELLP syndrome.

24. **Correct answer: D**

If the hospital has a labor and delivery unit, then the trauma nurse should obtain as thorough a history and physical as possible prior to transfer. This provides the labor nurse with a clearer picture of risk and urgency. If the hospital does not have a maternal unit, then the trauma nurse should obtain a history and physical, insert an IV for fluid resuscitation and medication administration, and obtain a CBC with liver enzymes.

25. **Correct answer: C**

Corticosteroids ordered for a 30-week gestation, gravida 5, para 2, 32 year old in labor are used to increase fetal lung maturity in case of premature delivery. Additional benefits include decreased inflammation in the mother's liver if she is at risk for HELLP syndrome.

26. **Correct answer: B**

Magnesium sulfate should be started as a 4–6 g bolus with a maintenance dose via an IV infusion of 2 g/hr to prevent seizures. The magnesium sulfate should be administered regardless of the presence or absence of hypertension. If hypertension is also present, then an additional goal is to keep the SBP 90–100. Antihypertensives may also be administered to decrease the systolic blood pressure.

27. **Correct answer: A**

Per the 2015 Neonatal Resuscitation Program guidelines, naloxone is not recommended to be administered during the first 15 minutes of neonatal life. Naloxone is used as an antagonist to opioid administration given to the mother within 4 hours of delivery. The primary goal, even if opioid use by the mother is known, is to provide resuscitation for the infant. The goal is to support the infant's heart rate and ventilation. Note that if the mother has a heroin addiction, naloxone should not be given to the neonate as it may cause seizures.

28. **Correct answer: D**

Any woman presenting to the emergency room with respiratory and/or circulatory compromise and pregnant with a viable fetus should have a fetal assessment completed before discharge. Prolonged respiratory distress and/or circulatory compromise could lead to fetal asphyxia and fetal death. Early assessment and intervention may save the baby's life. The nurse should also question discharge of this patient due to her presentation consistent with a diagnosis of tuberculosis. The patient may require further assessment.

29. **Correct answer: A**

If a woman of childbearing age presents to the emergency department with abdominal pain and vaginal bleeding, she should have an hCG test done. An hCG tests for pregnancy. Unilateral pelvic pain, palpable pelvic mass, and abnormal vaginal bleeding is indicative of an ectopic pregnancy. Underage females may be hesitant to report sexual activity if parents are present. Ectopic pregnancy occurs in approximately 2% of women. If ectopic pregnancy results in a rupture, additional symptoms include Kehr's sign (referred shoulder pain), tachycardia, hypotension, decreased level of consciousness, and cold, clammy skin. Failure to identify and intervene in the presence of ectopic pregnancy may lead to maternal death.

30. **Correct answer: C**

When managing the hemodynamics of a pregnant patient in a trauma, it is important to keep in mind that anemia is common and the hematocrit is usually around 35%. This can impair the oxygen-carrying capacity and despite a normal or high pulse oximetry reading, hypoxemia and hypoxia may be present. Additionally, blood volume for a singleton increases to 45% with cardiac output increasing by 30–35% to provide circulating volume to both mother and fetus. This increase in circulating volume contributes to dilutional anemia. To provide adequate fetal circulation, maternal systemic vascular resistance is decreased and may lead to a normal drop in blood pressure of approximately 10 mmHg. The overall impact to hemodynamic is masked hypovolemic shock. With multiple fetuses, circulating volume increases even more.

31. **Correct answer: A**

A woman, who is gravida 2, para 3, has been pregnant twice and delivered three viable children. Gravida refers to the number of times the woman has been pregnant. Para refers only to the number of viable children delivered and does not indicate that those children survived infancy. It is important to also ask about number of abortions (spontaneous and voluntary), to more accurately determine maternal history.

32. **Correct answer: C**

A woman noted to be a nullipara means that she has never delivered a viable fetus regardless of number of pregnancies. Null refers to zero and para refers to viable deliveries.

33. **Correct answer: B**

A female of childbearing age who presents with vaginal bleeding, severe abdominal pain with cramping, and cervical os dilated > 3 cm is experiencing an inevitable abortion. Treatment includes bed rest, pain control, RhoGAM administration, and uterine evacuation. The type of uterine evacuation depends on the gestational age of the fetus and patient–physician discussion. Social services should be notified to provide emotional support and community resources for grief counseling if desired.

34. **Correct answer: D**

Infusion of oxytocin 200 units per 1000 ml of Lactated Ringer's is contraindicated as the dosage is too high. The appropriate order would be for oxytocin 20 units per 1000 ml of Lactated Ringer's. This patient has experienced an incomplete abortion and will need urgent surgical intervention to completely evacuate the remaining tissue and avoid complications.

35. **Correct answer: D**

Embryonic chromosomal defects are the most common cause of spontaneous abortion in the 1st trimester. Late spontaneous abortions are commonly caused by maternal anatomic abnormalities, infection, and maternal endocrine disorders.

36. **Correct answer: C**

Complete abortions left untreated may result in a septic abortion in the presence of infection. Septic abortion may occur after incomplete abortions or after an unsuccessful uterine evacuation. Normal vaginal flora that becomes opportunistic can lead to profound infection and sepsis.

37. **Correct answer: D**

With the increase in circulating vascular volume, the maternal heart rate increases as cardiac output increases. The increase in heart rate may be confused as pregnancy-induced hypertension (PIH), hyperthyroidism, or pain. Expected tachycardia may also mask hemorrhagic blood loss and may not indicate hypovolemic shock until blood loss exceeds 2 L.

38. **Correct answer: D**

Candida albicans is not a normal vaginal flora. *Escherichia coli,* alpha-hemolytic *streptococci*, and beta-hemolytic *streptococci* are all normal vaginal flora. Each of these organisms is opportunistic and can lead to septicemia in mother and infant before and during delivery.

39. **Correct answer: A**

Contact a surgical consult and prepare the patient for surgery; this patient is experiencing septic abortion after a dilation and curettage. Severe abdominal distention, constant pelvic pain, fever, chills, and uterine tenderness indicate not only infection, but likelihood of infection of *Clostridium perfringens*. *Clostridium perfringens* is an anaerobic organism that produces gas gangrene, tissue necrosis, and uterine tissue sloughing. If the infection is severe enough, a hysterectomy is indicated. The trauma nurse will need to monitor for toxic shock and administer antibiotics as ordered. Spectinomycin hydrochloride is an antibiotic for gonorrhea and ganciclovir is an antiviral. Neither treatment is indicated for this patient.

40. **Correct answer: C**

Post-abortion discharge instructions should include avoiding intercourse, douching, and tampons for at least 2 weeks. This is to decrease exposure to infection. Other instructions include that vaginal bleeding should last for 1–2 weeks, and mild cramping will occur during the first few days. To monitor for infection, her temperature should be taken both in the morning and evening, and to report any temperature > 100°F to her obstetrician.

41. **Correct answer: D**

PIH stands for pregnancy-induced hypertension. Preeclampsia is a mild form of PIH. Eclampsia is a severe form of PIH and is life-threatening.

42. **Correct answer: C**

The primary difference between preeclampsia and eclampsia is that seizures are noted only with eclampsia. The presence of seizures indicates a life-threatening process for both mother and fetus.

Fetal bradycardia, particularly during a seizure, can lead to asphyxia and fetal neurologic deficits. Albuminuria is noted with both preeclampsia and eclampsia. HELLP syndrome can be seen with both disease processes. The systolic blood pressure in preeclampsia is less than 140 mmHg, and in eclampsia the systolic blood pressure is > 140 mmHg.

43. **Correct answer: D**

   A woman experiencing seizures and eclampsia should be positioned on the left side to improve blood flow to the fetus. This position also increases renal blood flow and urine output and decreases edema. Supine positioning places the fetus under the diaphragm and inhibits full lung expansion. Supine positioning inhibits blood flow from the legs, kidneys, and intestines and causes pressure on the lower back and spine. Prone position places pressure on the uterus and increases fetal distress. Right side positioning is less beneficial than left side.

44. **Correct answer: B**

   Placenta previa is a concern during late pregnancy because as the fetus grows and the cervical os thins, the placenta placement near or over the cervical os pulls away and leads to bleeding. During labor, the os also opens leading to more profound bleeding and increased maternal risk for hemorrhage. Complete placenta previa occurs when the placenta implants centered over the cervical os. Partial placenta previa has < 50% of the placenta over the cervical os. With a marginal placenta previa, only the margin is over the cervical os.

45. **Correct answer: A**

   Sudden painless bleeding of bright red blood, hypotension, tachycardia, and delayed capillary refill are consistent with a placenta previa presentation. Uterine rigidity, frank red blood, hypotension, tachycardia, and back pain are consistent with abruption. Foul vaginal discharge, constant pelvic pain, fever, and chills are consistent with septic abortion. Sharp abdominal pain without bleeding, tachycardia, and tachypnea can be seen with labor.

46. **Correct answer: C**

   This patient is at highest risk for abruption after the motor vehicle accident. The saturation of blood to her pants should be evaluated immediately to determine the source of the bleeding. Abruptions do not always present with bleeding after abdominal trauma, but should be considered whenever a pregnant woman suffers abdominal trauma. Preterm labor may result after an accident, but is not usually life-threatening to the mother. Infection is a concern, but it is not immediately life-threatening.

47. **Correct answer: B**

   Respiratory alkalosis is an expected finding when interpreting a blood gas of a pregnant patient due to the normal increase in minute ventilation and tidal volume. With the increase in energy needs, oxygen consumption increases by 15–20%, despite the decrease in oxygen reserves, total lung capacity, and functional residual capacity with fetal growth.

48. **Correct answer: D**

   Nursing priorities when caring for a mother experiencing abruption include marking and frequently assessing fundal height for changes indicating the severity of occult bleeding. Two large-bore IVs should be placed for infusions of normal saline, Lactated Ringer's, or O negative cross-matched blood. Continuous fetal monitoring should be initiated while surgical evaluation is performed. If the fetus is viable and maternal shock is severe, then immediate delivery is required to prevent loss of both mother and fetus.

49. **Correct answer: C**

   Fetal hemoglobin (HbF) improves fetal survivability until maternal oxygen drops below 50% of normal. This provides some compensatory mechanism for protecting the fetus from fluctuations in maternal oxygen levels. Fetal hemoglobin has a higher affinity for oxygen then adult hemoglobin. In the full-term infant, fetal hemoglobin is 60–80% of the total.

50. **Correct answer: C**

   The desire to void is not a sign of impending delivery. The desire is to bear down, presence of bloody show, bulging membranes, crowning, frequent contractions, and ruptured amniotic fluid are all indications of delivery.

51. **Correct answer: B**

Your immediate priority is to dry the infant and remove all wet linens from direct contact with the baby's skin. You do this first, to stimulate the baby to breath and to limit the negative effects of cold stress on the infant. Avoid the use of hot water bottles or gloves to warm the infant. Direct contact may cause serious burns to exposed skin. The best method to warm the infant is to use warmed blankets, a heat lamp, a radiant warmer, or place the baby on the mother's bare chest. Suctioning should include the use of a bulb syringe in the mouth and then nares, or use wall suction at 80-100 mmHg to the mouth. Avoid using a delee or large suction tubing in the nares. It may cause irritation and swelling, further impeding airflow and increase likelihood of respiratory distress. Although you will need to and want to call the NICU team or nursery to accept care of this infant, it is not the priority over providing resuscitation care to the infant.

52. **Correct answer: D**

Any initial newborn heart rate less than 100/min requires positive pressure ventilation (PPV) at a rate of 40–60 breaths per minute for 30 seconds with FiO_2 titrated to keep oxygen saturations via pulse oximetry greater than 85%. If after 30 seconds of effective PPV with visible chest rise, the heart rate is < 60 bpm, then chest compressions at a 3:1 ratio should be initiated for 60 seconds. The heart rate should be continuously monitored via ECG monitor while compressions are in progress. Suctioning should only be considered if the bulb syringe did not clear the airway of secretions and you cannot ventilate with chest rise.

53. **Correct answer: B**

If you are experiencing increasing difficulty obtaining chest rise when providing positive pressure ventilation (PPV) to an infant, reposition the mask and head, then insert an orogastric tube to aspirate stomach contents, and then place the OG open to air to vent the stomach. The vent will decrease pressures in the stomach and diaphragm to allow for increased lung expansion. Oral suctioning is indicated if secretions are noted, but the orogastric tube is the better choice. Low intermittent wall suction is indicated for gastric obstruction, diaphragmatic hernia, and ileus, not this scenario. PPV with positive inspiratory pressure (PIP) of 40 mmHg is excessive and likely to cause pneumothorax and sudden decompensation.

54. **Correct answer: B**

Narcan (naloxone) use is contraindicated to treat unknown drug exposure prior to delivery. If Narcan is used on an infant of a mother using methadone, the infant may begin to seize, impairing respiratory effort, and the seizures may lead to neurologic injury and death. Instead, provide positive pressure ventilation and titrate oxygen using pulse oximetry. For preterm infants under 28 weeks gestation or under 1000 g, use a polyethylene bag with a heat source such as a heat lamp or radiant warmer to stabilize temperature. If using a polyethylene bag, do not dry the infant first. The moisture helps to prevent fluid and electrolytes loss through thin, permeable skin.

55. **Correct answer: A**

Childbearing age for any female trauma victim is defined as a woman between the ages of 10–60. Due to genetic and environmental influences, ovulation with conception is possible for females as young as 10 years old to women believed to be in menopause. Err on the side of caution, and pregnancy tests should be administered for any female trauma victim to rule out an additional fetal patient(s).

56. **Correct answer: C**

Your patient is most likely suffering from endometritis. As bacteria infect the endometrial lining of the uterus, patients may present with low back pain, severe muscle spasms, malaise, and dysmenorrhea. Assessment reveals an enlarged uterus with serosanguineous or purulent, foul-smelling vaginal discharge and fever. Gonorrhea may present with fever in severe cases but not with an enlarged uterus. Chancroid presents with headaches and mucopurulent, foul-smelling discharge with vulvular lesions. Atrophic vaginitis presents with scant, watery, white discharge without abdominal pain.

57. **Correct answer: C**

Uterine rupture should be suspected of any pregnant female with history of abdominal trauma resulting in sudden deceleration or extreme abdominal compression. Patients present with severe abdominal pain and decreased or absent fetal heart tones and movement. Fetal parts or the entire fetus may be located in the abdominal cavity outside of the uterus, with minimal to no vaginal bleeding. Due to internal bleeding from the ruptured uterus and placental injury, the mother will become hypovolemic and hypotensive. Shock may develop, leading to both fetal and maternal death. Upon diagnosis, the mother should be treated immediately with volume replacement and prepared for surgery. Emergency cesarean delivery is indicated to save the fetus with probable hysterectomy to preserve maternal life.

58. **Correct answer: D**
A classical abdominal incision is the best method for postmortem cesarean delivery of a viable fetus. Delivery should occur within 4 minutes of maternal death to increase positive fetal neurologic outcome. Perimortem delivery may occur in the emergency department if indicated to save fetal life. The neonatal resuscitation team should be physically present, not on call, if postmortem cesarean delivery is indicated.

59. **Correct answer: B**
An infant's blood glucose should be assessed within 30 minutes of birth for high-risk infants that are unable to immediately feed. Illness, respiratory distress, and shock increase glucose consumption and can lead to hypoglycemia quickly. The condition is worsened if the infant is not consuming sufficient calories.

60. **Correct answer: B**
Paramedics just brought in a 30-year-old pregnant patient. She was a passenger in a rear-end MVA. She is brought in on a backboard. While waiting for a CT scan, she reports feeling light-headed. On monitor, her heart rate keeps dropping, her pulse oximetry is 88–92% and she is dyspneic. Repositioning the patient so the backboard is slightly angled to her left side would improve this patient's condition quickly. As the pregnancy progresses, the weight of the uterus and fetus places pressure on the vertebral column causing vasovagal symptoms and the vena cava leading to a drop in preload. Supine position also places increase pressure on the underside of the diaphragm decreasing lung expansion. Positioning with a slight left angle relieves pressure on both the vertebral column and the vena cava.

61. **Correct answer: D**
Hypotonia, jitteriness, poor suck, apnea, and seizures indicate a hypoglycemic state in the brain. The brain is extremely sensitive to fluctuations in oxygen and glucose. Most signs and symptoms of hypoglycemia initiate in the brain.

62. **Correct answer: D**
Initial IV fluids should be calculated at 80 ml/kg/d for an infant newly born.

63. **Correct answer: C**
Hypertonia, increased glucose and O_2 consumption, increased brown fat metabolism, and vasoconstriction are all physiological reactions to cold stress.

64. **Correct answer: A**
In response to cold stress, the body releases norepinephrine. The norepinephrine triggers an increase in metabolic rate, increased O_2 and glucose utilization, hypoxia, pulmonary constriction, and hypoxemia. If the cold stress continues, the infant is at risk for death as the body converts to anaerobic metabolism in the lack of oxygen.

65. **Correct answer: D**
Using a heat lamp at 6 inches away from the patient is too close and risks burning the infant's skin. The size and wattage of the bulb also determine how close the heat lamp should be without causing injury to skin. Please avoid using chemical heat gels or gloves filled with hot water against the skin. These methods may cause up to third-degree burns. Servo radiant warmer setting, using warmed, humidified oxygen, and warming stethoscopes all are appropriate to warm an infant or decrease risk of heat loss.

66. **Correct answer: B**
Tachypnea with a decreased PCO_2 is linked to congenital heart disease and other non-pulmonary disease processes. Pulmonary causes of tachypnea, such as respiratory distress syndrome, aspiration, and pneumothorax, lead to increased PCO_2.

67. **Correct answer: A**

The S.T.A.B.L.E. acronym can be used to remember what information should be prepared prior to transport of an infant aged 0–28 days from the emergency department to a high level of care within or outside the facility. S.T.A.B.L.E. stands for sugar, temperature, airway, blood pressure, lab work, and emotional support for family and patient. The speed at which the ED staff can stabilize an infant for transport improves patient outcomes by decreasing injury to tissues and lessening risk of complications. The transporting team is better able to quickly transport the infant for a higher level of care.

68. **Correct answer: D**

If an infant's head has been delivered with the cord wrapped tightly around the neck (nuchal cord), then clamp the cord in two places and use sterile scissors to cut between the two clamps. If the body is delivered without releasing the pressure of the cord around the neck, the pressures might strangle the infant or irregularly tear the cord causing bleeding in the infant and mother. Stretching the cord over the head without relieving the pull on the cord could also result in tearing of the cord. Once the head is delivered, especially with a nuchal cord, the infant does not receive oxygen from the mother or is able to take a breath. The anoxic episode may lead to profound neurologic compromise.

69. **Correct answer: B**

Actions should be taken to maintain an infant's blood glucose at 50–120 mg/dl. If unable to consume sufficient calories to maintain adequate glucose levels, insert an IV and provide dextrose boluses and maintenance fluids with dextrose. If the glucose is too high, decrease IV flow rate or the amount of glucose concentration. Some sources indicate a lower range to 40mg/dl. In asymptomatic infants, a value of 25mg/dl is acceptable. Use caution in accepting values under 45 mg/dl as patients have been noted to have longer term neurologic compromise and decreased IQ scores.

70. **Correct answer: A**

If an amniotic sac delivers with the infant inside, then rupture the sac and peel it away from the face to provide resuscitation by drying and suctioning the infant and initiate ventilation. Remember to suction the mouth first and then the nares. If the infant is estimated to be greater than 23 weeks gestation and weighs greater than 400 g, then continue resuscitation until neonatal staff can arrive. Remember to keep the infant warm and dry and continue to provide ventilation that produces visible chest rise.

71. **Correct answer: C**

As gestation progresses, risk for abdominal trauma increases. Small bowel injury is less common as organs are pressed up into the upper abdomen or downward into the pelvic inlet by the fetus. As the abdominal wall (rectus abdominis) is stretched along and away from the linea alba, the spleen and the liver trauma is common due to the decreased muscular protection. Both gastric motility and emptying is delayed, which increases absorption nutrient absorption. With the progression of pregnancy, gastroesophageal sphincter is looser resulting in more frequent gastroesophageal reflux as abdominal pressure increases with fetal growth.

72. **Correct answer: D**

Breech positioning during vaginal delivery is dangerous as risk of strangulation is increased. If the cord is wrapped around the neck during delivery or if the infant is pulled on while the neck is at the cervix without a contraction, the risk of strangulation also exists. Assisting delivery by pulling on the infant should only be done with contractions. The infant is also at risk for prolapsed cord if portions of the cord exit the vagina before the infant. This inhibits blood flow and oxygen to the infant during delivery and increases the risk for neonatal resuscitation. Breech positioning is called a frank breech if both feet are near the head, a full breech with feet near the abdomen, and a singling footling breech if only one foot presents through the vagina.

73. **Correct answer: C**

If you note that the umbilical cord precedes any portion of the infant in the vaginal canal, then use a sterile gloved hand to support the head or presenting part off the cord and leave your hand in place. This allows blood and oxygen to pass through the cord to the infant. You will need to leave your hand in place during transfer to the obstetrical unit or surgical suite for an emergency cesarean. Oxygen should be administered to the mother. Do not push the cord back into the vagina as this may result in further compression or kinking of the cord. If able, reposition the mother on her hands and knees with her buttocks in the air to decrease pressure on the vaginal canal and allow for gravity to release pressure on the cord.

74. **Correct answer: D**

Ectopic pregnancy, appendicitis, PID, diverticulitis, and ovarian torsion present with similar symptoms to those of ruptured ovarian cysts. Symptoms include sudden, sharp, unilateral lower back pain and peritoneal irritation. Patients may also complain of nausea and vomiting, low-grade fever, and hemoperitoneum.

75. **Correct answer: D**

Mothers should be discouraged to drink or consume ginkgo or ginseng preparations after delivery. Both substances have been identified as platelet anti-aggregators and may lead to additional bleeding. Oxytocin, fundal massages, and breastfeeding all release hormones and chemicals that result in uterine contractions and decreased bleeding.

76. **Correct answer: C**

Fetal bradycardia is classified as a fetal heart rate less than 100 bpm. Immediate interventions to increase fetal heart rate include providing oxygen, repositioning, IV fluids, and transfer to obstetrical unit.

77. **Correct answer: A**

Staphylococcus aureus is the organism to most likely cause toxic shock syndrome.

78. **Correct answer: D**

Removing identifiable sources of infection is an important step in effectively treating toxic shock syndrome. Potential sources of TSS include tampons, diaphragms, contraceptive sponges, and intimacy toys. Blood pressure should be stabilized with isotonic crystalloids, vasopressors, and inotropes. PaO_2 should be maintained over 60 mmHg with appropriate oxygen support devices. The patient does not need to be transferred to an isolation room, unless contact isolation cannot be maintained in her current location. In addition, antibiotics should be initiated as soon as available and the patient transferred to an intensive care unit.

79. **Correct answer: A**

As mandatory reporters, we have an obligation to report an alleged crime to police. Before providing any nonemergency care, thoroughly document injuries with pictures whenever possible. Your patient's injuries are consistent with sexual assault and should be investigated. Stigma of rape and fear if the assailant is known may hinder the victim from reporting the assault and filing charges. You cannot force a victim to file a complaint or to submit to forensic examination. Until the patient refuses forensic examination, continue collecting evidence according to policy.

80. **Correct answer: C**

Laboratory personnel are not considered to be members of the Sexual Assault Response Team (SART). However, their training includes specific techniques and policies for special handling of forensic evidence that could be later used in court.

81. **Correct answer: D**

The SART process for reporting and collection when sexual assault is known or suspected begins with police notification, a patient advocate and sexual assault nurse examiner (SANE) are notified, initial disclosure occurs between staff and police, and forensic evidence is collected. The patient's advocate and SANE may assist the patient through the hospital system to receive appropriate counseling, medical treatment, and follow-up care. Once evidence is collected, it is turned over to the appropriate authorities for judicial proceedings.

82. **Correct answer: D**

If the hospital does not have a designated patient advocate or counselor, then contact social services to have a worker sit with the victim. It is crucial not to leave the woman alone at this time. Not only may she inadvertently destroy forensic evidence, but she may be at risk for suicide or may walk away from treatment for fear or shame. A counselor as well as patient support, friends, and family should be included in providing support to the victim. Notify police as soon as sexual assault is suspected or determined to fully initiate appropriate SART processes. Should the case go to court, the district or city attorney represents the victim. The counselor, advocate, or social worker can explain appropriate procedures and provide community resources and compensation programs to the victim. Medical personnel should continually explain the purpose of all medical procedures and provide support as needed.

83. Correct answer: B

Pelvic fracture type and severity have no impact on maternal or fetal mortality. The risk for hemorrhage is not increased with fetal gestation, but due to the increase in circulating vascular volume to the uterus and the impaired autonomic control of the uterine spiral arteries during pregnancy. Should a hemorrhage be present, risk for fetal death is high when the gestation is <20 weeks or with delayed treatment and fetal hypoxia occurs. Even still, maternal mortality is approximately 9% and fetal loss is approximately 35%. Overall the risk for pelvic fractures in the pregnant patient is rare, but increases when injury is associated with motor vehicle accidents (either as a pedestrian or passenger) or with falls from great heights.

84. Correct answer: A

Clothing collected as forensic evidence should be removed via unbuttoning or unzipping if possible; if clothing must be cut, avoid cutting through bullet holes, knife cuts, tears, or button holes. Cutting though any existing hole, tear, or break in fabric can damage evidence and impede future investigation. All collected evidence should be labeled with patient name, hospital name, collection site (ED), date and time of collection, description of specimen, and collector's full name. All items released to police should be documented on the medical chart as well as in the police report. Any biohazard materials related to the victim's care should be turned over to police for documentation; this includes weapons, bullet or knife fragments, fibers, blood samples, and clothing.

85. Correct answer: B

It is not true that a consent for or against must be signed before an official forensic examination. Additional consents include a general consent for medical assessment and specific consents for disposition of physical and diagnostic evidence to police. Consents should be specific regarding types of evidence collected and disposition, such as DNA sampling, fibers, clothing, weapons, photographs, and all written documentation.

86. Correct answer: A

Chest rise is the fastest way to determine if ventilations with a bag-mask-valve are effective followed by immediate improvement in heart rate. Additional methods are to observe for improvement in color and audible breath sounds are auscultated.

87. Correct answer: B

This baby is in secondary apnea as the baby did not respond to previous stimulation while drying and suctioning. Immediate action should include providing positive pressure ventilation with 21% oxygen for 30 seconds. As research becomes available, the concentration of FiO_2 recommended is to begin at 21% FiO_2 and titrate oxygen to remain within the recommended range for minutes of life. By 1 minute of life, pulse oximetry should be at least 65% and increase by 5% minimum every minute of life. By 5 minutes of life, pulse oximetry should be between 85 and 95%.

88. Correct answer: A

Immediate intubation is indicated when a neonate cannot be ventilated effectively via positive pressure ventilation. Additional indicators for intubation include a neonate who has extreme low birth weight, an infant requiring prolonged positive pressure ventilation, an infant not responding to resuscitation efforts, or an infant who requires surfactant therapy. Intubation is also indicated for infants with a diaphragmatic hernia.

89.   **Correct answer: D**

A T-piece resuscitator or flow-inflating bag-mask-valve would be appropriate methods for providing continuous positive airway pressure (CPAP). A self-inflating bag-mask-valve requires the user to squeeze the bag to provide oxygen. Current NRP guidelines recommend that the initial oxygen begin at 21–30% FiO_2 during resuscitation of a premature neonate and that oxygen be titrated for saturation via pulse oximetry. Because the infant has a heart rate $>$ 100 and has spontaneous respiratory effort, positive pressure ventilation (PVV) is not indicated at this time.

90.   **Correct answer: C**

Deciding factors when transporting a pregnant trauma patient should include gestational age and that the facility offers both maternal and neonatal emergency services. If the fetus is greater than 20 weeks gestation, the patient should be transferred to a trauma center to increase the rate of fetal survival. If the fetus in less than 20 weeks gestation, then fetal viability is not possible and maternal life takes precedence, and facility choice shifts to maternal needs only.

91.   **Correct answer: C**

Transition from fetal circulation to independence requires two major changes in circulation. The first change requires that the infant's lungs fill with air, resulting in pulmonary vascular bed dilation and a subsequent drop in pulmonary vascular resistance. The second change occurs when the cord is clamped. Cord clamping initiates an increase in systemic vascular resistance, thus, beginning the closure of fetal right-to-left shunts. Complete circulatory transition may take hours or days depending on gestation at delivery.

92.   **Correct answer: A**

If a flow-inflating bag-mask-valve does not inflate during use, follow MR SOAPA. First verify the mask seal and reposition the baby's head. Next, suction the mouth to clear the airway, then open the mouth. Then check pressures by verifying that the tubing is connected to oxygen, not air, and the valve is turned to between 8 and 10 lpm. Finally increase the PIP with each ventilation. Assess the problem from the baby toward the wall connections. Use suction to clear oral and nasal secretions and reposition the head to the sniffing position. Check that the manometer is connected properly and see if the flow-control valve is not open fully. Next, check for any kinks or breaks in the bag or tubing. If you are unable to rapidly determine the cause of the bag failure, immediately obtain and use another bag or bag-mask-valve device. Many equipment complications can be avoided during resuscitation by checking the bag, connections, and oxygen flow prior to delivery.

93.   **Correct answer: B**

Childhood vaccinations are not an important part of history assessment. The nurse should obtain a complete sexual history including last menstrual period, contraception used, sexual activities within the last 72 hours, reproductive history, and sexually transmitted diseases. General and mental health histories should also be obtained. Make sure to document data regarding the assault including abuser's actions, weapons or items used in the assault, location, abuser's description, and post-assault activities. Any post-assault activities, including showering, voiding, eating, drinking, and changing of clothing, can damage forensic evidence collection.

94.   **Correct answer: A**

A 1mg/10ml concentration of epinephrine should be administered at 0.1–0.3 ml/kg via the umbilical vein and 0.3–1 ml/kg via the endotracheal tube. Absorption rates of epinephrine via the endotracheal tube are unreliable in the neonate and may not be as effective. Umbilical venous administration of epinephrine is the preferred route of administration. Epinephrine increases oxygen demand within tissues. To prevent ischemia and infarction of cardiac tissue, it is critical that oxygen be correctly delivered and confirmed prior to epinephrine administration. If the patient is intubated, use both primary and secondary assessment tools to verify endotracheal tube placement.

95.   **Correct answer: D**

If neonatal circulation is compromised, the lungs may not have exhaled adequate quantities of CO_2 to register a change in the device. The resuscitation team must use primary confirmation (equal chest rise, audible breath sounds in all lung fields, absent air movement over the stomach, rise in heart rate, and visualization of the tube between the vocal cords) to determine positive endotracheal tube placement.

96. **Correct answer: A**

    The steps of resuscitation are the same regardless of location. Upon delivery of the infant, begin drying, stimulating, and clearing the airway using available articles of clothing. The cord should be clamped using a tie, shoelace, or other material that clamps, but does not cut, the cord. Do not cut the cord as this may provide an entry of bacteria into neonatal circulation. Wait for EMS personnel to cut the cord using sterile equipment. Clamping the cord is instrumental in transitioning neonatal circulation. The infant should be placed skin to skin with the mother and face up on the mother's chest, then covered to maintain temperature. The floor is cold and the infant would lose heat via conduction if placed on the floor. Drying the infant prior to placing the infant on the mother's chest will decrease the risk of evaporative heat loss and cold stress.

97. **Correct answer: B**

    According to current NRP 2015 guidelines from the American Academy of Pediatrics, if, after 10 minutes of resuscitation, there is no heartbeat and each resuscitation step has been completed correctly and verified, then the team may stop resuscitation efforts. More time may be needed to ensure that each step of resuscitation was completed correctly and effectively. Additional time may also be needed to fully treat identified causes of fetal arrest such as hemorrhagic or hypovolemic shock and asphyxia. Ethical dilemmas challenge resuscitation providers to balance legal, ethical, and moral elements in delivering care. If the prognosis is unknown, continual communication with the parents by the physician is critical in determining best outcome for the infant, even if that choice is to withdraw support. After any resuscitation, it is vital for staff members to discuss the resuscitation to identify team strengths and opportunities for improvement and any ethical challenges. Discussion may identify more effective ways to communicate and improve competence among various disciplines, departments, and ancillary staff.

98. **Correct answer: C**

    Politely refuse the order, notify your transport neonatologist and follow standard stabilization protocol of using Dextrose 10% at 2 ml/kg IV. The ED physician may not be aware of or current to the standards of care in newborn stabilization. It would be appropriate to politely decline the order and to verify with a neonatologist while following standard stabilization practice. Dextrose concentrations of 25% and 50% provide a bolus of glucose that would cause profound hyperglycemia followed by rebound hypoglycemia, as well as severe damage to the vessels.

99. **Correct answer: B**

    Infants experiencing severe hypothermia are dying from a lack of sufficient oxygen supply for demand by the tissues and hypoglycemia related to an increase in glycogen metabolism with diminishing supply. In the absence of both oxygen and glucose, anaerobic metabolism is used to create energy at great cost to tissues as lactic acid builds up in the body. As pH decreases and lactic acid increases, tissues throughout the body are destroyed. Bradycardia, apnea, renal failure, and altered neurologic function worsen as tissues are destroyed, and hypoxia and hypoglycemia continue.

100. **Correct answer: B**

    The safest method for temperature assessment is using the thermometer in the axilla for 3–5 minutes with skin touching skin. Many hospitals have halted rectal temperatures as a standard method for assessing temperature in most neonates because of the danger of inserting the tip too far into the colon, resulting in perforation where the sigmoid colon angles sharply and/or vaginal stimulation. Because of its flexibility, a temperature probe may be inserted into the anus up to 5 cm to obtain core temperatures. A tympanic thermometer is difficult to use and less reliable in the neonatal population because the ear canal is often smaller than the tympanic tip and cannot make a complete seal with the skin.

101. **Correct answer: B**

    Blood pooling into the retroperitoneal space is expected with a pelvic fracture for any pregnant trauma patient. The increase in blood flow related to fetal development increases the risk of hemorrhage. With pelvic fractures, the mechanism of injury may result in rupture of the amniotic sac, leading to pooling of amniotic fluid in the vagina, which would be noted on slide evaluation as positive ferning and a positive nitrazine test.

102. **Correct answer: C**

The infant assessment indicates a neonate who is less than 23 weeks gestation weighing under 400 g. Per NRP guidelines, this infant is not viable and resuscitation measures should be withheld. Estimated gestational dates provided by the mother may be inaccurate by plus or minus 2 weeks. The findings are more consistent with the ultrasound assessment of 21 weeks. Care should now be focused on family grieving and emotional support.

103. **Correct answer: D**

The bladder in a pregnancy trauma patient is at higher risk when the mechanism of injury involves a shearing force that may tear the ureters from the bladder. Due to hormonal influence of progesterone, estrogen, and relaxin, the ureters stretch between the kidneys and the bladder with fetal growth. As the bladder is moved anteriorly and superiorly in the abdomen to outside of the pelvic inlet, the increasing tension within the urinary tract from increased GFR increases the risk of injury and rupture.

104. **Correct answer: B**

Glycosuria is normal in the pregnant patient due to the increase in GFR and insulin-resistant receptors. The increase in GFR will also result in a decrease in creatinine and BUN to as much as 50% pre-pregnancy values. Proteinuria and hematuria would indicate injury to the glomerulus and requires further investigation.

105. **Correct answer: B**

Neonatal Resuscitation Provider 2015 guidelines focus care around the continual assessment and management of airway, breathing, and circulation.

106. **Correct answer: A**

Any female trauma patient of childbearing age is assumed pregnant until proven otherwise. Pregnancy may not be obvious due to patient age, size, or skeletal build, and failure to assess for pregnancy may result in abortion or miscarriage. Drugs, alcohol, and energy drinks should not be always assumed unless situation or circumstances indicate involvement.

107. **Correct answer: D**

Candidiasis infections present with profuse, white curd-like vaginal discharge that may be yeasty or sweet smelling. Vulvular inflammation, redness, and dermatitis to inner thighs are also symptoms of this infection. Complaints often include itching, burning, and painful urination. The history includes sudden onset, recent or current antibiotic use, or coincides with menses. Frequent candidiasis infections should be assessed for causes such as frequent douching, sexual activity, hygiene habits, and work environment of both patient and sexual partners.

108. **Correct answer: A**

Placental function and inherent maternal resources are critical maternal factors to consider when planning care of the neonate prior to and after delivery. Placental function determines the rate and flow of nutrients and oxygen to the fetus as well as cellular waste products flowing away from the fetus. The placenta also plays a critical role in the physiologic changes within the mother that increase glucose and essential elements to the fetus during development. Maternal resources comprise the mother's ability to obtain and maintain adequate and appropriate nutrition, cardiovascular and respiratory function in order to transport oxygen, carbohydrates, fats, vitamins, minerals, amino acids, and more to the fetus. If maternal resources are compromised, then fetal health becomes compromised. Additional complications to adequate maternal resources include preexisting medical and mental health conditions, drug ingestion, and exercise.

109. **Correct answer: A**

Due to the greater surface to body ratio of infants, heat loss is three to four times greater or faster for infants than for adults. Evaporative heat loss is the primary and most likely cause of heat loss in the newly born infant.

110. **Correct answer: B**

Paramedics are en route with a 21 week pregnant patient that was thrown 20 feet due to a car bombing. She has first-degree burns to her legs and arms, scattered bruising to her arms and torso, and a scalp abrasion. Paramedics are providing oxygen via a nonrebreather mask. On arrival to your ED, the patient reports that it is difficult to breathe. The first action that should be taken is to preserve an airway, thus, the trauma nurse should prepare for intubation with a slightly smaller ETT to prevent pulmonary injury. Progesterone release results in vascular edema, including in the airway. This increases the risk of airway closer with injury. Priority is given to protecting airway patency, positioning the mother left lateral to prevent pressure on the vena cava and vertebral column that would drop maternal blood pressure, then placement of a NGT to decrease the risk of aspiration due to delayed gastric emptying. Should vasopressors be needed, levophed and epinephrine should be avoided due to a link to decreased uterine perfusion. Ephedrine and mephentermine are better choices, as there is no impact to uterine perfusion.

111. **Correct answer: B**
Paramedics are en route with a 35-week pregnant gunshot victim. On arrival, CPR has been in progress for the past minute. After primary survey, the trauma attending determines that maternal resuscitation is not likely and the obstetrician agrees. To improve fetal survival, a postmortem cesarean section should occur within 4 minutes of life-threatening maternal rhythm. The 4-minute timeframe includes the maximum 1 minute cut to delivery time. A neonatal team, including neonatologist, should be present to manage the neonate.

112. **Correct answer: C**
The number one cause of fetal death when trauma is involved is due to maternal shock. As maternal perfusion decreases, gradients in oxygen, glucose, and carbon dioxide shift, preventing the fetus from drawing oxygen and nutrients from maternal circulation and diffusion of carbon dioxide and waste from fetal circulation. The result is fetal hypoxemia, hypoglycemia, and acidosis that progress to result in fetal arrest. Priority management of a pregnant trauma victim is to aggressively manage maternal shock, thus, supporting fetal survival.

113. **Correct answer: A**
A pregnant trauma victim has an estimated 1,750 ml blood loss (moderate with approximately 25–25% blood loss). Maternal physiologic compensatory actions you should expect to see include mild tachycardia (100–120) with restlessness, MAP of 50–60 mmHg, and oliguria. For mild blood loss at 20–25% or 1200–1500 ml, tachycardia is less than 105, peripheral vasoconstriction is noted (cold, pale extremities), and a MAP of 70–75 mmHg. Should blood loss exceed 2 L, the loss is considered severe and the patient is in hemorrhagic hypovolemic shock. Untreated severe blood loss may result in DIC, anuria, and altered LOC due to hypoxia.

Abunnaja, S., Marshall, C., Cuviello, A., Brenes, R. A., & Tripodi, G. (2014). Concomitant deep venous thrombosis, femoral artery thrombosis, and pulmonary embolism after air travel. *Case Reports in Vascular Medicine, 12*(3), 675–678.

Albertine, P., Borofsky, S., Brown, D., Patel, S., Lee, W., Caputy, A., & Taheri, M. R. (2016). Small subdural hemorrhages: Is routine intensive care unit admission necessary? *American Journal of Emergency Medicine, 34*(3), 521–524.

American Association of Critical-Care Nurses (AACN). (2006). *Core curriculum for critical care nursing* (6th ed.). St. Louis, MO: Elsevier Saunders.

American Burn Association. (2011). *Advanced burn life support course provider manual.* Chicago, IL: American Burn Association.

American College of Obstetricians and Gynecologists. (2013). FAQs: The Rh Factor: How it can affect your pregnancy. Retrieved from http://www.acog.org/Patients/FAQs/The-Rh-Factor-How-It-Can-Affect-Your-Pregnancy#already

American College of Surgeons (ACS). (2014). Resources for the optimal care of the injured patient. Chicago, IL: American College of Surgeons.

American College of Surgeons Committee on Trauma. (2012). *Advanced trauma life support student course manual* (9th ed.). Chicago, IL: American College of Surgeons.

American Heart Association. (2016). *Advanced cardiovascular life support provider manual 2015 guidelines.* Dallas, TX: American Heart Association.

American Heart Association. (2016). *Pediatric advanced cardiovascular life support provider manual 2015 guidelines.* Dallas, TX: American Heart Association.

Anderson M. L., Peterson, E. D., & Peng, S. A. (2013). Differences in the profile, treatment, and prognosis of patients with cardiogenic shock by myocardial infarction classification: A report from NCDR. *Circulation of Cardiovascular Quality Outcomes, 6*(6), 708–715.

Andrejaitiene, J., & Sirvinskas, E. (2012). Early post-cardiac surgery delirium risk factors. *Perfusion, 27*(2), 105–112.

Anticoagulant reversal agent nets FDA approval. (2015). *Cardiology Today, 18*(11), 19.

Antonopoulos C. N., Sfyroeras, G. S., Kallinis, A., Kakisis, J. D., Liapis, C.D., & Petridou, E. T. (2014). Epidemiology of concomitant injuries in traumatic thoracic aortic rupture: A meta-analysis. *Vascular, 22*(6), 395–405. doi: 10.1177/1708538113518205

Arikanoglu, Z., Taskesen, F., Gül, M., Aliosmanoglu, I., Önder, A., & Kapan, M. (2015). Full-thickness isolated small intestine injury due to blunt trauma. *Journal of Academic Emergency Medicine, 14*(4), 204–206.

Aristotelis, V. K., Liouta, E., Komaitis, S., Anagnostopoulos, C., & Stranjalis, G. (2016). Idiopathic intracranial hypertension: Epidemiology, pathophysiology, clinical features and contemporary management. *Hospital Chronicles, 11*(2), 77–84.

Arti, H., Khorami, M., & Ebrahimi-Nejad, V. (2016). Comparison of negative pressure wound therapy (NPWT) & conventional wound dressings in the open fracture wounds. *Pakistan Journal of Medical Sciences Quarterly, 32*(1), 65–69.

Asadi, F. (2015). NSG 532: Advanced Human Physiology—Immunology Online Lecture Slides. [Charts Source].

Banti, M., Walter, J., Hudak, S., & Soderdahl, D. (2016). Improvised explosive device-related lower genitourinary trauma in current overseas combat operations. *Journal of Trauma Acute Care Surgery, 80*(1), 131–134.

Batchelor, J. S. (2015). A meta-analysis to determine the effect of coagulopathy on intracranial haematoma progression in adult patients with isolated blunt head trauma. *Trauma, 17*(4), 243–249.

Battle, C. E., & Evans, P. A. (2015). Predictors of mortality in patients with flail chest: A systematic review. *Emergency Medicine Journal, 32*(12), 961.

Binenbaum, G., & Forbes, B. J. (2014). The eye in child abuse: Key points on retinal hemorrhages and abusive head trauma. *Pediatric Radiology, 44*, 571–577.

Bissell, B. D., Erdman, M. J., Smotherman, C., Kraemer, D. F., & Ferreira, J. A. (2015). The impact of endocrine supplementation on adverse events in septic shock. *Journal of Critical Care, 30*(6), 1169–1173.

Blackburn, S. (2013). *Maternal, fetal, & neonatal physiology: A clinical perspective* (4th ed.). Maryland Heights, MO: Elsevier.

Bosse, G. M. (2014). Hot asphalt burns: A review of injuries and management options. *American Journal of Emergency Medicine, 32*(7), 820.e1–820.e3.

Brennan J. (2013). Head and neck trauma in Iraq and Afghanistan: Different war, different surgery, lessons learned. *Laryngoscope, 123*(10), 2411–2417.

Brorsen, A. J., & Rogelet, K. R. (2014). *PCCN certification review* (3rd ed.). Sudbury, MA: Jones & Bartlett Learning.

Burns, S. (Ed.). (2014). *AACN essentials of critical care nursing* (3rd ed.). New York, NY: McGraw-Hill Education.

Campbell, R. L., Bashore, C. J., Lee, S., Bellamkonda, V. R., Li, J. T. C., Hagan, J. B., . . . Bellolio, M. F. (2015). Predictors of repeat epinephrine administration for emergency department patients with anaphylaxis. *Journal of Allergy and Clinical Immunology in Practice, 3*(4), 576–584.

Chaari, A., Chtara, K., Toumi, N., Bahloul, M., & Bouaziz, M. (2015). Neurogenic pulmonary edema after severe head injury: A transpulmonary thermodilution study. *American Journal of Emergency Medicine, 33*(6), 858. e1–858.e3.

Chen, J., Lv, J., Ma, K., & Yan, J. (2014). Assessment of internal mammary artery injury after blunt chest trauma: A literature review. *Journal of Zhejiang University, 15*(10), 864–869.

Christensen, M. (2014). An exploratory study of staff nurses' knowledge of delirium in the medical ICU: An Asian perspective. *Intensive & Critical Care Nursing, 30*(1), 54–60.

Christoffersen, J. K., Hove, L. D., Mikkelsen, K. L., & Krogsgaard, K. R. (2017). Well leg compartment syndrome after abdominal surgery. *World Journal of Surgery, 41*(2), 433–438.

Clarke, S., & Santy-Tomlinson, J. (2014). *Orthopedic and trauma nursing: An evidence-based approach to musculoskeletal care.* Chichester, West Sussex, UK: Wiley Blackwell.

Cleary, M. A., Nottingham, S. L., Kasamatsu, T. M., & Bennett, J. P. (2016). Using a continuing education workshop to facilitate implementation of evidence-based practices for recognition and treatment of exertional heat stroke in secondary school athletic trainers. *Athletic Training & Sports Health Care, 8*(3), 100–111.

Critical Care Nurse. (2012). Delirium assessment and management. *Critical Care Nurse, 32*(1), 79–82.

Day, S., & Fearnley, C. (2015). A classification of mitigation strategies for natural hazards: Implications for the understanding of interactions between mitigation strategies. *Natural Hazards, 79*(2), 1219–1238.

Dean, K., Jenkinson, C., Wilcock, G., & Walker, Z. (2014). The development and validation of a patient-reported quality of life measure for people with mild cognitive impairment. *International Psychogeriatrics, 26*(3), 487–497.

Delano, M. J., & Ward, P. A. (2016). Sepsis-induced immune dysfunction: Can immune therapies reduce mortality? *Journal of Clinical Investigation, 126*(1), 23–31.

Delpachitra, S. N., & Rahmel, B. B. (2016). Orbital fractures in the emergency department: A review of early assessment and management. *Emergency Medicine Journal: EMJ, 33*(10), 727.

Denton, J. S., Segovia, A., & Filkins, J. A. (2006). Practical pathology of gunshot wounds. *Archives of Pathology & Laboratory Medicine, 130*(9), 1283–1289.

deRegloix, S. B., Baumont, L., Daniel, Y., Maurin, O., Crambert, A., & Pons, Y. (2016). Comparison of penetrating neck injury management in combat versus civilian trauma: A review of 55 cases. *Mil Medicine, 181*(8), 935–940. doi: 10.7205/MILMED-D-15-00434

Dong, N., Luo, L., Wu, J., Jia, P., Li, Q., Wang, Y., . . . Shen, B. (2015). Monoclonal antibody, mAb 4C13, an effective detoxicant antibody against ricin poisoning. *Vaccine, 33*(32), 3836–3842.

Duma, S. (2011). *Pregnant occupant biomechanics: Advances in automobile safety research.* Warrendale, PA: SAE International.

Eby, D. W., Molnar, L. J., Zhang, L., St Louis, R. M., Zanier, N., Kostyniuk, L. P., & Stanciu, S. (2016). Use, perceptions, and benefits of automotive technologies among aging drivers. *Injury Epidemiology, 3*(1), 1–20.

Echeverria, A. B., Branco, B. C., Goshima, K. R., Hughes, J. D., & Mills, J. L. (2014). Outcomes of endovascular management of acute thoracic aortic emergencies in an academic level 1 trauma center. *The American Journal of Surgery, 208*(6), 974–980.

Emergency Nurses Association (ENA). (2012). *Emergency nursing pediatric course provider manual* (4th ed.). San Diego, CA: Emergency Nurses Association (ENA).

Emergency Nurses Association. (2014). *Trauma nurse core course provider manual* (7th ed.). San Diego, CA: Emergency Nurses Association.

En-Pei, L., Shao-Hsuan Hsia, Lin, J., Chan, O., Jung, L., Chia-Ying, L., & Han-Ping, W. (2017). Hemodynamic analysis of pediatric septic shock and cardiogenic shock using transpulmonary thermodilution. *BioMed Research International, 2017,* 3613475. doi: 10.1155/2017/3613475

Eshraghi, B., Torabi, H., Masoomian, B., & Akbari, M. R. (2014). Prevalence of intraocular injuries in patients with orbital blow-out fractures. *Iranian Journal of Ophthalmology, 26*(3), 160–165.

Etz, C. D., Weigang, E., Harter, M., Lonn, L., Mestres, C. A., DiBartolomeo, R., . . . Czerny, M. (2015). Contemporary spinal cord protection during thoracic and thoracoabdominal aortic surgery and endovascular aortic repair: A position paper of the vascular domain of the European Association for Cardio-Thoracic Surgery. *European Journal of Cardiothoracic Surgery, 47*(6), 943–957. doi: 10.1093/ejcts/ezv142

Feldt, B. A., Salinas, N. L., Rasmussen, T. E., & Brennan, J. (2013). The joint facial and invasive neck trauma (J-FAINT) project, Iraq and Afghanistan 2003–2011. *Otolaryngol Head Neck Surgical, 148*(3), 403–408.

Fitzgerald, C. A., Morse, B. C., & Dente, C. J. (2014). Pelvic ring fractures: Has mortality improved following the implementation of damage control resuscitation? *The American Journal of Surgery, 208*(6), 1083–1090.

Floresca, D., Dupree, L., Basile, S., & Tan, P. (2012). Evaluation of appropriate serologic testing for suspected heparin-induced thrombocytopenia. *American Journal of Health-System Pharmacy, 69*(18), 1581–1587.

Fowler, T. T., Taylor, B. C., Bellino, M. J., & Althausen, P. L. (2014). Surgical treatment of flail chest and rib fractures. *Journal of American Academy of Orthopedic Surgery, 22*(12), 751–760. doi: 10.5435/JAAOS-22-12-751.

Freeman, J. F., Ciarallo, C., Rappaport, L., Mandt, M., & Bajaj, L. (2016). Use of capnographs to assess quality of pediatric ventilation with 3 different airway modalities. *American Journal of Emergency Medicine, 34*(1), 69–74.

Garner, M. R., Taylor, S. A., Gausden, E., & Lyden, J. P. (2014). Compartment syndrome: Diagnosis, management, and unique concerns in the twenty-first century. *HSS Journal: The Musculoskeletal Journal of Hospital for Special Surgery, 10*(2), 143–152.

Ghane, M., Gharib, M., Ebrahimi, A., Saeedi, M., Akbari-Kamrani, M., Rezaee, M., et al. (2015). Accuracy of early rapid ultrasound in shock (RUSH) examination performed by emergency physician for diagnosis of shock etiology in critically ill patients. *Journal of Emergencies, Trauma and Shock, 8*(1), 5–10.

Gillman, L. M., Brindley, P. G., Blaivas, M., Widder, S., & Karakitsos, D. (2016). Trauma team dynamics. *Journal of Critical Care, 32*, 218–221.

Goodwin Veenema, T. (2013). *Disaster nursing and emergency preparedness* (3rd ed.). New York, NY: Springer Publishing Company.

Gul, E. E., Abdulhalikov, T., Aslan, R., & Aydogdu, I. (2011). A rare and undesirable complication of heparin-induced thrombocytopenia: Acute massive pulmonary embolism. *Clinical and Applied Thrombosis/Hemostasis, 17*(5), 546–548.

Hall, J. E. (2015). *Guyton & Hall textbook of medical physiology* (13th ed.). Philadelphia, PA: Elsevier.

Han, G., Wang, Z., Du, Q., Xiong, Y., Wang, Y., Wu, S., . . . Wang, A. (2014). Damage-control orthopedics versus early total care in the treatment of borderline high-energy pelvic fractures. *Orthopedics (Online), 37*(12), e1091–1100.

Hernandez, D. J., Jatana, K. R., Hoff, S. R., & Rastatter, J. C. (2014). Emergency airway management for pediatric blunt neck trauma. *Clinical Pediatric Emergency Medicine, 15*(3), 261–268.

Hickey, J. (2013). *Clinical practice of neurological & neurosurgical nursing* (7th ed.). New York, NY: LWW.

Higashi, H., Kanki, A., Watanabe, S., Yamamoto, A., Noda, Y., Yasokawa, K., . . . Ito, K. (2014). Traumatic hypovolemic shock revisited: The spectrum of contrast-enhanced abdominal computed tomography findings and clinical implications for its management. *Japanese Journal of Radiology, 32*(10), 579–584.

Hsuan, C. (2016). *Hospital responses to the Emergency Medical Treatment and Labor Act (EMTALA): Noncompliance, hospital utilization and readmissions, and strategic ambulance diversions* (Order No. 10159186). Available from ProQuest Dissertations & Theses Global: Health & Medicine. (1824385772). Retrieved from https://search.proquest.com

Hu, J., Flannagan, C. A., Bao, S., McCoy, R. W., Siasoco, K. M., & Barbat, S. (2015). Integration of active and passive safety technologies - A method to study and estimate field capability. *Stapp Car Crash Journal, 59*, 269–296. Retrieved from https://search.proquest.com

Irwin, A. L., Crawford, G., Gorman, D., Wang, S., & Mertz, H. J. (2016). Thoracic injury risk curves for rib deflections of the SID-IIs build level D. *Stapp Car Crash Journal, 60*, 545–580.

Ivancic, P.C. (2012). Biomechanics of sports-induced axial-compression injuries of the neck. *Journal of Athletic Training, 47*(5), 489–497. doi: 10.4085/1062-6050-47.4.06

Ivatury, R. R. (2012). Thin chest wall is an independent risk factor for the development of pneumothorax after chest tube removal. *American Surgeon, 78*(4), 478–480.

Janzing, H. M., & Broos, P. L. (2001). Routine monitoring of compartment pressure in patients with tibial fractures: Beware of overtreatment! *Injury, 5*: 415–421.

Jesmin, S., Gando, S., Wada, T., Hayakawa, M., & Sawamura, A. (2016). Activated protein C does not increase in the early phase of trauma with disseminated intravascular coagulation: Comparison with acute coagulopathy of trauma-shock. *Journal of Intensive Care, 4*(1), doi: 10.1186/s40560-015-0123-2

Jones & Bartlett Learning. (2016). *2016 nurse's drug handbook* (15th ed.). Sudbury, MA: Jones & Bartlett Learning

Kashani, A. T., Rabieyan, R., & Besharati, M. M. (2016). Modeling the effect of operator and passenger characteristics on the fatality risk of motorcycle crashes. *Journal of Injury and Violence Research, 8*(1), 35–42.

Kautza, B., Zuckerbraun, B., & Peitzman, A. B. (2015). Management of blunt renal injury: What is new?. *European Journal of Trauma and Emergency Surgery, 41*(3), 251–258.

Kearns, R., Sugarman, S., Cairns, B., Holmes, J, & Rich, Preston B. (2016). Radiation injury, burns and illness: A review of best practices. *EMS World, 45*(10), 52–60.

Keller, M., Han, P. P., Galarneau, M. R., & Gaball, C. W. (2015). Characteristics of maxillofacial injuries and safety of in-theater facial fracture repair in severe combat trauma. *Military Medicine, 180*(3), 315–320.

Kemper, A. R., Kennedy, E. A., Mcnally, C., Manoogian, S. J., Stitzel, J. D., & Duma, S. M. (2011). Reducing chest injuries in automobile collisions: Rib fracture timing and implications for thoracic injury criteria. *Annals of Biomedical Engineering, 39*(8), 2141–2151.

Khan, M., Azfar, M., & Khurshid, S. (2014). The role of inhaled nitric oxide beyond ARDS. *Indian Journal of Critical Care Medicine, 18*(6), 392–395.

Kivanc, S. A., Budak, B. A., Cevik, S. G., Baykara, M., Yasar, S., & Ozmen, A. T. (2016). Occupational-related chemical ocular injuries: An analysis of 82 patients. *The European Research Journal, 2*(2), 143–146.

Kizior, R. J., & Hodgson, B. B. (2016). *Saunders nursing drug handbook 2017.* St Louis, MO: Saunders.

Kizior, R. J., & Hodgson, B. B. (2016). *Saunders nursing drug handbook, 2017 Kindle edition.* St. Louis, MO: Elsevier.

Klinngam, N., Sittipunt, C., Poonyathawon, S., Chatrkaw, P., Tachaboon, S., & Srisawat, N. (2015). The neutrophil function in severe Sepsis/Septic shock patients with mods. *Intensive Care Medicine Experimental, 3*, 1.

Kon, A. A., Shepard, E. K., Sederstrom, N. O., Swoboda, S. M., Marshall, M. F., Birriel, B., & Rincon, F. (2016). Defining futile and potentially inappropriate interventions: A policy statement from the society of critical care medicine ethics committee. *Critical Care Medicine, 44*(9), 1769–1774. doi: 10.1097/CCM.0000000000001965

Krausz, A. A., Krausz, M. M., & Picetti, E. (2015). Maxillofacial and neck trauma: A damage control approach. *World Journal of Emergency Surgery, 10*, 31. doi: 10.1186/s13017-015-0022-9

Lance, R. M., Capehart, B., Kadro, O., & Bass, C. R. (2015). Human injury criteria for underwater blasts. *PLoS One, 10*(11).

Lavingia, K. S., Collins, J. N., Soult, M. C., Terzian, W. H., Weireter, L. J., & Britt, L D. (2015). Torso computed tomography can be bypassed after thorough trauma bay examination of patients who fall from standing. *The American Surgeon, 81*(8), 798–801.

LaVole, L., & Mena, K. (2016). What is hypovolemic shock? symptoms and treatment. *Medical News Today.* Retrieved from http://www.medicalnewstoday.com/articles/312348.php

Lawrence, E., & Li, F. (2015). Foot burns and diabetes: A retrospective study. *Burns & Trauma, 3*(24). doi: 10.1186/s41038-015-0024-6

Leviskaia, T. G., Thrall, K. D., Peterson, J. M., Fryxell, G. E., Timchalk, G. A., & Tarasevich, B. J. (2014). Topical applicator composition and process for treatment of radiologically contaminated dermal injuries. *US patent 20140249102.*

Levy, B., Bastien, O., Karim, B., Cariou, A., Chouihed, T., Combes, A., . . . Kuteifan, K. (2015). Experts' recommendations for the management of adult patients with cardiogenic shock. *Annals of Intensive Care, 5*(1), 1–10.

Lin, L. (2015). Understanding EMTALA. *Reimbursement Advisor, 30*(10), 3–6.

Lippincott. (2016). *Nursing 2017 drug handbook* (37th ed). Philadelphia, PA: Walters Kluwer

Loubani, O. M., & Green, R. S. (2015). A systematic review of extravasation and local tissue injury from administration of vasopressors through peripheral intravenous catheters and central venous catheters. *Journal of Critical Care, 30*(3), 653.e9–653.e17.

Low, G. M. I., Inaba, K., Chouliaras, K., Branco, B., Lam, L., Benjamin, E., . . . Demetriades, D. (2014). The use of the anatomic "zones" of the neck in the assessment of penetrating neck injury. *The American Surgeon, 80*(10), 970–974.

Lui, N., & Wright, C. (2015). Intraoperative tracheal injury. *Thoracic Surgery Clinic, 25*(3), 249–254.

MacQueen, I. T., Dawes, A. J., Hadnott, T., Strength, K., Moran, G. J., Holschneider, C., . . . Maggard-Gibbons, M. (2015). Use of a hospital-wide screening program for early detection of sepsis in general surgery patients. *American Surgeon, 81*(10), 1074–1079.

Majercik, S., Vijayakumar, S., Olsen, G., Wilson, E., Gardner, S., Granger, S. R., . . . White, T. W. (2015). Surgical stabilization of severe rib fractures decreases incidence of retained hemothorax and empyema. *American Journal of Surgery, 210*(6), 1112–1117.

Marmo, L. (2013). *Compact clinical guide to critical care, trauma and emergency pain management.* St. Louis, MO: Springer Publishing Company.

Masini, B. D., Racusin, A. W., Wenke, J. C., Gerlinger, T. L., & Hsu, J. R. (2013). Acute compartment syndrome of the thigh in combat casualties. *Journal of Surgical Orthopedic Advances, 22*(1), 42–49.

McCully, B. H., Fabricant, L., Geraci, T., Greenbaum, A., Schreiber, M. A., & Gordy, S. D. (2014). Complete cervical spinal cord injury above C6 predicts the need for tracheostomy. *American Journal of Surgery, 207*(5), 664–668; discussion 668–669.

McGuigan, A., & Brown, R. (2016). Early and delayed presentation of traumatic small bowel injury. *BMJ Case Reports, 2016.*

Mcqueen, M. M., & Duckworth, A. D. (2014). The diagnosis of acute compartment syndrome: A review. *European Journal of Trauma and Emergency Surgery, 40*(5), 521–528.

McQuillan, K., Flynn Makic, M. B., & Whalen, E. (2009). *Trauma nursing: From resuscitation through rehabilitation* (4th ed.). St. Louis, MO: Elsevier Saunders.

Mohr, N. M., Harland, K. K., Shane, D. M., Ahmed, A., Fuller, B. M., & Torner, J. C. (2016). Inter-hospital transfer is associated with increased mortality and costs in severe sepsis and septic shock: An instrumental variables approach. *Journal of Critical Care, 36*, 187–194.

Moore, K. (2015). Hot topics: Chemical burns in the emergency department. *Journal of Emergency Nursing, 41*(4), 364–365.

Morimura, N., Takahashi, K., Doi, T., Ohnuki, T., Sakamoto, T., Uchida, Y., . . . Ikeda, H. (2015). A pilot study of quantitative capillary refill time to identify high blood lactate levels in critically ill patients. *Emergency Medicine Journal, 32*(6), 444.

Morsy, M., Efeovbokhan, N., & Jha, S. K. (2015). Complete heart block and asystole following blunt cardiac trauma. *Journal of Community Hospital Internal Medicine Perspectives, 5*(5). doi: 10.3402/jchimp.v5.28423

Mourelo, M., Galeiras, R., Pértega, S., Freire, D., López, E., Broullón, J., & Campos, E. (2015). Tracheostomy in the management of patients with thermal injuries. *Indian Journal of Critical Care Medicine, 19*(8), 449–455.

Mullins, T. L. K., Miller, R. J., & Mullins, E. S. (2015). Evaluation and management of adolescents with abnormal uterine bleeding. *Pediatric Annals, 44*(9), e218–222.

Napolitano, L. M., Biester, T. W., Jurkovich, G. J., Buyske, J., Malangoni, M. A., Lewis, F. R., . . . Spain, D. A. (2016). General surgery resident rotations in surgical critical care, trauma, and burns: What is optimal for residency training? *The American Journal of Surgery, 212*(4), 629–637.

National Association of Emergency Medical Technicians (NAEMT). (2016). *Prehospital trauma life support* (8th ed.). Burlington, MA: Jones & Bartlett Learning.

Nayduch, D. (2009). *Nurse to nurse: Trauma care.* New York, NY: McGraw-Hill.

Nielsen, J. S., Sally, M., Mullins, R. J., Slater, M., Groat, T., Gao, X., . . . Malinoski, D. J. (2017). Bicarbonate and mannitol treatment for traumatic rhabdomyolysis revisited. *The American Journal of Surgery, 213*(1), 73–79.

Nursing Drug Handbook. (2017). *Nursing 2017 drug handbook.* New York, NY: Lippincott, Wolters, Kluwer.

Okumura, E., Tsurukiri, J., Oomura, T., Tanaka, Y., & Oomura, R. (2016). Partial resuscitative endovascular balloon occlusion of the aorta as a hemorrhagic shock adjunct for ectopic pregnancy. *The American Journal of Emergency Medicine, 34*(9), 1917.e1–1917.e2.

Oyston, P. C. F., & Williamson, E. D. (2013). Prophylaxis and therapy of plague. *Expert Review of Anti-Infective Therapy, 11*(8), 817–829.

Peterkin, N. D., Atkin, J. S., & Coris, E. E. (2016). What is the best practice for the treatment of exertional heat illnesses (heat cramps, heat syncope, heat exhaustion, and exertional heat stroke)? *Athletic Training & Sports Health Care, 8*(3), 97–99.

Prasad, P., Dalmotas, D., & Chouinard, A. (2015). Side impact regulatory trends, crash environment and injury risk in the USA. *Stapp Car Crash Journal, 59*, 91–112.

Proehl, J. (2008). *Emergency nursing procedures* (4th ed.). St. Louis, MO: Elsevier Saunders.

Puzio, T., Shah, M., Dineen, H., Chen, J., Caddell, K., & Charles, A. (2016). A case of iliac crest avulsion with peritoneal disruption and bowel herniation after blunt trauma. *The American Surgeon, 82*(7), 655–658.

Quick, J. A., & Barnes, S. L. (2015). Correct coagulopathy: Quickly and effectively. *Lancet, 385*(9982), 2024–2026.

Radenkovic, D. V., Johnson, C. D., Milic, N., Gregoric, P., Ivancevic, N., Bezmarevic, M., . . . Bajec, D. (2016). Interventional treatment of abdominal compartment syndrome during severe acute pancreatitis: Current status and historical perspective. *Gastroenterology Research and Practice.* doi: 10.1155/2016/5251806

Rahmani, S. H., Faridaalaee, G., & Jahangard, S. (2015). Acute transient hemiparesis induced by lightning strike. *American Journal of Emergency Medicine, 33*(7), 984.e1–984.e3.

Rasmussen, K. C., Hoejskov, M., Johansson, P. I., Kridina, I., Kistorp, T., Salling, L., . . . Secher, N. H. (2015). Coagulation competence for predicting perioperative hemorrhage in patients treated with lactated ringers vs. dextran—A randomized controlled trial. *BioMed Central Anesthesiology, 15*(178). doi: 10.1186/s12871-015-0162-1

Ray, A., Suri, J., Chakarborty, S., & Bhattacharya, D. (2014). Authors' reply. *Lung India, 31*(3), 316.

Redelmeier, D. May, S. C., Thiruchelvam, D., & Barrett, J. F. (2014). Pregnancy and the risk of a traffic crash. *Canadian Medical Association Journal, 186*(10), 742–750.

Rentea, R. M., Lam, V., Biesterveld, B., Fredrich, K. M., Callison, J., Fish, B. L., . . . Otterson, M. F. (2016). Radiation-induced changes in intestinal and tissue-nonspecific alkaline phosphatase: Implications for recovery after radiation therapy. *The American Journal of Surgery, 212*(4), 602–608.

Ricci, Z. J., Mazzariol, F. S., Kaul, B., Oh, S. K., Chernyak, V., Flusberg, M., . . . Rozenblit, A. M. (2016). Hollow organ abdominal ischemia, part II: Clinical features, etiology, imaging findings and management. *Clinical Imaging, 40*(4), 751–764.

Richards, J. E., Morris, B. J., Guillamondegui, O. D., Sweeney, K. R., Tressler, M. A., Obremskey, W. T., & Kregor, P. J. (2015). The effect of body mass index on posttraumatic transfusion after pelvic trauma. *The American Surgeon, 81*(3), 239–244.

Riehl, J. T., Sassoon, A., Connolly, K., Haidukewych, G. J., & Koval, K. J. (2013). Retained bullet removal in civilian pelvis and extremity gunshot injuries: A systematic review. *Clinical Orthopaedics and Related Research, 471*(12), 3956–3960.

Rodriguez, R. M., Hendey, G. W., Mower, W., Kea, B., Fortman, J., Merchant, G., & Hoffman, J. R. (2011). Derivation of a decision instrument for selective chest radiography in blunt trauma. *Journal of Trauma, 71*(3), 549–553.

Rondon-berrios, H., Agaba, E. I., & Tzamaloukas, A. H. (2014). Hyponatremia: Pathophysiology, classification, manifestations and management. *International Urology and Nephrology, 46*(11), 2153–2165.

Rowley-Conwy, G. (2014). Management of major burns: Rehabilitation and recovery. *Nursing Standard (2014+), 28*(25), 65.

Rural Trauma Committee of the American College of Surgeons Committee on Trauma. (2011). *Rural trauma team development course* (3rd ed.). Chicago, IL: American College of Surgeons Committee on Trauma.

Russell, J. L., Wiles, D. A., Kenney, B., & Spiller, H. A. (2014). Significant chemical burns associated with dermal exposure to laundry pod detergent. *Journal of Medical Toxicology, 10*(3), 292–294.

Salinas, N. L., & Faulkner, J. A. (2010). Facial trauma in Operation Iraqi Freedom casualties: An outcomes study of patients treated from April 2006 through October 2006. *Journal of Craniofacial Surgery, 21*(4), 967–970.

Schaefer, N., Griffin, A., Gerhardy, B., & Gochee, P. (2014). Early recognition and management of laryngeal fracture: A case report. *The Ochsner Journal, 14*(2), 264–265.

Singla, A., Amini, M. R., Alpert, M. A., & Gornik, H. L. (2013). Fatal anaphylactoid reaction associated with heparin-induced thrombocytopenia. *Vascular Medicine, 18*(3), 136–138.

Smalls, N., Obirieze, A., & Ehanire, I. (2015). The impact of coagulopathy on traumatic splenic injuries. *American Journal of Surgery, 210*(4), 724–729.

Society of Trauma Nurses. (2013). *Advanced trauma care for nurses student manual.* Lexington, KY: Society of Trauma Nurses.

Society of Trauma Nurses (STN). (2013). Trauma outcomes and performance improvement course (TOPIC). Lexington, KY: Society of Trauma Nurses.

Society of Trauma Nurses. (2015). Optimal trauma center organization & management course. Lexington, KY: Society of Trauma Nurses.

Stephenson, J. A., Gravante, G., Butler, N. A., Sorge, R., Sayers, R. D., & Bown, M. J. (2010). The systemic inflammatory response syndrome (SIRS): Number and type of positive criteria predict interventions and outcomes in acute surgical admissions. *World Journal of Surgery, 34*(11), 2757–2764.

Tajima, K., Zheng, F., Collange, O., Barthel, G., Thornton, S. N., Longrois, D., . . . Mertes, P. M. (2013). Time to achieve target mean arterial pressure during resuscitation from experimental anaphylactic shock in an animal model. A comparison of adrenaline alone or in combination with different volume expanders. *Anaesthesia and Intensive Care, 41*(6), 765–773.

Talebi-Taher, M., Babazadeh, S., Barati, M., & Latifnia, M. (2014). Serum inflammatory markers in the elderly: Are they useful in differentiating sepsis from SIRS? *Acta Medica Iranica, 52*(6), 438–442.

TCAR Education Programs. (2014). *Pediatric care after resuscitation course (PCAR).* Scappoose, OR: TCAR Education Programs.

TCAR Education Programs. (2014). *Trauma care after resuscitation (TCAR).* Scappoose, OR: TCAR Education Programs.

Toliyat, M., Singh, K., Sibley, R. C., Chamarthy, M., Kalva, S. P., & Pillai, A. K. (2017). Interventional radiology in the management of thoracic duct injuries: Anatomy, techniques and results. *Clinical Imaging, 42*, 183–192.

Towe, C., Solomon, B., Donington, J. S., & Pass, H. I. (2014). Treatment of recalcitrant subcutaneous emphysema using negative pressure wound therapy dressings. *BMJ Case Reports, 2014.*

Vahidi, E., Shakoor, D., Aghaie Meybodi, M., & Saeedi, M. (2015). Comparison of intravenous lidocaine versus morphine in alleviating pain in patients with critical limb ischaemia. *Emergency Medicine Journal, 32*(7), 516.

Winters, B. A., & Nuttall, C. (2015). Evaluation and management of spinal column fractures in adults. *The Journal for Nurse Practitioners, 11*(10), 1043–1047.

Yelon, J. & Luchette, F. (2014). *Geriatric trauma and critical care.* New York, NY: Springer.

Zaets, S. B., Xu, D. Z., Feketova, E., Berezina, T. L., Malinina, I. V., Deitch, E. A., & Olsen, E. H. (2014). Does recombinant factor XIII eliminate manifestations of multiple-organ injury after experimental burn similarly to gut ischemia-reperfusion injury or trauma-hemorrhagic shock? *Journal of Burn Care Resuscitation, 35*(4), 328–336. doi: 10.1097/BCR.0b013e3182a228ee

Zarar, A., Khan, A. A., Adil, M. M., & Qureshi, A. I. (2014). Anaphylactic shock associated with intravenous thrombolytics. *American Journal of Emergency Medicine, 32*(1), 113.e3–113.e5.

Zhang, Z., Su, X., & Liu, C. (2015). Cardiac arrest with anaphylactic shock: A successful resuscitation using extracorporeal membrane oxygenation. *American Journal of Emergency Medicine, 33*(1), 130.e3–130.e4.